Genetics, Health Care and Public Policy

An Introduction to Public Health Genetics

By

Alison Stewart
Philippa Brice
Hilary Burton
Paul Pharoah
Simon Sanderson
Ron Zimmern
Public Health Genetics Unit, Cambridge

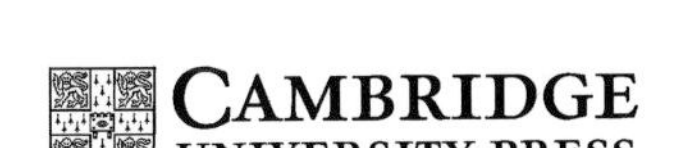

CAMBRIDGE UNIVERSITY PRESS
Cambridge, New York, Melbourne, Madrid, Cape Town, Singapore, São Paulo

Cambridge University Press
The Edinburgh Building, Cambridge CB2 8RU, UK

Published in the United States of America by Cambridge University Press, New York

www.cambridge.org
Information on this title: www.cambridge.org/9780521529075

First published 2007

Printed in the United Kingdom at the University Press, Cambridge

A catalogue record for this publication is available from the British Library

ISBN 978-0-521-52907-5 paperback

Contents

Foreword

It is a privilege to introduce this new book on public health genetics. Advances in genetic research have created unprecedented tools for understanding human health. The new knowledge arising from this research has the potential to transform disease prevention and management, and public health genetics is a new field poised to harness the insights of this knowledge for the benefit of population health.

To accomplish the task, public health genetics must take a comprehensive approach. It must bring together traditional public health principles, a meaningful evaluation of the combined effects of genetics and environment on health, and attention to the social implications of genetic risk information. Integration of knowledge across a broad array of subject areas will be needed, to support appropriate public policy, health services, mechanisms for communication and stakeholder engagement, and education and training programmes.

This important effort will require the participation of professionals from diverse disciplines. All will have essential expertise to offer the emerging field of public health genetics, yet many will have had little exposure to the full range of issues it must address. Working together will require a common language, based on the underlying science, principles, and goals. For everyone who wishes to participate in the exciting new venture of public health genetics, this book is the right place to start.

Wylie Burke MD PhD
University of Washington

Acknowledgements

We thank Ooonagh Corrigan, Helen Firth, Alison Hall, Julian Higgins, Stuart Hogarth, Kathy Liddell, Andrew Read, Martin Richards and Susan Wallace for comments on the manuscript, and all our colleagues for their advice and support.

1

Introduction

Public health genetics is a new discipline. It brings together the insights of genetic and molecular science as a means of preventing disease and of protecting and improving the health of the population. Its scope is wide, and requires an understanding of genetics, epidemiology, public health, the principles of ethics, law and the social sciences and much else besides.

At the core of public health genetics is the notion that genes, like the classic environmental factors that have been shown over many decades to be causally implicated in disease, are themselves important determinants of health; and that they play as important a role as exposures to physical and biological agents or to social and structural factors such as poverty and unemployment. But, as with environmental determinants, genes act not on their own but in combination with other factors. Every gene interacts with others in the genome and with a host of external exposures to produce the full range of human characteristics. The complexities of these relationships mean that, while genetic factors are at work in all diseases, no single genetic variant (except in the case of relatively rare 'genetic diseases', discussed further below) will be predictive of when or whether disease will strike, or of its severity.

The health and social policy issues that form much of the practice of public health genetics are equally complex, including legal and regulatory frameworks in genetic testing; science funding and policy; consent, confidentiality and data protection; the pharmaceutical and biotechnology industries; the patenting of genes and genetic sequences; and the education and training of health professionals and of the public in the implications of genetic science.

The definition of public health genetics

Two widely used definitions of public health genetics come from the United States. The University of Washington in Seattle defines it as *the application of advances in human genetics and molecular biotechnology to improve public health and prevent disease*. The University of Michigan tells us that it provides an opportunity for public health professionals to gain *an understanding of the effects of genes on health and disease and to apply genetic information to public health practice.*

In the United Kingdom we have built on the well respected Acheson definition of public health and defined it *as the impact of genetics on the art and science of promoting health and preventing disease through the organised efforts of society.*

The broad scope implied by this definition was endorsed recently, as discussed further later in this chapter, by an international expert group that defined public health genetics as *the effective translation of genome-based knowledge and technologies for the benefit of population health.*

All of these formulations emphasise that the subject matter of public health genetics is how the health of the population and individuals within it, and the way in which public health and clinical medicine are practised will be affected by genetic science and technology.

A detailed analysis of the modified Acheson definition that we have used in the UK brings out a number of points:

1. It is important to note the different meanings that can be attached to the word 'genetics': genetics as the study of inheritance and inherited diseases, and genetics as the study of DNA, molecular and cellular biology. The discipline of public health genetics uses 'genetics' in the second of these senses, moving beyond inherited and congenital diseases and dealing, in addition, with the role of genetic factors in the complex disorders, such as coronary heart disease, cancers, diabetes, asthma, stroke or dementia, that contribute most to mortality and morbidity.
2. The definition of public health genetics makes clear that its aim is to promote health and to prevent disease, both for individuals and for the population as a whole. The public health perspective is in essence one that asks of scientific advances, technological interventions, policy and legislation whether they add to or detract from improvements in human health.
3. The word 'prevention', as used in public health, includes not just measures designed to prevent the onset of disease but, in addition, clinical interventions that lead to the reduction of disability and the progression of disease.
4. The definition states that the practice of public health genetics is both an art and a science, implying that it requires not just technical competencies, but also a sensitivity to the plural views that exist in society about genetic science and its consequences, and an ability to work across a whole range of disciplines and cultures.
5. The sphere of influence of public health genetics goes far beyond health service boundaries. The phrase 'organised efforts of society' refers to a panoply of health determinants that includes not just the practices of health services

themselves but factors as diverse as fiscal policy, patent law, educational curricula, data protection, genetic test regulation, the funding of science and many others besides. Ethical, legal and social perspectives run across all these activities and contribute to a key aspect of public health genetics practice.

Genetic and environmental factors as determinants of health

Environmental exposures and social factors have provided much of the material for classical analytical epidemiology. Using case–control and cohort observational study designs, epidemiologists have sought to demonstrate associations between various exposures and the incidence or prevalence of disease, and to determine those that might be causal. The association of smoking and lung cancer; of the human immunodeficiency virus (HIV) and acquired immunodeficiency syndrome (AIDS); of unemployment and all-cause mortality; of fat consumption and coronary heart disease; and of social isolation and depression are classical examples of associations that have emerged from such studies. The implicit assumption in all these studies was that the population was homogeneous. The investigators did not, of course, actually believe that this was so, but they analysed the results as if genetic heterogeneity between individuals in the population under study did not exist. The public health community, in turn, saw little in genetics to interest them, and did not regard genetic variation as an important matter that contributed to public health practice.

Public health genetics seeks to remedy this incomplete characterisation of health determinants by showing how genes play a major role. Figure 1.1 is a conceptual diagram of health determinants. It is set out in that particular way to illustrate a number of points. First, genetic factors are included explicitly as a health determinant. Second, the arrows demonstrate that the determinants interact in a complex way. For example, the presence of radon in the natural environment will

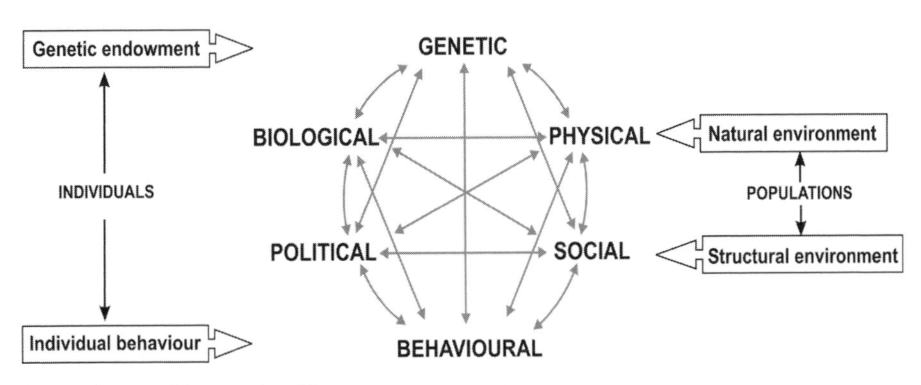

Figure 1.1 Determinants of human health

increase the mutation rate in exposed populations; genetic factors can affect certain aspects of human behaviour; the hepatitis virus and aflatoxins will affect the somatic genome and predispose exposed individuals to cancer.

Third, it brings out the point that natural environmental and structural determinants are external factors best influenced by interventions at the population level, while, by contrast, genetic factors and behaviour are essentially individual. In other words, how an individual chooses to behave, whether to smoke or indulge in other harmful behaviours, can only be changed or affected by the will of that particular individual, albeit that external or structural factors have an influence on such individual decisions.

The fourth point is that the multiple interactions in the figure can be reduced to a more simple representation, which simply shows a mutual relationship between genes and environment. Determinants of health and disease can only be genetic or environmental, since an 'environmental factor' is defined as anything that is not genetic. Genes and the environment interact with each other such that the risk of disease differs from individual to individual depending on their genetic constitution and environmental exposure. We normally call this 'gene–environment interaction', but it is probably more accurate to speak about the combined effects of genetic and environmental factors. The reason is that the term gene–environment interaction has a technical meaning for the statistician (see Chapter 3 for further discussion). The statistician takes the term interaction to refer to a risk estimation that does not conform to a pre-stated statistical model. No such assumption is made in our use of the term. All that we wish to imply is that genetic and environmental factors combine to influence risk.

Fifth and finally, the categorisation of determinants into those that are primarily population determined and those that are determined at an individual level reflects a distinction that is crucial to the understanding of preventive strategies and interventions. The epidemiologist Geoffrey Rose (1985) pointed out that there were two ways of preventing disease:

- by identifying those at greatest risk and directing preventive interventions at those individuals; and
- by trying to reduce the risk across the population as a whole through structural or environmental change that affects the whole population.

Blood pressure provides a good example. It is a risk factor for stroke. The high-risk approach identifies and treats individuals with blood pressure levels above a given threshold. The population approach seeks to reduce the mean blood pressure in the population through the reduction of salt consumption. Figure 1.2 is a conceptual diagram of the distribution of blood pressure levels across the population; it also shows the risk of stroke according to blood pressure levels. What Rose argued was that although treatment of high blood pressure in individuals at

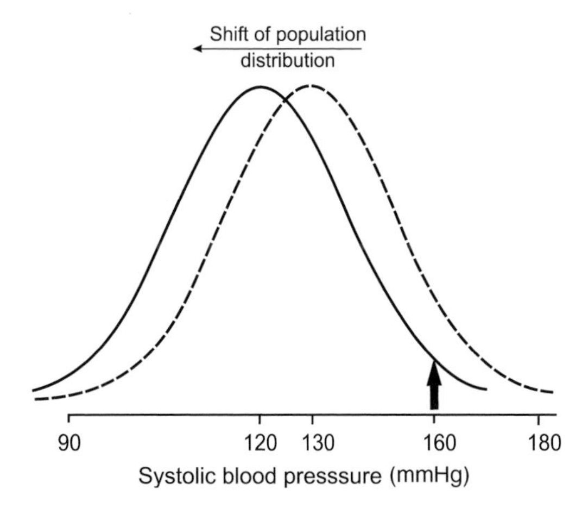

Figure 1.2 Population blood pressure levels and risk of stroke. Systolic blood pressure is shown in mmHg; 160 mmHg is used as a cut-off point (see arrow) above which individuals are considered to be at a significantly increased risk of stroke. The height of the curve at a given point represents the number or proportion of individuals within the population with that blood pressure level

the far end of the distribution brought about a much greater absolute risk reduction for each individual, a far greater number of strokes would be prevented in the population if the distribution curve could be shifted to the left by small reductions in mean blood pressure levels, by lowering the mean population salt consumption.

That genetic and environmental factors work together provides a key insight for public health genetics. The distribution of a risk factor such as blood pressure or cholesterol level across a population is determined by genetic, environmental and stochastic (random) factors. These factors between them are responsible for the shape and position of the frequency distribution of risk factors across the population. If we envisage a theoretical situation where all the individuals are exposed to exactly the same environmental factors, the variance of the resulting distribution will be reduced and will be a function of only the genetic variation in the population under study. The shape of the residual distribution will be due entirely to genetic factors, to the interaction between the genetic factors and the common environment, and to stochastic (random) variation. The position of the curve along the risk axis will in turn be determined by the nature of the environment – with some environments providing a greater, and others a lesser, health risk.

Rose's analysis has been used by some to argue that the targeting of preventive interventions at individuals who are at high genetic risk is not a defensible public health strategy. Rose himself did not draw this conclusion, however, stating that the whole-population and high-risk approaches were complementary and should both be pursued.

Genetic disease, complex disease and the combined effects of genetic and environmental factors

We have seen that genetic and environmental components both contribute to the development and risk of disease. However, we designate some diseases, cystic fibrosis or Duchenne muscular dystrophy for example, as 'genetic diseases'. What do we mean by this term and how do such diseases differ from those that we do not place in this category? All genetic factors are transmitted across generations in patterns that conform to the laws of inheritance first formulated by Mendel. The details of this mechanism are discussed in Chapter 2. The important point to appreciate here is that, in most cases, the physical manifestations that are influenced by these genetic factors – the diseases or physiological traits themselves – do not show such a pattern across generations and between family members, even though some traits and diseases have a tendency to cluster within families. A genetic disease is one where, in contrast to most, the manifestations of the disease show a pattern of transmission that is seen to conform to Mendel's laws.

The question then is why some diseases have these characteristics and not others. The diseases that pass across generations, genetic diseases, are usually single-gene disorders where the presence of the genetic abnormality is sufficient (on its own or with environmental factors) to give rise to the observable features of the disease. Most diseases, including those that are of greatest public health importance such as heart disease, diabetes, cancer or schizophrenia, are much more complex and come about as a result of the combined effects of multiple genes and their interaction with each other and with a range of environmental factors. For these reasons they are often referred to as complex or multifactorial diseases.

In multifactorial diseases, individual genes may make a contribution to the disease but each is insufficient in itself to cause the disease. The disease only manifests itself if other factors, such as other genetic variants and/or environmental factors, are also present such that together the factors comprise a sufficient cause of the disease. Suppose an individual possesses a set of genetic variants, and is exposed to a range of environmental factors, that together are sufficient to cause a specific disease. What are the implications for his or her offspring? Each gene only has a 50% chance of being passed on to the next generation (see Chapter 2 for further explanation). It is unlikely, therefore, that the full constellation of genetic components associated with the disease in that individual will be passed on; nor may it be assumed that the individual in the next generation is exposed to the same raft of environmental factors. Examples such as this illustrate why complex diseases do not conform to simple patterns of inheritance.

The manifestation or expression of genetic factors as disease or physiological traits is referred to by geneticists as the phenotype. The genetic factors themselves

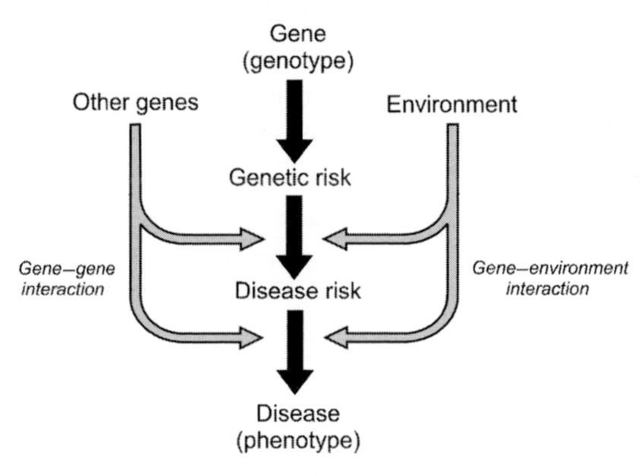

Figure 1.3 Penetrance. The penetrance of a genetic variant is the probability that traits or characteristics associated with that variant will manifest within a stated period of time

are called the genotype. Geneticists refer to the likelihood that a genetic variant will manifest its traits or characteristics within a stated time interval as penetrance (Figure 1.3). Penetrance refers to phenotype and is a property not just of the gene in question but of the genetic and external environment. Diseases such as cystic fibrosis or Duchenne muscular dystrophy are conditions whose penetrance is virtually 100% and may therefore be described as genetic diseases. If the genetic variant is inherited then it is certain that the individual will develop the disease (though, as discussed further in Chapter 2, even highly penetrant single-gene diseases may show variability in factors such as age of onset or range and severity of symptoms).

At the other end of the spectrum, is it possible to establish that there are diseases or traits that are entirely environmental, without any genetic influence at all? Accidental injury, for example as a result of a motor vehicle accident, may on first sight appear to be entirely environmental in origin, but a little reflection might lead one to question that initial impression. We know that there are certain conditions that predispose to sudden loss of consciousness, some of which are due to single-gene disorders. These include, for example, long QT syndrome, cardiomyopathies and certain forms of epilepsy. There is also reasonable evidence that certain genes are involved in traits such as impulsiveness, risk-taking behaviours or clumsiness, all of which could have an impact on the probability of being injured in a motor vehicle accident. The epidemiology of such accidents shows a huge sex difference; this is again evidence of a genetic factor at work.

The genetic disorder phenylketonuria (PKU; Box 1.1) provides another instructive example of the combined effect of genetic and enviromental factors: both a genetic mutation *and* a phenylalanine-containing diet are needed for the disease to

Box 1.1 Phenylketonuria: both a genetic and an environmental disease
Phenylketonuria (PKU) is a disease of the newborn and causes profound mental retardation. The disease is due to an abnormality in the gene that produces the enzyme phenylalanine hydroxylase. The enzyme converts the amino acid phenylalanine to tyrosine. Its absence allows the build up of phenylalanine which is toxic for the developing brain. The treatment is to restrict phenylalanine in the diet of the infant. The genetic abnormality *and* the presence of the environmental factor, phenylalanine, are both required for the disease PKU to develop. Neither one nor the other factor is sufficient on its own. The penetrance of the disease is 100% if phenylalanine is present but 0% if it is absent from the diet.

develop. We refer to PKU as a genetic disease because the dietary factor, phenylalanine, is ubiquitous while the genetic defect is rare, occurring in around 1 in 10 000 births. If, in an alternative world, a population all had the genetic abnormality that we associate with PKU but phenylalanine was not found in the diet of that population, the few cases of PKU observed in that world would be deemed to be toxic or nutritional in origin.

The phenylalanine-free world is obviously a hypothetical one. Real examples can also be found, however, to illustrate the point that whether we choose to label a disease as genetic or environmental in origin is dependent on the relative prevalence of those factors. If the genetic factor is rare against a common set of environmental factors we label the disease genetic, and vice versa if the environmental factor is rare. The relationship between smoking and lung cancer provides one example. If we study a population in which everyone smoked 60 cigarettes a day, the variation in lung cancer among individuals would by and large be determined by genetic factors, an insight due to Geoffrey Rose. When the tubercle bacillus was ubiquitous, medical students of the time were taught that individual constitution was a prime determinant of whether or not one developed tuberculosis and of its severity. They also learnt that rickets was a disease of vitamin D deficiency. But now, at least in the developed world, the few cases of rickets that we see are more often than not due to a plethora of individually rare genetic disorders of vitamin D metabolism, and very infrequently to dietary deficiency. These examples show that, as a general rule, to question whether a disease is genetic or environmental is meaningless; both contribute to the disorder and any attempt to segregate one set of factors from the other is conceptually unsound.

Public health genetics does not attempt to argue against the importance of environmental exposures as determinants of health – quite the reverse. Both genetic and environmental factors play a role in disease risk but in terms of prevention, a central goal of public health, it is generally only the environmental part of this interaction that can be altered. The high incidence of diabetes mellitus in Pima Indians has been explained as the result of exposure of a particularly 'thrifty' genotype to a Western diet. Genetic factors are clearly at work but in practical terms the dietary exposure is much more important, as it is only by changing the diet that it will be possible to reduce the incidence of diabetes mellitus in this population.

The emergence and development of public health genetics

Public health genetics as a recognised and separate discipline of public health emerged only in the mid 1990s. It represented a coming together of insights and influences from several quarters: the increasing power and sophistication of epidemiology, the burgeoning discipline of genetic epidemiology, the excitement generated by the human genome project, and the recognition that there was a need to understand and resolve the many ethical, legal and social issues raised by advances in genetic science.

Advances in epidemiology and its application to public health

Epidemiology is now recognised as the core science that underpins the work of public health practitioners. In the last five decades it has developed beyond recognition. Basic concepts such as disease incidence and prevalence, relative and absolute risks and rates have been refined; the nature of causation and of how multiple factors interact in a web of causative factors are now better understood. Major methodological developments in study design have taken place, for cohort and case–control studies, and for randomised clinical trials.

Descriptive studies, documenting the relation of disease to person, place and time, have given way to analytical studies designed to elucidate association between exposures and disease, and causative pathways. Understanding the roles of bias, confounding and random factors in the interpretation of epidemiological data is now fundamental to epidemiological training, and advanced biostatistical techniques such as multiple logistic regression are now commonplace for the professional epidemiologist.

The approaches of epidemiology have also had an impact on mainstream clinical medicine, as clinical epidemiology and evidence-based medicine, both placing emphasis on numeracy, measurement and statistics in the evaluation of medical interventions, have been integrated into medical curricula.

The rise of genetic epidemiology

Genetic epidemiology began to be recognised as a separate subset of epidemiological research in the 1950s. In its early decades, most of its practitioners focused on the genetic analysis of pedigree data. They carried out studies on families and siblings, on twins and adoptees, and their interests lay mainly in the single-gene disorders and chromosomal abnormalities. Their background was mathematical and the techniques that they used were highly complex and statistical, involving tools such as segregation analysis and linkage. This branch of epidemiology is still a robust and active one that has contributed much to the understanding of genetic diseases and the pinpointing of causative genes.

Another approach to genetic epidemiology, one that stresses its role in studying genetic–environmental interactions in disease aetiology, began to emerge during the 1970s and 1980s. The epidemiologists who took this approach regarded genetic factors in the same way as environmental exposures. They took the view that each played a role in the determination of disease risk and that the exposures, whether genetic or environmental, could be analysed using the same techniques derived from classical epidemiology such as case–control studies. The populations they studied were not family members or pedigrees but community-based population samples. Publications in the mid to late 1980s and early 1990s started to use the paradigms of genetic epidemiology to underpin public health work. Its techniques were applied to improve the estimation of disease risk for diseases such as familial breast and ovarian cancer; to evaluate screening programmes for genetic diseases; to study the role of folic acid in the pathogenesis of neural tube defects and much else besides.

The growth of genetic science

New approaches to genetics also began to emerge during the last two decades of the twentieth century. Since the re-discovery of Mendel's work in 1900, and the recognition by Boveri, Bateson and others of the chromosomal basis of inheritance, the emphasis had been largely on single-gene diseases. It was William Bateson who first coined the word 'genetics', defining it as the study of heredity and variation. The 1940s and 1950s saw the first demonstrations that defects in specific proteins were responsible for diseases including glycogen storage disease type 1 and sickle cell anaemia. By 1966, Victor McKusick was able to document a catalogue of 1500 single-gene disorders or traits; this formed the basis of the first edition of his book *Mendelian inheritance in man.*

The discovery of the structure of DNA by Watson and Crick in 1953, and the subsequent elucidation of the genetic code through which the DNA sequence specifies the sequence of proteins paved the way for a new molecular era in genetics. Recombinant DNA technology was developed during the 1970s and methods for sequencing DNA were reported independently in 1977 by Fred Sanger, and by Walter Gilbert and Alan Maxam. The polymerase chain reaction – a means of amplifying tiny quantities of DNA – was invented in 1983.

These technical tools allowed much greater progress in elucidating the genetic mechanisms of disease during the 1980s and 1990s, particularly in determining the location and sequence of genetic variants responsible for single-gene disorders. These studies relied on the construction of genetic and physical maps of chromosomes, and the use of genetic linkage in families (discussed further in Chapters 2 and 3) to narrow the search down to a chromosomal region that could then be examined in more detail to pinpoint the causative gene. Early successes of this approach included the discovery of the genes that, when mutated, gave rise to cystic fibrosis, Duchenne muscular dystrophy and Huntington's disease.

In the latter half of the 1990s, the development of automatic sequencers and robotics enabled the cheap and rapid sequencing of DNA on an industrial scale. With these developments, the human genome project, begun as an international collaborative effort in 1989, entered an exponential phase with the result that, in 2003, two years ahead of schedule, the completion of a 'reference sequence' covering around 99% of the gene-containing regions was announced (see Chapter 2 for further information). Alongside the human genome project, other genome projects achieved the sequencing of the complete genomes of a variety of organisms including important pathogens, and organisms (such as the fruit fly and the mouse) used as models in research on genetics and developmental biology.

The complete human genome sequence provides the raw material for elucidating the relationships between genetic factors and human characteristics. But it is only the first step. Attention has turned to the far more complex task of analysing its composition and function and, most importantly, charting the variation that contributes to individual human characteristics including susceptibility to disease. The 'post-genomic challenge' is discussed further in Chapter 2.

The impetus for public health genetics

Against the background of accelerating output from the human genome project, and increasing interest in its implications for medicine and for society more generally, 1996 saw the publication of a paper by Muin Khoury entitled 'From genes to public health: application of genetics in disease prevention' in the *American Journal of Public Health*. Khoury observed that the scientific advances of the previous decade and the output from the human genome project would have a profound impact on the practice of medicine. Most importantly this would require a detailed public health response necessitating application of the core functions of public health to genetic technologies in disease prevention.

These core functions were, as set out in the 1998 publication *The Future of Public Health*, by the Institute of Medicine's Committee for the Study of the Future of Public Health:

- assessment using the tools of epidemiological analysis
- policy development, taking into account ethical, legal and social considerations and
- assurance, through the implementation and evaluation of interventions and programmes.

Preventive strategies were to embrace primary, secondary and tertiary interventions that would respectively bring about modification of environmental/ lifestyle factors, early detection and intervention, and the prevention of complications and deterioration. Epidemiological principles needed to be applied to genetics; a new paradigm of disease prevention had to be established, requiring knowledge of the interaction of genetic and environmental factors in disease, of the validity of genetic tests, and of how disease might be prevented through the 'identification and interruption of environmental cofactors that lead to clinical disease among persons with susceptibility genotypes'.

In the mid 1990s, academics within Schools of Public Health in the United States were beginning to see the need for more formal education in the public health implications of genetics. The University of Michigan was the first to plan specific training programmes in the subject; 17 students enrolled in their course in the autumn of 1996. The University of Washington established a similar course a year later, involving seven different Schools that included Law, Medicine, Arts and Science, Pharmacy, Nursing and Public Policy.

The year 1996 also saw the development of interest at government level as the Director of the Centers for Disease Control and Prevention (CDC) in Atlanta established a Task Force on Genetics and Disease Prevention with a remit, among others, to develop a strategic plan for CDC-wide genetic activities. The Task Force's report, *Translating Advances in Human Genetics into Public Health Action: A Strategic Plan*, was published in October 1997. The document provided some impetus for the first annual conference on Genetics and Public Health in Atlanta in May 1998, organised by CDC, the Health Resources and Services Administration in Maryland, the National Human Genome Research Institute and the Association of State and Territorial Health Officials and Affiliates (ASTHO). The aim of the conference was to address 'the public health opportunities and challenges presented by advances in human genetics research'.

Discussions took place on both sides of the Atlantic about the funding of a specialist centre for genetics and public health. These resulted in the establishment in 1997 of the Office of Genetics and Disease Prevention (now the Office of Genomics and Disease Prevention) at CDC in Atlanta, USA and of the Public Health Genetics Unit in Cambridge, UK. As if mirroring the academic developments at Michigan and Washington, the American Medical Association (AMA), the American Nurses Association (ANA) and the National Genome Research

Institute (NGRI) established the National Coalition for Health Professional Education in Genetics (NCHPEG) to enable exchanges of information and coordination of genetics educational activity among health professionals.

Since then, much has happened on both sides of the Atlantic. The Office of Genomics and Disease Prevention at CDC has continued to provide leadership in the field within the US and to develop a thriving programme of genetic epidemiological reviews under the title HuGENet (see Chapter 3 for further details). It has also recently funded three Centers for Genomics and Public Health at the Universities of Washington, Michigan and North Carolina and has established as its priorities: contributions to the knowledge base on genomics and public health – focusing on chronic diseases; technical assistance to local, state and regional public health organisations; and development and training of the current and future public health workforce.

In the UK, the Public Health Genetics Unit has continued to develop with national funding from the Wellcome Trust, the Department of Health and the Department of Trade and Industry. In April 2001, the importance of genetics for health services was recognised by the then Secretary of State for Health, Alan Milburn, in a speech in which he announced the establishment of a number of Genetics Knowledge Parks in England and Wales. Significant resources were provided for this endeavour at Cambridge, Cardiff, London, Manchester, Newcastle and Oxford. The Cambridge Genetics Knowledge Park took the lead on public health genetics and policy issues, emphasising the importance of integrating insights from genetic and molecular science, the population sciences, social sciences, arts and the humanities.

Community genetics

Some of the same forces that gave rise to public health genetics also provided the impetus for the development of a sub-discipline of clinical genetics that has come to be known as 'community genetics', largely since the establishment of a journal of that name in 1998.

Leo ten Kate (1998) defines community genetics as 'bringing genetic services to the community as a whole'. Community genetics practitioners have tended to come largely from within a genetic service background, but the discipline draws heavily on public health concepts and practice, emphasising, for example, the need for sound epidemiological data to underpin population genetic screening programmes, and for evaluation of the importance of psychological, social, ethical and legal issues arising out of such programmes.

Community genetics has made important contributions in several areas, including community-based approaches to genetic services for populations affected by haemoglobin disorders, and consideration of the role of primary care providers in the delivery of clinical genetic services.

The main difference between community genetics and public health genetics is the latter's broader perspective, embracing the whole of genetic science rather than concentrating on inherited disorders, and endeavouring to contribute to and influence public policy in many spheres including not just health service practice but also strategy for research and development, industry policy, science communication, the role of the media, and formulation of the legal and regulatory framework for science and medicine.

Attitudes to public health genetics

The growing emphasis, spurred by the human genome project, on discovering and characterising genetic determinants of health and disease has not been universally welcomed. Two highly influential publications in the late 1980s and early 1990s set out some of the contentious issues. The first, entitled *Proceed with Caution: Predicting Genetic Risks in the Recombinant DNA Era*, by American geneticist Tony Holtzman (1989), sought to point out the dangers of predictive and susceptibility testing without appropriate regulatory controls. The second, by Lori Andrews (1994) and colleagues on behalf of the Institute of Medicine, *Assessing Genetic Risks: Implications for Health and Social Policy*, fulfilled a similar function. Social scientists, fearful of the 'geneticisation' of medicine and society, also joined in to warn of the dangers of unbridled devotion to genetic science with books such as *Genethics* by David Suzuki and Peter Knudson (1990), *Exploding the Gene Myth* by Ruth Hubbard and Elijah Wald (1997), and *The DNA Mystique: The Gene as a Cultural Icon* by Dorothy Nelkin and Susan Lindee (1995). Even geneticists and other biologists appeared to feel the need to warn of the dangers of genetics: *Not in our Genes*, by Richard Lewontin, Steven Rose and Leon Kamin (1984) serves as an example.

Interest in genetics on the part of public health practitioners has also aroused some disquiet. There appear to be two main reasons for this reaction. The first reflects a general and long-standing schism between public health and clinical medicine. Despite the advent of evidence-based medicine and awareness of the importance of a population perspective in health care, public health continues to be a Cinderella specialty within the medical disciplines. The fascination of the basic sciences, the thrill of genetics and molecular biology, and the greater understanding of disease mechanisms at a cellular level continue to attract the best and most able medical graduates. At the other end of the spectrum, individuals working in the sphere of public health and social services have tended to embrace the importance of social and environmental determinants of disease and to beat a retreat away from the reductionist approach of science.

In our view, such tensions are unhelpful and potentially damaging. A public health paradigm of health and disease must take into account all determinants – biological and physical, political, economic, social and behavioural. It is the place of genetic epidemiology and public health genetics to dissect out the contribution of each component in this complex aetiology of human variation and disease and to show that the only appropriate model is one that takes in to account the full range of exposures and determinants.

Some clinical genetics professionals and others have also been suspicious of the motivation for public health genetics, fearing that the hard-won recognition of clinical genetics as a champion of individual choice and non-directive information would be undermined by a public-health-driven emphasis on using genetic diagnosis to reduce the birth prevalence of genetic diseases. We believe that public health genetics, with its emphasis on the interlocking influences of genetic and environmental factors on health, its broad perspective encompassing the humanities and social sciences as well as biology and medicine, and its focus on environmental determinants as the targets for preventive action, has done much to allay these fears in the years since its inception.

An international public health genetics network: the Bellagio initiative

During the decade since the establishment of the Office of Genomics and Disease Prevention (OGDP) in Atlanta and the Public Health Genetics Unit (PHGU) in Cambridge, other initiatives in public health genetics, varying in focus but with similar overall aims, have been taking shape in several countries, and have begun to have an impact. Knowledge resources have been developed at several locations, programmes of research and policy analysis have been initiated, and the expertise of those taking the approach of public health genetics/genomics has become influential in the advisory and policy-making framework of some countries.

The sheer volume and complexity of emerging genomic knowledge, however, and the speed of technological development are such that the goals of public health genetics cannot be achieved by individual groups or institutes, or even by individual countries. Although the full benefits of genomic research are probably still several decades away, some potential applications are emerging already. A need has therefore been identified to create an international infrastructure to ensure that new developments can be evaluated as they emerge, that robust but flexible regulatory policies are in place to maintain public confidence, and that the health professional workforce has the necessary education and training to be able to integrate new knowledge and interventions successfully into their professional practice. There is a need, too, to ensure that any benefits from developments in genomics are available not only to rich countries but also to those in the developing world.

With these challenges in mind, an expert meeting was convened with funding from the Rockefeller Foundation at their conference centre in Bellagio, Italy in

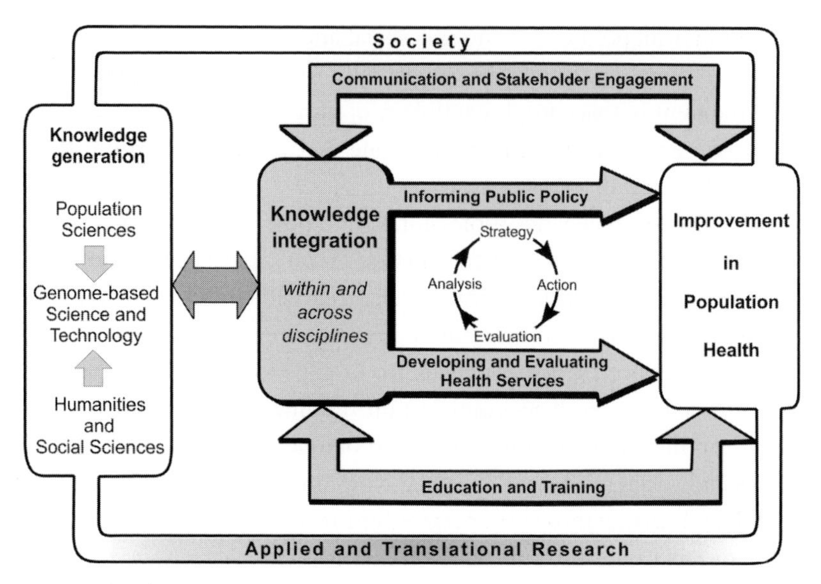

Figure 1.4 Strategy for the effective translation of genome-based knowledge and technologies for the benefit of population health

April 2005. The workshop was attended by a multidisciplinary group of experts from the UK, US, Canada, France and Germany. The key outcome was that the participants unanimously agreed first the vision for and the scope of the enterprise covered by the field that has come to be known as 'public health genetics/genomics' and, second, to establish an international forum for its promotion, to be known as the Genome-based Research and Population Health International Network or GRaPH *Int*. The use of the term *Int* signifies that the collaboration is not only *international* but also *interdisciplinary* and *integrated.*

The goal of GRaPH *Int* is the effective translation of genome-based knowledge and technologies for the benefit of population health. Figure 1.4 sets out the strategy, developed at the workshop, for achieving this goal. The functions and activities shown in the centre of the figure define the scope of the enterprise. On the left of the figure is the generation of knowledge through research; on the right is the desired output: improvement in public health. Overarching all these activities are the activities, people, institutions and views that make up society in its widest sense.

Figure 1.4 highlights:

1. The fundamental role of genome-based science and technology. The term *genome-based* is used in preference to *genomics* or *genetics* to refer to the knowledge, science, research or technologies that derive from an understanding of the genome. The word *genome* is not confined to the human genome.

Improvements in human and population health that come about through a greater understanding of, for example, bacterial or viral genomes come within the scope of the enterprise.

2. The need to incorporate research and knowledge from the population sciences and from the humanities and social sciences as relevant inputs to the enterprise.
3. The central role of knowledge integration (both within and across disciplines).
4. The use of that integrated and interdisciplinary knowledge to underpin four core sets of activities used by the enterprise to effect improvements in population health:
   - informing public policy
   - developing and evaluating health services – both preventive and clinical
   - communication and stakeholder engagement
   - education and training.
5. The importance of programmes of applied and translational research, which contribute to the goal of improved population health and also identify gaps in the knowledge base that need to be addressed by further basic research. It is acknowledged that the boundaries between 'basic' and 'applied' research are indistinct.
6. The dynamic and interactive nature of the enterprise (represented by double-headed arrows): it is informed by societal priorities, generates knowledge as well as using it, and is modulated by the effects of its own outputs and activities.
7. The cycle of analysis – strategy – action (implementation) – evaluation that represents an approach to public health practice. It is equivalent (but uses different terminology) to the Institute of Medicine's cycle of assessment – policy development – assurance.

The activity described as 'knowledge integration' is the driving force of the enterprise. It is defined as the process of selecting, storing, collating, analysing, integrating and disseminating information both within and across disciplines for the benefit of population health. It includes methodological development. It is the means by which information is transformed into knowledge.

The scope of the four activities that form the core of the enterprise is set out in Box 1.2. The role of GRaPH *Int* is to take on a leadership role by providing an international forum for dialogue and collaboration; promoting relevant research; supporting the development of an integrated knowledge base; promoting education and training; encouraging communication and engagement with the public and other stakeholders; and informing public policy.

GRaPH *Int* aims to engage and enlist all individuals and organisations, in any country, who have an interest in helping to achieve its goals. The hope is that an international and collaborative approach will bring advantages of coherence and synergy to the field.

Box 1.2 Genome-based knowledge for the benefit of population health: the four core activities

Informing public policy
- Legal, philosophical and social analysis
- Regulatory frameworks
- Engagement in the policy process
- Promoting relevant research
- International comparisons
- Working with governments

Education and training
- Genetic literacy for health professionals
- Specific training of public health specialists
- Educational materials
- Courses, workshops and conferences

Developing and evaluating health services
- Includes both preventive and clinical services
- Strategic planning
- Service organisation, manpower planning and capacity building
- Service review and evaluation
- Guideline development

Communication and stakeholder engagement
- General genetic literacy
- Public engagement
- Marketing the enterprise
- Engaging with industry

About this book

This book sets out the basic principles of public health genetics. It is written from a public health perspective but is aimed at all health professionals including specialists in genetics and genetic counselling.

This first chapter has set out some basic concepts. It defines public health genetics, outlines its history and sets out the scope and breadth of the subject. It introduces readers to the notion of genes as causative factors in disease and stresses the importance of their interaction with environmental determinants.

Chapter 2 is a primer of basic genetics and genetic technology. It aims to introduce a reader with no prior knowledge of genetics to the concepts required for the practice of public heath genetics. It discusses the relationships between genetic variants and disease, and the impact of the human genome project.

Chapter 3 provides an introduction to epidemiology, emphasising measures of incidence and prevalence and the quantification of the relative and absolute effects of exposures to genetic and environmental factors. It introduces genetic approaches to epidemiology and explains linkage, the role of twin and adoption studies and the concept of heritability. It moves on to describe approaches based on association studies and sets out how gene–environment interactions may be analysed.

Chapter 4 is about genetics in medicine and introduces the reader to the different types of genetic disorders and to genetic tests and their use. It discusses the role of genetics in disease prevention, in diagnosis and screening, and in new therapies, such as pharmacogenetics, gene therapy and stem cell therapy.

Chapter 5 is about the place of genetics in health services. It concentrates on the situation in the UK and deals with existing services, both clinical and laboratory, for genetic disorders. It outlines screening programmes for genetic diseases and discusses the options for integration of genetics into 'mainstream' medicine and primary care.

Chapter 6 sets out the ethical, legal and social implications of genetic science and deals with topics such as genetic determinism, eugenics, reproductive choice, embryo research, discrimination and genetic enhancement. It also discusses issues arising from the establishment of genetic databases, and the ethical and legal context of clinical genetics practice.

The seventh and final chapter discusses public policy options and the current policy framework for a number of key issues including use of genetics in reproductive decision-making, consent and confidentiality, protection against unfair discrimination, regulation of genetic tests, regulation of pharmacogenetics and advanced gene-based and cellular therapies, and intellectual property and patents. General policy concerns including science and public health policy, the role of the commercial sector, genetic literacy and the general public, and education and training for health professionals are also discussed.

In a book covering such a huge and fast-moving field it is virtually impossible to provide a reference list that is both comprehensive and up-to-date, and we have not attempted to list specific citations for every piece of information included. Instead, at the end of each chapter we provide a guide to 'further reading' for readers who wish to investigate specific topics in more detail. We have concentrated on recent reviews and also point out websites and web pages that provide high-quality information. The books, papers, reports and other resources referred to in the further reading sections are listed at the end of the book.

Further reading and resources

Principles of public health

The *Oxford Handbook of Public Health Practice* (Pencheon *et al.* 2006) gives a useful introduction to the basic principles and themes of public health. In his book *Healing the Schism: Epidemiology, Medicine, and the Public's Health*, Kerr White (1991) discusses the long-standing divisions between public health and clinical medicine, mentioned in this chapter as a barrier to the development of an effective, modern view of public health.

The emergence of public health genetics

The book *Genetics and Public Health in the 21st Century*, edited by Khoury, Burke and Thomson (2000), provides an excellent overview of the conceptual framework of public health genetics and its early development during the 1990s, with chapters by many of the leaders in the field. *Translating Advances in Human Genetics into Public Health Action: A Strategic Plan*, from the US Centers for Disease Control and Prevention (1997), is an example of an early attempt to make the case for public health leadership in genetics. Robert Fineman was one of the first to point out the breadth of the knowledge base for public health genetics, in his paper 'Qualifications of public health geneticists?' (1999).

The concepts and agenda of public health genetics have been further developed in many papers and reviews published over the last five years. For example, Gwinn and Khoury set out the research priorities for public health sciences in the genomics era, in a 2002 paper published in the journal *Genetics in Medicine*. The potential for using genetic information in disease prevention is assessed in Khoury (2003) 'Genetics and genomics in practice. The continuum from genetic disease to genomic information in health and disease' and in 'An epidemiologic assessment of genomic profiling for measuring susceptibility to common diseases and targeting interventions' by Khoury and colleagues (2004c). Zimmern's chapter on 'Public health genetics' in the 2003 *Encyclopedia of the Human Genome* presents a succinct overview of the very broad policy agenda for public health genetics.

The human genome project and 'genomic medicine'

The mainstream medical and science journals have monitored the development of ideas about 'genomic medicine' and its potential impact. Examples of the enthusiasm generated in the late 1990s by the prospect of the completion of the human genome project include Francis Collins's 1999 'Shattuck lecture' and John Bell's 1998 paper 'The new genetics and clinical practice'. (For an accessible introduction to the human genome and genomic science, Matt Ridley's (1999) book *Genome* is excellent though now somewhat dated. Further pointers to readings on basic genomics are given in Chapter 2.) In 2002–2003, the *New England Journal of Medicine* ran a useful series on *Genomic medicine*, which began with a 'primer' by Guttmacher and Collins (2002), and included reviews by Burke (2002) on 'Genetic testing' and 'Genomics as a probe for disease biology' (Burke 2003), by Khoury *et al.* (2003) on 'Population screening in the age of genomic medicine', and by Clayton (2003) on 'Ethical, legal, and social implications of genomic medicine'.

For a flavour of the controversy surrounding the potential of genomics to 'transform' medical practice, the first port of call is Holtzman and Marteau's 2000 paper 'Will genetics revolutionise medicine?'. The controversy over what genomics can 'deliver' for medicine has not entirely died away; for example, Merikangas and Risch, writing in *Science* in 2003, proposed that genetics research should not be directed at complex diseases that are wholly or largely preventable by environmental modification, prompting a detailed rebuttal by Khoury *et al.* in their 2005 paper 'Do we need genomic research for the prevention of common diseases with environmental causes?'. The case for a balanced approach has also been made by Willett in a 2002 paper in *Science* and by Haga and colleagues in their 2003 paper 'Genomic profiling to promote a healthy lifestyle: not ready for prime time'. A similarly cautious view of the potential for genomic profiling is taken in a 2005 report from the Human Genetics Commission. Holtzman has continued to voice scepticism about the agenda for public health genetics, in a 2006 paper published in *Community Genetics*.

Key enthusiasts for the 'genomic revolution', while not dampening their enthusiasm, have in recent years modified their estimates of the time scales involved. See, for example, Guttmacher and Collins's 2005 commentary in *JAMA*, and John Bell's 2004 review in *Nature*. In a masterful review published in the *Lancet*, Davey Smith and colleagues (2003) take stock of the current 'state of the art' in genetic epidemiology and assess realistically the prospects for public health benefits from an increased understanding of genetics and genomics.

Community genetics

Community genetics is defined in Leo ten Kate's 1998 editorial in *Community Genetics* and discussed further in his 2005 paper 'Community genetics: a bridge between clinical genetics and public health'. An editorial by ten Kate published in *Community Genetics* in 2000 makes comment on the relationship between community and public health genetics; a different view is provided by Zimmern in his 2001 review of the Khoury, Burke and Thomson book, also published in *Community Genetics*. Modell and Kuliev's 1998 article on 'The history of community genetics: the contribution of the haemoglobin disorders' illustrates the concepts of community genetics using the haemoglobinopathies as an example.

Current developments in public health genetics

For up-to-date information on current developments in public health genetics, and guides to the latest publications, the websites of the PHGU in Cambridge UK and the OGDP at the CDC in Atlanta USA are useful sources. Information about activities in public health genetics/genomics is also available from the websites of the three US centres (Michigan, North Carolina and University of Washington) designated as Centers for Genomics and Public Health.

Recent reviews on public health genetics include 'Genetics and public health – evolution, or revolution?' by Halliday *et al.* (2004), and 'Genomics and the prevention and control of common chronic diseases: emerging priorities for public health action', by Khoury and Mensah (2005). The latter is published in the April 2005 issue of the online journal *Preventing Chronic Disease*, hosted on the CDC website, which contains several articles setting out a US perspective for integrating genomics into state health programmes. A 2005 report from a Committee of the Institute of Medicine (edited by Lyle Hernandez) summarises the current 'state of the art' and prioritises issues that need to be addressed.

The new international consensus on the scope and aims of public health genetics, developed at the 2005 Bellagio meeting, is set out in a report of the meeting available on the PHGU website. It is also summarised briefly in Zimmern and Stewart's chapter in the latest edition of the *Oxford Handbook of Public Health Practice*. A paper in *Genetics in Medicine* by Burke, Khoury, Stewart and Zimmern (2006), on behalf of the Bellagio participants, develops the concepts in more detail. The GRaPH *Int* and PHGEN websites provide information about the development of international networks for public health genetics.

Genomics and global health

The role of genomics in global health, particularly in developing countries, is a huge topic that is not covered explicitly in this book. Readers interested in this field will find an excellent overview in the 2002 book *Genomics and World Health*, by the World Health Organisation's Advisory Committee on Health Research. Other WHO publications and fact sheets are available in the Genomics Resource Centre on the WHO website. Christianson and Modell (2004) have published an excellent review on 'Medical genetics in developing countries'. The 2003 report *Genomics and Global Health*, by the Genomics Working Group of the Science and Technology Task Force of the United Nations Millennium Project (based at the University of Toronto), takes a broader view of the field that includes biotechnology as well as genetics and genomics. Key goals for the genomics and global health agenda are set out in articles by Singer and Daar (2001) and Daar and colleagues (2002) in *Science* and *Nature Genetics*.

2

Genetic science and technology

Practitioners of public health genetics need a working knowledge of the basic principles of genetic science, including not just the classical rules of inheritance but also how the genetic 'programme' is played out in the functions of cells, tissues and whole organisms. They also need an understanding of how genetic changes may be related to the development and progression of disease. The first part of this chapter is devoted to laying the groundwork in genetic science and medical genetics.

In this chapter we also introduce some of the basic features of deoxyribonucleic acid (DNA) technology, which has enabled scientists to study and manipulate the genetic material. The development of this technology has been the driving force behind the human genome project, which has now delivered a complete 'reference sequence' for the human genome and is rapidly moving forward in the task of assigning functions to genes and their products. It is the explosion of information arising from the human genome project, and from the 'post-genomic' sciences such as proteomics, functional genomics, comparative genomics and bioinformatics, that is providing the raw material and the impetus for the development of new approaches to the diagnosis, treatment and prevention of disease. These new opportunities for genetics in medicine will be discussed in Chapter 4.

Basic molecular genetics

In most organisms, the genetic material in each cell is the chemical DNA. The DNA molecule acts as a code to specify the synthesis of different proteins, which are responsible for carrying out the functions of the cell. The total DNA content of an organism is called its genome. Essentially all the different cell types in the body (for example, muscle, skin or liver cells) carry the same genome, but they acquire their differences by decoding different subsets of the information it contains.

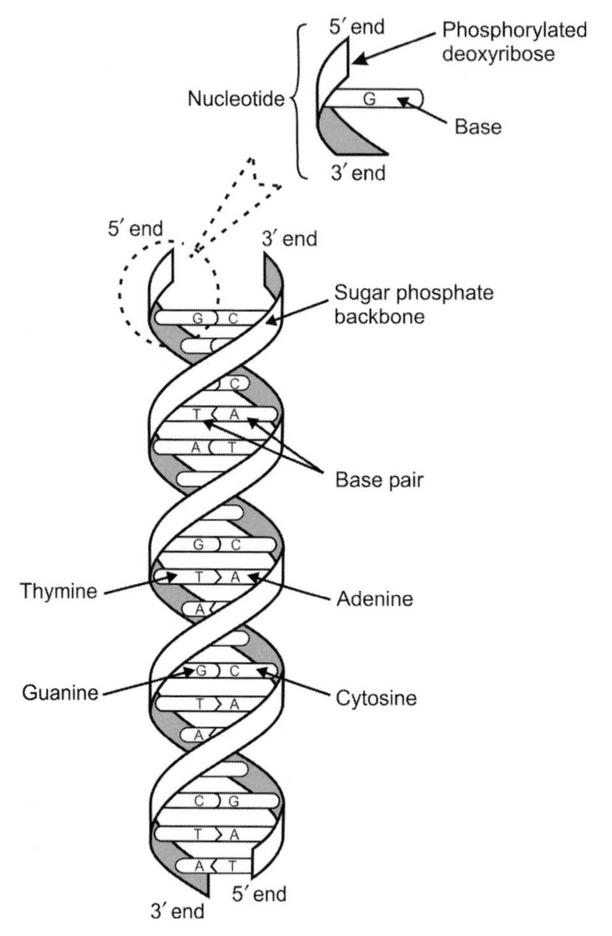

Figure 2.1 Structure of DNA

The DNA molecule has certain unique structural features that enable it to perform its function of carrying genetic information. DNA consists of two strands of linked chemical units called nucleotides, each of which is made up of a molecule known as a 'base' linked to a phosphorylated molecule of the sugar deoxyribose (Figure 2.1). The strands are wound around each other to form the famous double-helical structure elucidated by Watson and Crick in 1953. The 'rungs' connecting the two strands of this ladder-like structure are formed by pairs of bases. There are four different bases in DNA: adenine (A), thymine (T), cytosine (C) and guanine (G). The bases can only pair in specific combinations: A with T and C with G. As a result, the sequence of bases on one strand of the molecule exactly specifies the sequence on the other strand and the strands are said to be 'complementary'. From Figure 2.1 it can be seen that each strand of the DNA molecule has a direction. The phosphorylated end of the strand is called the 5′ end and the non-phosphorylated end is the 3′ end. The two strands pair in a 'head to tail' (antiparallel) fashion.

Genes and the genome

The information content of the DNA molecule lies in the sequence of bases along its length: sets of three bases (codons) act as a code to specify different amino acids, the building blocks of proteins. A sequence of DNA that contains the information to code for a protein is known as a gene. Surprisingly, less than 2% of the human genome is accounted for by genes; the function of the remainder, sometimes called 'junk DNA', is largely unknown.

There is no simple correlation between the complexity of an organism and the size of its genome, mainly because the amount of non-coding DNA varies widely in different species. The human genome consists of about three billion base pairs of DNA and contains around 22 000 protein-coding genes.

Chromosomes

Within the cell, each long DNA molecule is packaged with specific proteins to form chromatin. Complex higher-order winding and folding of the chromatin forms the structures called chromosomes, which reside within the nucleus of the cell. Each chromosome contains a particular set of genes arranged in a specific order and the set of chromosomes in a cell is known as the karyotype. The position of a particular gene on a chromosome is called its locus. Every species has a characteristic normal karyotype; the normal human karyotype consists of 46 chromosomes (Figure 2.2).

In sexually reproducing 'diploid' organisms, including humans, chromosomes come in pairs; the two members of a pair have the same length and shape and are said to be homologous (Figure 2.2). One member of each homologous pair was inherited from the individual's father and the other from the mother. Homologous chromosomes contain the same set of genes in the same order, so every individual has two copies of every gene. However, the two copies may vary slightly from each other. Genetic variation is discussed further later in this chapter.

Mammals such as humans also have two sex chromosomes, called X and Y. Females carry two X chromosomes while males have an X and a Y. The X and Y chromosomes contain different sets of genes from one another. The other 22 pairs of chromosomes are known as autosomes.

Although most of the DNA is stored in the 46 chromosomes in the nucleus, a small amount is found in other subcellular structures called mitochondria, which act as the cell's power houses. All of an individual's mitochondrial DNA is inherited from his or her mother, in the cytoplasm of the egg cell.

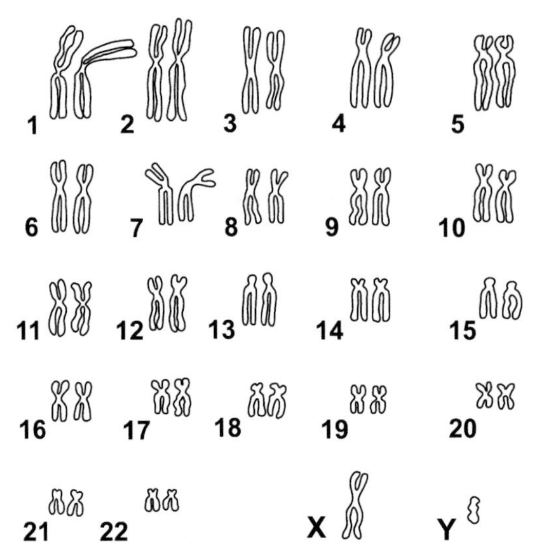

Figure 2.2 Human karyotype. Depiction of full set of chromosomes from a human male: 22 homologous pairs of autosomes and one pair of sex chromosomes, one X and one Y. A female karyotype would have two X chromosomes and no Y

The 'central dogma': DNA makes RNA makes protein

The DNA sequence of a gene has to be read by the cell and translated into the amino acid sequence of a protein. Decoding requires the participation of an intermediary called messenger ribonucleic acid RNA (mRNA). RNA is also a nucleic acid, but unlike DNA it is single-stranded, and the nucleotide base thymine is replaced by uracil (U), while the sugar ribose replaces deoxyribose. When a gene is expressed in a cell, a molecule of mRNA is synthesised that has a sequence of bases complementary to one strand of the gene's DNA (Figure 2.3). The DNA strand that acts as the template is read in the 5′ to 3′ direction. Sets of three bases (triplets) along the mRNA – known as codons – specify each of the 20 amino acids found in proteins. There are also codons that signal the end of the gene (stop codons). Some amino acids are specified by more than one codon; for example, phenylalanine is encoded by the codons UUU or UUC, while proline is specified by any of four codons, CCU, CCC, CCA or CCG.

Gene expression is a two-part process. In the first stage, known as transcription, mRNA is made using a DNA template (Figure 2.3). In the second stage, translation, the order of codons on the mRNA specifies the order in which amino acids are joined together. The amino acid chain (also known as a polypeptide chain) that emerges from translation arranges and folds itself to acquire a characteristic three-dimensional shape: the protein. The protein molecule may be modified by

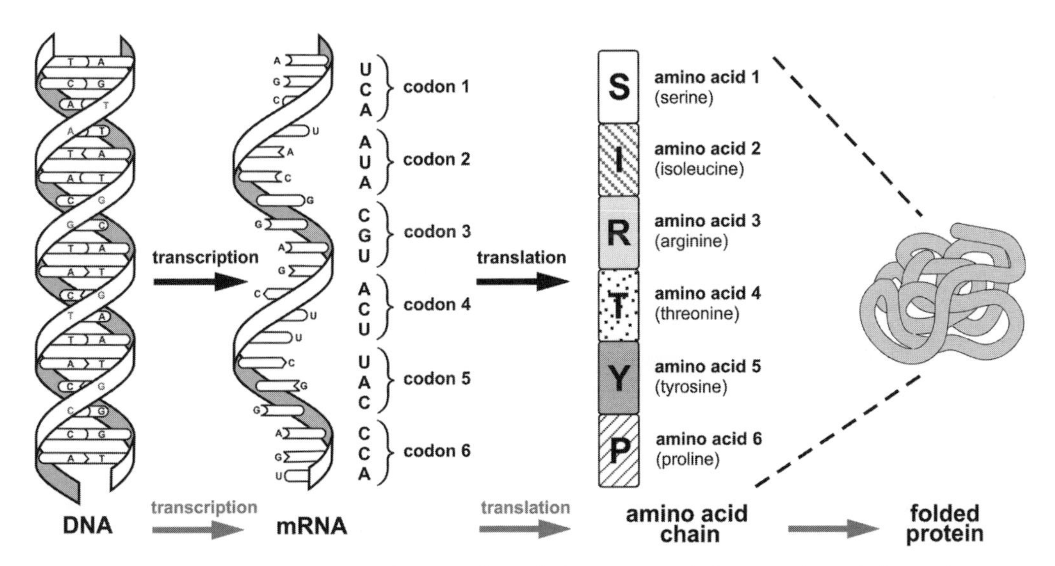

Figure 2.3 Gene expression: transcription and translation. In transcription, DNA is copied to make mRNA; in translation, the mRNA codons direct the formation of a chain of amino acids. The amino acid chain folds itself to form a protein molecule

the addition of various chemical groups such as sugars, phosphate groups or lipids (fats) and transported to the compartment of the cell where it carries out its function. In order to be functionally active it may need to act together with other proteins in a complex.

Gene structure and expression in more detail

The picture of the gene as a string of bases that maps exactly to the amino acid sequence of a protein is an oversimplification. In fact the coding sequence of a gene is interrupted by stretches of non-coding DNA called introns; the stretches of coding DNA are called exons (Figure 2.4). There are also specialised sequences of DNA, outside the coding sequence, that have a role in the control of gene expression: in determining when, where (that is, in which cells) and for how long a gene is switched on. These regulatory sequences are known as promoters and enhancers. Promoters tend to be fairly close to the transcriptional start site of the gene, while enhancers may be many hundreds or even thousands of base pairs away, on either side of the coding sequence or even sometimes within an intron.

A more detailed look at gene expression shows that the process is compartmentalised between the nucleus of the cell and the cytoplasm. Transcription takes place in the nucleus, then the introns are removed (spliced) out of the primary RNA transcript to form a mature mRNA. The mRNA leaves the nucleus and translation is carried out by a large molecular machine called the ribosome, which contains

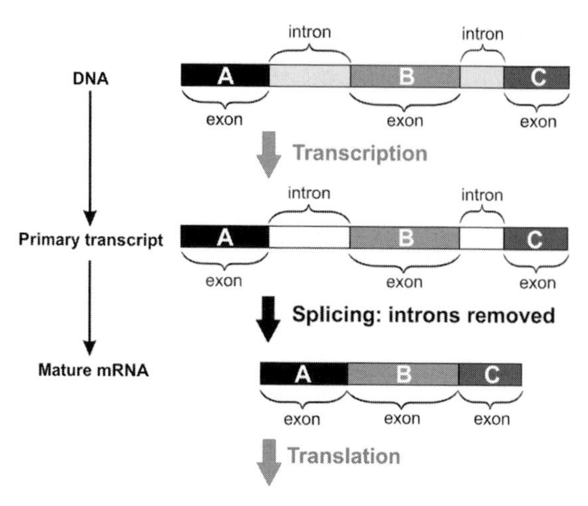

Figure 2.4 Introns and exons. Introns are regions of non-coding DNA interspersed with regions of coding DNA (exons) within genes. Introns are removed from mRNA in a process called splicing, to create mature mRNA transcripts

specific ribosomal proteins and a set of specific RNA molecules called ribosomal RNA. The role of the ribosome is to assemble a string of amino acids in the order specified by the mRNA codons. Another type of RNA molecule, transfer RNA (tRNA), also plays a part in this process, acting as a molecular adaptor between the amino acid and the corresponding mRNA codon. There are different tRNAs specific for each of the 20 amino acids found in protein.

It is important to appreciate that gene expression is not an autonomous function of DNA. In fact the same applies to every aspect of DNA and RNA metabolism. All of these functions require the participation of large protein complexes and complex regulatory mechanisms. For example, the initiation of transcription alone requires the function of a huge protein complex that consists of the basic transcriptional machinery (proteins responsible for functions such as recognition of the start site and polymerisation of the RNA nucleotides) and a battery of regulatory proteins that bind to specific sequences in promoters and enhancers. The chromatin proteins also play a role, for example by regulating the accessibility of gene sequences to the transcriptional machinery. Intron splicing, translational initiation, translation itself and post-translational processing similarly all depend on the function of a large repertoire of proteins.

The complexity of the genetic programme

Every cell of the body (apart from the sex cells: sperm or eggs) contains a full complement of DNA – a full diploid genome. Different types of cells have different

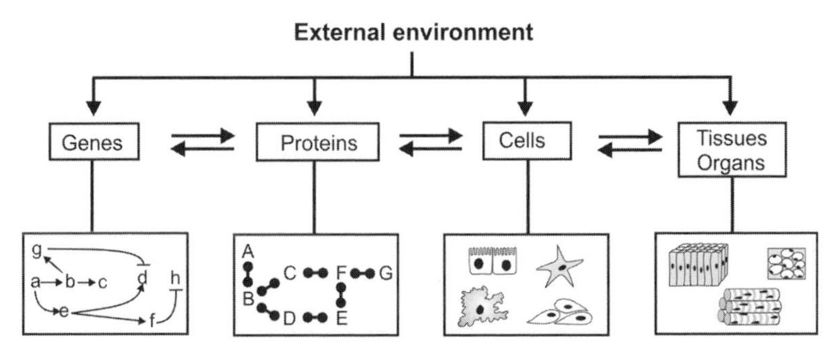

Figure 2.5 Gene regulation. Complex regulatory systems involving genes, proteins, cells, tissues and organs, and influenced by the external environment, control the expression of genes in growth, development and maintenance of the body. The system is hierarchical, with genes representing the lowest level of the hierarchy, and tissues and organs the highest level. Two-way arrows indicate interactions between components of adjacent levels. Interactions may be stimulatory or inhibitory. For example, in the simple gene regulation diagram shown at the left of the figure, arrows indicate stimulation (gene switched on) and blunt-ended lines indicate inhibition (gene switched off). Adapted from Martinez Arias, A. and Stewart, A. (2002). *Molecular Principles of Animal Development*, Figure 2, by permission of Oxford University Press

functional characteristics because they have expressed different subsets of the genome in a specific temporal pattern as the organism developed.

The process by which a single fertilised egg grows and develops into an organism with a wide variety of cell and tissue types, integrated into a functional whole, involves far more than a simple, linear decoding of the organism's DNA. The decoding process itself is regulated and carried out by proteins, which in this way feed information back to the genome, selecting the next batches of genes to be decoded as development proceeds (Figure 2.5).

As cells of a specific type develop and multiply, they must transmit their developmental state to the cells they give rise to. That is, the new cells arising from a cell division must somehow 'know' which sets of their genes should be active or inactive. This is achieved by modifications to the DNA that are heritable from one cell generation to the next but do not involve changes to the primary DNA sequences. These modifications are termed 'epigenetic'.

A common epigenetic modification is methylation of DNA. Methylation tends to silence gene expression by promoting an inactive configuration of chromatin that prevents the initiation of transcription. Other epigenetic modifications include chemical changes (such as acetylation and deacetylation) to chromatin proteins. Epigenetic mechanisms are an important source of variation in gene function that does not involve variation in the DNA sequence itself.

As cell numbers grow, groups of cells communicate with one another, sending and receiving signals that help to direct and coordinate the unfolding of the genetic programme. Some signals are spatially restricted so that they act only among neighbouring groups of cells whereas others (for example, hormones) have much longer-range effects. In this way, each cell of the organism acquires its final characteristics both as a result of its developmental history (the constellation of proteins and mosaic of active and inactive genes it acquired from the earlier cells that gave rise to it) and the signals it receives and sends.

Even a very 'simple' genetic regulatory circuit reveals a remarkable degree of complexity, with multiple control points where regulation is mediated by multi-subunit protein complexes whose composition and function may themselves be variable and responsive to regulation. The combinatorial nature of gene regulation – the fact that different combinations of proteins can be used to achieve different regulatory outcomes – means that a relatively small number of proteins (and therefore genes) can be used to build an exquisitely complex regulatory system.

Extra complexity is also achieved at the level of individual genes and proteins. For example, the use of alternative splicing patterns can enable different cells to produce different proteins from the 'same' gene, by using different sets of exons. Alternative splicing is a characteristic feature of, for example, many genes that encode the structural proteins of muscle. Even the 'same' protein – that is, a protein with a specific amino acid sequence – may acquire different post-translational modifications in different cell types, altering its function.

Mechanisms such as these, which enable complexity to be achieved using a limited set of genes, appear to be the explanation for the relatively small size of the human genome: it had been thought that the sophisticated brain functions of human beings would be associated with a genome of well over 100 000 genes, but with only about 22 000 genes our genome is not appreciably larger than those of organisms such as fruit flies or nematode worms.

The complex, interconnecting web of regulatory processes functions not only during development but throughout the life of the organism, maintaining the body's basic metabolic systems and carrying out the specialised physiological processes of different tissues and organs. We are beginning to discover some of the genetic and cellular pathways that operate during these processes: although common types of mechanisms emerge, the ways in which these mechanisms are deployed and combined add layer upon layer of complexity.

It follows that it is almost always over-simplistic to speak in terms of a 'gene for' a particular characteristic (or disease): no gene acts in isolation. The genome does not work in a direct, instructive way to build and maintain an organism, but unfolds its programme in stages as part of an interactive system involving a functional hierarchy of genes, proteins, cells, tissues and organs (Figure 2.5).

At every stage, this internal system is connected to, and influenced by, the external environment.

Genetic variation: mutation and polymorphism

With the exception of identical twins or clones, every individual is genetically unique. Sequence variation in DNA arises by the process of mutation. Mutations can be caused by environmental factors such as certain chemicals or radiation, or by errors in DNA processing, for example during replication. Most mutations are repaired by the DNA repair apparatus of the cell, but some may survive and be passed on when the cell divides. If an unrepaired mutation occurs in a sex cell, it may be inherited by the offspring of the individual in whom it arose.

There are several different types of mutation (Box 2.1). Point mutations (also known as single base substitutions) change the DNA sequence at a single nucleotide. A point mutation may have no functional effect or only a very subtle effect if, for example, the mutation occurs in the 'junk' DNA or if it changes a codon sequence to one that still encodes the same or a similar amino acid (Figure 2.6). However, if a point mutation has the effect of substituting a different amino acid or of introducing a stop signal, for example, it may lead to the production of a very different protein or even no protein at all. A mutation in a regulatory sequence may lead to mis-expression of the gene or prevent expression altogether. Such mutations may have a profound effect on the individual harbouring them.

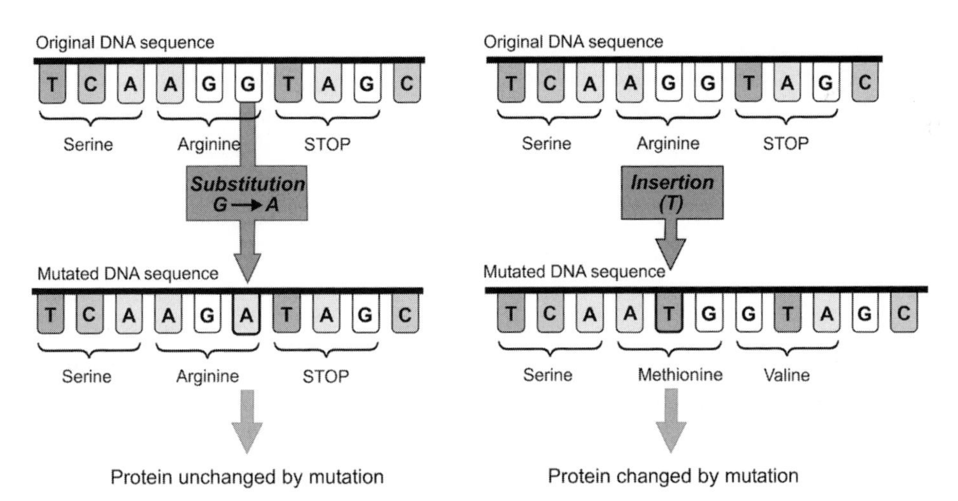

Figure 2.6 Point mutations. Two different point mutations may have very different effects. In this example, a substitution mutation does not change the coding sequence but an insertion mutation alters the whole reading frame of the DNA sequence and alters the protein it encodes

Box 2.1 Types of mutations

1. Point mutations (single base substitutions)

- **Missense mutations** alter the codon to one encoding a different amino acid and may change the function of the protein.
- **Nonsense mutations** replace an amino acid-encoding codon with a stop codon so that the protein chain is terminated prematurely.
- **Silent mutations** have no effect on protein sequence because they occur in the 'junk' DNA or because they change the codon sequence to one that encodes the same amino acid (Figure 2.6).
- **Splice site mutations** alter the sequence at a splice site so that an intron is no longer removed correctly and an abnormal protein is produced.
- **Regulatory** mutations disrupt the control sequence of the gene so that it is expressed inappropriately.

2. Insertions and deletions

- **Frameshift insertions and deletions** insert or delete one or two bases so that the reading frame (the sequence of triplet codons) of a protein is disrupted. The result is an abnormal protein or one that is terminated prematurely.
- **In-frame insertions and deletions** insert or delete sets of three bases so that the reading frame is not altered. A small in-frame insertion or deletion may not have a serious effect but larger changes are likely to be deleterious.

3. Chromosomal mutations (alterations of large blocks of DNA)

- **Translocations** involve transfer or exchange of chromosomal material between two chromosomes.
- **Inversions** reverse the orientation of a chromosome piece.
- **Deletions and duplications** remove or duplicate large segments of DNA.
- **Chromsome non-disjunction** results from abnormal chromosome separation during meiosis and can lead to a whole chromosome being duplicated or lost (known as aneuploidy).

Other types of mutation, including insertions, deletions, inversions and translocations, may alter blocks of DNA ranging from just one or a few nucleotides to large segments of the chromosome, affecting from one to many hundreds of genes. Their effects vary, depending, for example, on the size and site of the alteration and whether it leads to further genetic changes. Examples of diseases caused by different types of mutations are discussed later in this chapter and in Chapter 4.

One interesting type of mutation, which has been implicated in several genetic diseases including Huntington's disease, fragile X syndrome and myotonic dystrophy, involves expansion of blocks of repeated sequence present in the coding or regulatory regions of some genes. Depending on the gene and the position of the triplet repeat, expansion may lead to production of an altered protein or to no functional product at all. Huntington's disease is caused by expansion of a tract of repeated CAG triplets in the DNA sequence of the huntingtin gene on chromosome 4. The normal number of repeats is between 11 and 30 but people with Huntington's disease may have between 36 and 125 repeats and produce an altered huntingtin protein with abnormal function. Triplet repeats have a tendency to be unstable; that is, they can increase in length from one generation to the next. This can lead to increasing severity of disease and/or earlier onset, a phenomenon known as 'anticipation'. For this reason, triplet repeat expansions are sometimes described as 'dynamic mutations'.

Although all sequence variation must arise initially by mutation, the term is usually reserved for rare and often deleterious variants. 'Normal' sequence variants that are found at a frequency of at least 1% in a population are termed polymorphisms.

Different variants of the same gene are known as alleles. An individual who has two identical alleles of a particular gene is said to be homozygous for that gene, while a person who carries two different alleles is said to be heterozygous. The specific set of alleles or sequences carried by an individual is known as his or her genotype. The observable characteristics of an individual are known as the phenotype. As discussed in Chapter 1, the phenotype results from interactions between the individual's genetic make-up and environmental influences. Few characteristics are attributable to genetic factors alone.

Cell division and the maintenance of the genome

When an ordinary somatic cell divides, its whole genome must be faithfully passed on to each of the two new cells (Figure 2.7, left panel). This type of cell division is called mitosis. First, the DNA of the cell is replicated. This process takes advantage of the fact that the sequence of one strand of the DNA molecule is complementary to the sequence on the other strand: the helix essentially 'unzips' and, in a process catalysed by specific proteins, each of the two strands acts as a template for the synthesis of a new complementary strand. The result is two new DNA molecules identical to the original one. When each chromosome has replicated in this way, the two new chromosomes can be seen to be attached to one another in a region called the centromere, giving them a characteristic cross-shaped structure. The membrane that surrounds the cell nucleus dissolves and the replicated chromosomes then line up in a plane through the middle of the cell. As the cell divides they pull apart at the centromere so that one copy of each chromosome passes into each of the two new cells. A new nucleus forms around the chromosomes of each of the cells. Cell division is a tightly regulated process that requires the participation of specialised proteins at every stage.

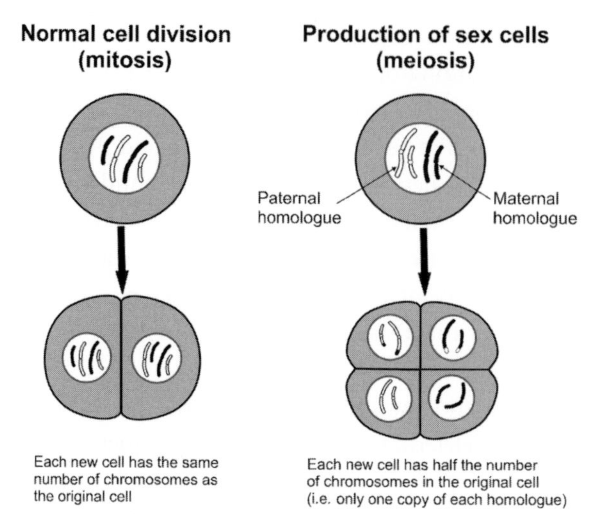

Figure 2.7 Mitosis and meiosis. Mitosis is the normal form of cell division, a process of replication that produces daughter cells with diploid genomes (two sets of chromosomes). Meiosis is a specialised form of cell division that creates sex cells with haploid genomes (one set of chromosomes)

Meiosis and recombination: the formation of sex cells

As mentioned previously, when sex cells (sperm or eggs) are produced, the genome must be halved so that each parent passes on only one copy of each chromosome to each of its offspring. The formation of sex cells, also called gametes, is achieved by a specialised cell division called meiosis (Figure 2.7, right panel). Meiosis is a two-stage process. In the first stage, the chromosomes are replicated as in mitosis, but instead of lining up individually through the middle of the cell, they line up as homologous pairs, so that when the cell divides, the members of each pair segregate from one another. Each of the resulting two cells then undergoes a mitosis-like division that separates the replicated chromosomes. The end result is four haploid sex cells, each of which contains only one member of each homologous chromosome pair and therefore only one allele of each gene (Figure 2.7). Fertilisation restores the diploid genome.

Meiosis has a very important additional feature: when homologous chromosome pairs line up during the first phase of meiosis, chromosome segments – in other words, sets of alleles – may be exchanged between adjacent members of a pair, in a process known as crossing over (Figure 2.8). The number of exchanges varies in different meioses but is typically around one to two per chromosome pair. The positions along the chromosome at which the exchanges take place can also vary. These exchanges shuffle alleles between the homologues, a process called

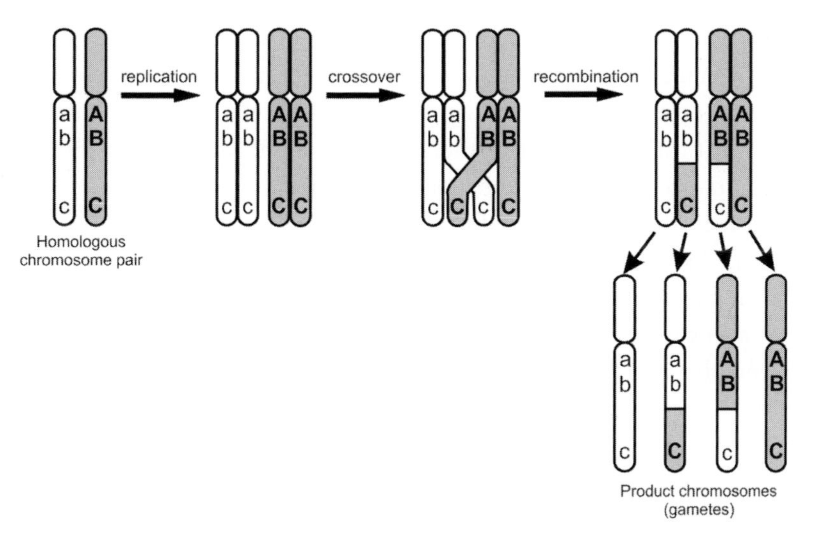

Figure 2.8 Recombination. Exchange of alleles between homologous chromosomes during meiosis creates genetic variation among the daughter chromosomes. Adapted with permission from *Crossing-over and Recombination During Meiosis*. Access Excellence @ the National Health Museum Available at www.accessexcellence.org/RC/VL/GG/comeiosis.html

genetic recombination. Genes located on different chromosomes will segregate at random from each other and so alleles at those loci will be separated during meiosis approximately 50% of the time. However, genes on the same chromosome will have a greater tendency to be inherited together and are said to be linked. The degree of linkage depends roughly on the physical distance between the genes: the closer they are together, the tighter the linkage. Analysis of linkage, discussed in more detail in Chapter 3, has been a mainstay of research aimed at mapping, on the chromosomes, the genes associated with genetic diseases.

Sexual reproduction has several features that enhance the genetic variation that arises by sequence mutation. At the first meiotic division, the orientation of each homologous pair is independent of the orientation of all the other pairs so each sex cell is likely to end up with a different haploid set of chromosomes. This is known as independent assortment of chromosomes. Further variation arises when recombination shuffles sets of alleles between homologous chromosomes, then fertilisation brings together genes from two different individuals to create a unique new individual.

Inheritance patterns

Until the end of the nineteenth century, it was generally thought that inheritance was a process of blending of the characteristics of two different parents. However, the work of Mendel, largely unrecognised during his lifetime but rediscovered early in the twentieth century, showed that genetic factors (which we now know as genes) do not blend at fertilisation but persist in the offspring as discrete units that are in turn transmitted to the next generation. Mendel also showed that these factors occur in pairs, and that the members of the pairs segregate from one another when sex cells are formed.

As discussed briefly in Chapter 1, there are some phenotypic characteristics, including some genetic diseases, that are determined solely or largely by the alleles at a single genetic locus, and in these cases it is possible to see Mendel's laws at work directly. An example is the ABO blood group system in humans (Figure 2.9). The ABO blood group is determined by three alleles (*A*, *B* and *i*) at a single locus. The *A* and *B* alleles each encode a distinct protein expressed on the surface of red blood cells. The *i* allele is non-functional, producing no protein. If an individual has the genotype *AA* or *Ai*, he or she has the blood group (phenotype) A. Similarly, individuals with the genotypes *BB* or *Bi* have blood group B. Only individuals with the genotype *ii* show the effects of carrying the *i* allele, and have blood group O. In this situation, both the A and B traits are said to be dominant over O, and O is said to be recessive. Individuals with the genotype *AB* have blood group AB (that is, they produce both the A and B proteins); in this situation, the A and B traits are said to be co-dominant.

Knowing the ABO blood group genotypes of two parents makes it possible to predict the probability that their children will have a particular genotype, and therefore a particular blood group. For example, suppose two parents both have the genotype *Ai*. Because these alleles separate at meiosis when sex cells are formed, each parent will transmit only the *A* allele or the *i* allele, but not both, to each child. It follows (Figure 2.9) that there is a 75% chance that a child of theirs will have blood group A (genotypes *Ai* or *AA*) and a 25% chance that the child will have blood group O (*ii* genotype).

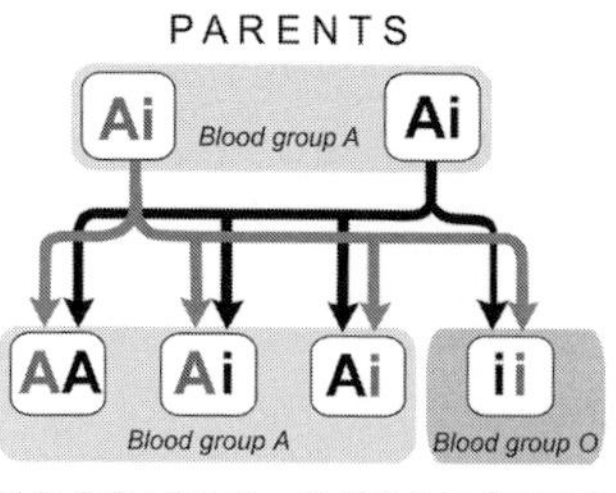

Figure 2.9 AO blood group inheritance. The red blood cell surface marker A allele is dominant over the i allele, so that heterozygous individuals (Ai) have blood group A. The offspring of parents who are both heterozygous may have blood groups A or O

Genes and disease

Mutations in the DNA sequence of a gene can cause disease. If a disease-causing mutation is present in the sex cells of an individual it can be passed on to his or her children. About 4000 heritable diseases are known to be associated with mutations in single genes. These diseases are known as single-gene or Mendelian disorders, because they show patterns of inheritance consistent with those discovered by Mendel.

Some genetic diseases are caused not by mutations in single genes but by larger-scale alterations involving whole chromosomes or large pieces of chromosomes. Perhaps the best known of these disorders is Down syndrome, which is caused by the presence of an extra copy of chromosome 21 (Figure 2.10). Chromosomal disorders usually arise as a result of mistakes that occur during the meiosis divisions that give rise to sperm and egg cells.

Individually, genetic diseases caused by chromosomal alterations or single-gene mutations are rare, but collectively these disorders are relatively common. The combined birth prevalence for single-gene diseases and chromosomal abnormalities is around 1–2%, and it has been estimated that within a population of 250 000 there will be about 1000 living patients suffering from such diseases.

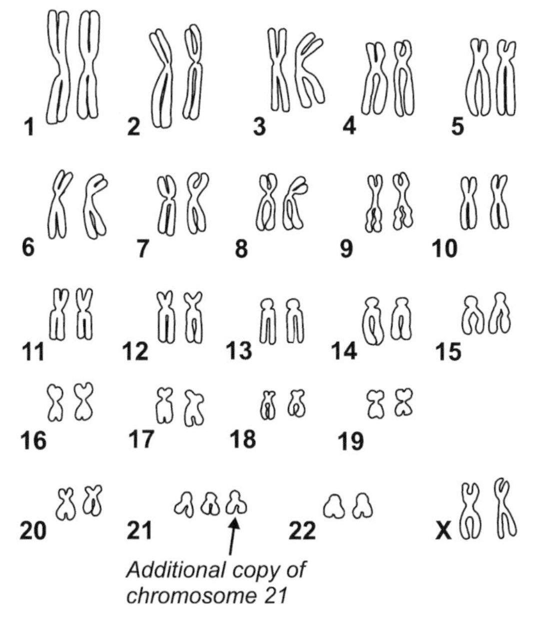

Figure 2.10 Down syndrome karyotype. Down syndrome is caused by trisomy 21, the presence of an additional copy of chromosome 21

In addition, as we have emphasised in Chapter 1, susceptibility to the common diseases of middle and later life is known to have a genetic component. In this case, the association between gene variants and disease is less clear-cut: more than one gene may be involved and the genes interact in complex ways with each other and with environmental and lifestyle factors to determine whether and how disease will develop.

Recent advances in genetics and molecular biology have begun to elucidate both the genetic mutations underlying many single-gene diseases, and some of the genetic variants (or polymorphisms) associated with susceptibility to common diseases.

Mendelian ('single-gene') diseases

Cystic fibrosis, Huntington's disease and haemophilia are all examples of Mendelian disorders caused by alterations in single genes.

Cystic fibrosis is an autosomal recessive disorder (Figure 2.11); that is, an individual will only develop the disease if he or she has two mutant alleles. An individual with one normal and one CF allele will be an unaffected carrier. Although a carrier does not develop disease, he or she has a 50% chance of passing on the mutant allele to each child; if two carriers conceive a child, there will be a

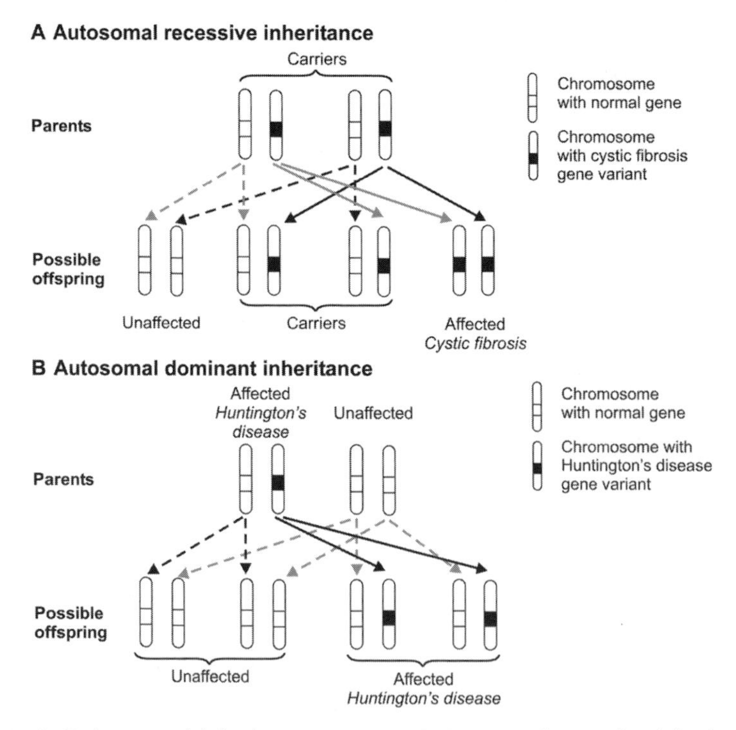

Figure 2.11 **A, B** Autosomal inheritance patterns. **A** Autosomal recessive inheritance; **B** autosomal dominant inheritance

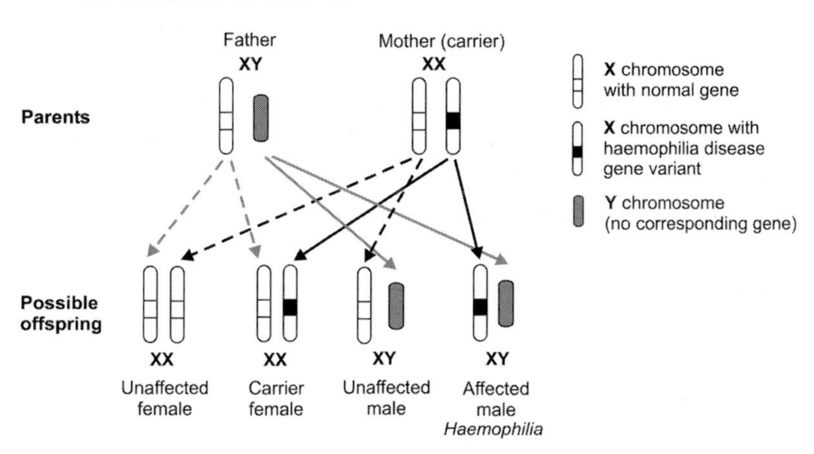

Figure 2.12 X-linked inheritance

25% chance of the child inheriting a mutant allele from both parents and of therefore being born with the disease.

In the case of Huntington's disease, the mutant allele is autosomal and dominant (Figure 2.11). This means that individuals with the disease may have either one or two copies of the mutant allele. A person with one parent who has Huntington's disease has a 50% chance of having inherited the mutant gene.

Haemophilia is an example of a sex-linked genetic disease (Figure 2.12). This means that the gene associated with the disease is on one of the sex chromosomes, almost invariably (as in the haemophilia example) the X chromosome. Females have two X chromosomes, so a female with one normal and one haemophilia mutant allele, which is recessive, will be a normal carrier. If her partner is unaffected, all their daughters will also be unaffected (either normal or carriers) but each son has a 50% chance of carrying the mutant allele on his single X chromosome, and therefore of being affected because he carries no normal allele for the gene.

Many Mendelian diseases are congenital; that is, they are clinically apparent at birth or soon after. Some, however, are later in onset and an individual carrying the mutation may have no symptoms until he or she reaches adulthood or middle age.

Mitochondrial disorders

Some single-gene diseases are caused by mutations not in nuclear DNA, but in the DNA of the mitochondria. An example is Leber's hereditary optic neuropathy, in which blindness results from damage to the optic nerve. Because the mitochondria are passed on via the cytoplasm of the egg, mitochondrial diseases show maternal inheritance. The severity of mitochondrial diseases can vary depending on the proportion of the mitochondria that carry the mutation.

Chromosomal disorders

Chromosomal abnormalities can affect either the total number of chromosomes, or their structure. These abnormalities occur at a surprisingly high frequency in human reproduction, affecting perhaps as many as 25% of all conceptions.

Most numerical chromosomal abnormalities affecting the autosomes (that is, chromosomes other than the sex chromosomes) are incompatible with life and are a major cause of spontaneous abortion. Those that are not always lethal, such as Down syndrome (also known as trisomy 21), usually cause major disability. After Down syndrome, which has an overall birth prevalence of about 1 in 1000 but is substantially more common in babies conceived by women over 35, the two most common trisomies seen in newborn infants are trisomies 13 and 18, affecting about 1 in 15 000 and 1 in 10 000 newborn infants respectively. Most babies with trisomy 13 or 18 die before birth or in early infancy.

Abnormalities of the number of sex chromosomes (for example, XXY, XYY, XXX) are much less likely to be lethal and indeed some individuals with these anomalies are unaware that their chromosomal constitution is not normal. Most, but not all, changes in the number of sex chromosomes cause infertility and can be associated with abnormalities of sexual development.

Structural chromosomal abnormalities include deletions, duplications, inversions and translocations affecting large segments of specific chromosome(s) in an individual. Large deletions or duplications are usually lethal or associated with severe birth defects; smaller lesions may have relatively mild effects. Cri du chat syndrome, a rare disease with a birth prevalence of about 1 in 50 000, is an example of a condition caused by a deletion, in this case deletion of part of chromosome 5. Individuals with this deletion have severe learning disability, abnormal larynx development (causing a characteristic cry that gives the syndrome its name), and may also suffer from respiratory problems.

A translocation, in which part of a chromosome has become detached from its correct location and has either joined on to a different chromosome or exchanged with part of a different chromosome, may cause no problem to the individual if it is balanced (that is, no chromosomal material is missing), and it has not disrupted an important gene at the translocation breakpoint. However, meiosis in an individual carrying such a translocation can lead to the production of sex cells in which the chromosomal material is not balanced, so that after fertilisation the fetus carries either a deletion or a duplication, which may be lethal. The existence of a balanced translocation in a family may be suggested by a family history of spontaneous abortion, and/or of the birth of babies with serious congenital defects. Balanced translocations are relatively common, occurring at a frequency of about 1 in 500 in live newborns.

Diseases caused by disorders in epigenetic mechanisms

For most genes, the alleles inherited from the mother and the father are functionally equivalent. However, some genes carry an epigenetic 'imprint', established at some point during the development of the sperm and the egg, which labels one allele as either paternally or maternally inherited (Figure 2.13). The imprint may affect whether the allele is expressed during development, and mutations that disrupt normal imprinting may result in disease.

An example is Prader–Willi syndrome, a rare disease with a birth prevalence of around 1 in 10 000. Most people with this disease have been found to have a small deletion in a specific region of one of their copies of chromosome 15. Strikingly, the deletion always affects the copy of chromosome 15 inherited from the patient's father. The region of chromosome 15 implicated in this syndrome carries certain genes that are active when inherited from the father but imprinted and inactive when inherited from the mother. As a result, individuals with Prader–Willi syndrome have no active copy of these genes during early development and show various clinical features associated with abnormal development, such as short stature, learning difficulties and feeding difficulties in infancy followed by massive over-eating and obesity during early childhood.

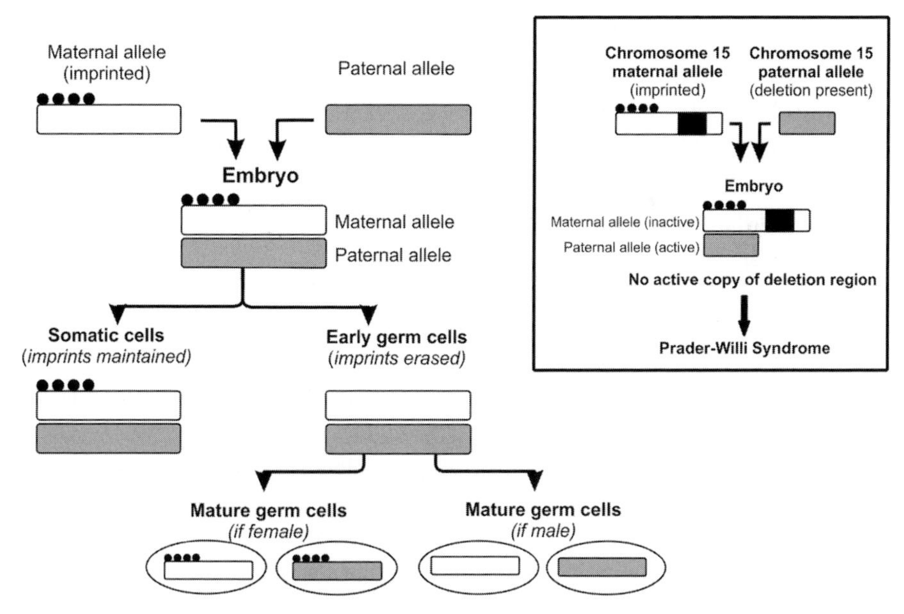

Figure 2.13 Imprinting. Imprinting is a form of labelling such as DNA methylation, which controls the expression of alleles in somatic (non-sex) cells according to whether they were maternally or paternally inherited. Paternal inheritance of a deleted region of chromosome 15 causes Prader–Willi syndrome in offspring

In the mouse, more than 70 protein-coding genes have been found to show genomic imprinting but it is not known whether, in all of these cases, the imprinting is essential for normal development. Imprinting is associated with epigenetic modifications of the genome, such as methylation, that inhibit gene expression. The genomic imprint inherited by an individual must be erased at some point, perhaps during the early stages of gamete development, and then the correct imprint for that individual's sex is established at a later stage of sperm or egg differentiation.

Epigenetic changes are also thought to be important in the development of cancer, discussed later in this chapter.

Mendelian subsets of common diseases

Most common disease is caused by the combined effects of many genes interacting with environmental factors. However, sometimes there are families in which several family members are affected by the same disease, often at an early age, and the disease shows a Mendelian inheritance pattern through the family, suggesting the existence of a single mutation that confers a high risk of disease. In these Mendelian (single gene) subsets of common disease, genotype can be used with a fairly high degree of certainty to predict the development of disease (the phenotype) (Table 2.1).

Table 2.1. Some multifactorial diseases with Mendelian subsets

Multifactorial disease	Mendelian subset
Atherosclerosis	Familial hypercholesterolaemia due to low-density lipoprotein receptor mutations
Cirrhosis of the liver	Hereditary haemochromatosis due to *HFE* mutations
Emphysema	$Alpha_1$-antitrypsin deficiency
Diabetes	Maturity-onset diabetes of the young due to mutations in the hepatocyte nuclear factor-4α, glucokinase or hepatocyte nuclear factor-1α genes
Breast cancer	Autosomal dominant hereditary breast cancer due to mutations in the *BRCA1*, *BRCA2*, *p53* or *PTEN* gene
Colorectal cancer	Familial adenomatous polyposis coli (FAP) due to mutations in the *APC* gene
	Hereditary non-polyposis colorectal cancer (HNPCC) due to mismatch repair gene mutations
Alzheimer disease	Autosomal dominant hereditary Alzheimer disease due to mutations in the amyloid precursor protein, presenilin 1 or presenilin 2 genes

Table reproduced from Rose, P. and Lucassen, A. (1999). *Practical Genetics for Primary Care*, Table 9.1, with permission from Oxford University Press.

An example is familial hypercholesterolaemia, a dominantly inherited condition that is characterised by a build-up of cholesterol and a high risk of premature cardiovascular disease. The disease is caused by mutations in a gene encoding a cell-surface receptor for a blood lipoprotein. About 1 in 500 people are thought to carry the mutant gene and virtually all will develop symptoms of the disease at some stage of their life. In the population as a whole, only about 1 in 20 people who develop hypercholesterolaemia carry a strongly predisposing single-gene mutation; in general, single-gene subsets of common diseases account for a maximum of 5–10% of the total burden of disease. In the rest of the population, disease results from the combined effects of several common gene variants, each of weak effect, together with environmental and lifestyle factors.

Multifactorial disease

As discussed in Chapter 1, most – perhaps even all – disease has at least some genetic input. Even infectious disease, for example, can be influenced by genetic factors that affect susceptibility to infection or the effectiveness of the body's disease-fighting mechanisms. Many common diseases, such as coronary heart disease, Alzheimer's dementia and diabetes, have been known for a long time to have a tendency to run in families, suggesting the possibility of a genetic contribution, though the shared environment experienced by most families also contributes to familial clustering of disease.

Some congenital diseases, such as neural tube defects or cleft lip and palate, also show a tendency to run in families but are not associated with a single genetic mutation. These diseases are also thought to result from a combination of genetic and environmental factors; for example, spina bifida may be due to a genetic predisposition that is only manifested when there is insufficient folate in the pregnant mother's diet.

It has proved difficult to pinpoint the genetic components of multifactorial disease, except for the rare Mendelian subsets of these diseases mentioned earlier. Problems include the involvement of more than one gene, each of which may have only a small effect on disease susceptibility; uncertainties in disease diagnosis (for example, Alzheimer's disease may be confused with other types of dementia); different genetic polymorphisms underlying disease in different populations, and the large effects of environment and lifestyle on the development of disease. Although each of the underlying genes is inherited according to Mendel's rules, the disease itself is not inherited in any simple Mendelian way. Strategies to identify genes associated with multifactorial disease are discussed in Chapter 3.

Cancer

Cancer is often described as a 'genetic disease', in the sense that it is caused by genetic alterations. However, the genetic alterations that characterise cancerous cells are somatic alterations. That is, they occur in the somatic cells of the body and are not passed on to the next generation.

Cancer is thought to be initiated when the DNA instructions in a cell are damaged or altered in such a way that the cell escapes the normal regulatory mechanisms that should control its behaviour (Figure 2.14). Such cells may multiply unchecked to form tumours, and acquire further genetic changes that give them the ability to migrate to, lodge and grow in distant sites of the body (metastasis).

Cancer-associated genetic alterations (Box 2.2) may be caused by a variety of factors including un-repaired errors in DNA replication or external carcinogenic factors such as ionising radiation or certain chemicals. 'Classical' models for the initiation and development of cancer focus on mutational changes to the DNA sequence. However, recent research suggests that epigenetic changes, which affect the expression of genes but not their DNA sequence, also play an important role in the development of the cancerous phenotype. The chance that genetic alterations will accumulate and lead to cancer increases with the age of the individual; hence, most cancers arise in people over the age of about 50.

Although chance certainly plays an important role in cancer development, and most cancers are classed as 'sporadic' for this reason, there is evidence that inherited characteristics also affect an individual's risk of developing cancer. In some cases the inherited risk is very high and can be attributed to a single inherited (germ-line) mutation; a well-known example is breast cancer due to mutation of the *BRCA1* or *BRCA2* genes. In these cases, the cancer often occurs at an earlier age

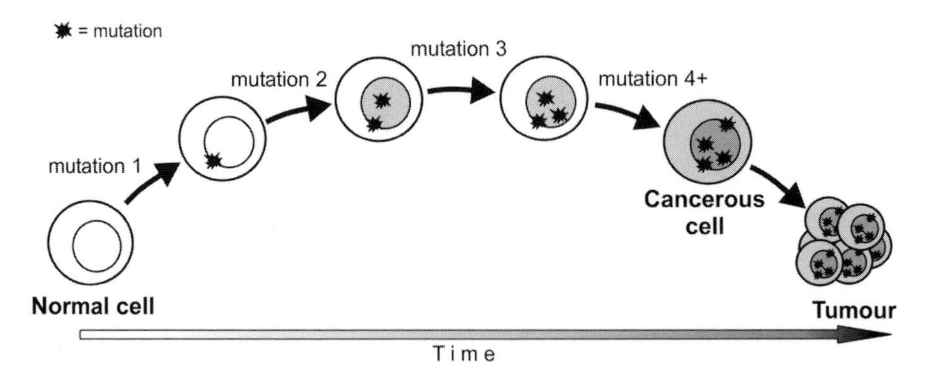

Figure 2.14 Cancer is a genetic disease. The accumulation of certain mutations and epigenetic changes in a cell over time may lead to a loss of control over normal cellular functions, uncontrolled replication and tumour formation

Box 2.2 Types of genetic changes implicated in carcinogenesis

The genes that are implicated in the development of cancerous cells are often classified as oncogenes or tumour suppressor genes, though this is likely to be an oversimplification of the range of ways in which cancer-causing genes can act.

- **Oncogenes**, when mutated, stimulate abnormal cell survival and division (the normal non-mutated form of the gene is known as a proto-oncogene). They generally act in a dominant fashion within a cell. This means that a mutation in only one of a cell's two copies of the gene is sufficient to change the cell's behaviour.
- **Tumour suppressor genes** hold back unrestrained growth and division, so inactivation of these genes (often due to epigenetic modifications such as methylation of their promoter regions) releases cells from their controlling functions. Tumour suppressor genes usually act recessively within a cell; that is, both copies need to be lost or inactivated to release the cell from growth control. The *BRCA1* and *BRCA2* genes associated with familial breast cancer are examples of tumour suppressor genes.
- **DNA repair genes**. Inactivation of these genes impairs the ability of the cell to repair any further mutations, thus accelerating the progression to malignancy.
- **Mismatch repair genes** are a class of DNA repair gene that are frequently mutated in colon cancer cells. Individuals who carry rare inherited mutations in these genes suffer from the hereditary colon cancer syndrome known as hereditary non-polyposis colorectal cancer (HNPCC).

than in the general population and the cancer risk is inherited in a Mendelian fashion. Because of the inherited mutation, all the cells in the individual's body have essentially 'taken the first step' towards becoming cancerous, making development of cancer – although not certain – much more likely. Hereditary cancers and cancer syndromes, like all Mendelian disease, are rare and account for a maximum of a few per cent of the cancer incidence in the population as a whole.

In most cases, cancer can be thought of as a multifactorial disease, such as coronary heart disease or diabetes; that is, predisposition to cancer is affected by multiple inherited and environmental/lifestyle factors. Expert opinion is divided about the extent to which inherited genetic polymorphisms contribute to cancer risk: some think that chance plays the major role, while others think that many, if not most, cancers in a specific tissue or organ arise in people with a genetic predisposition to that type of cancer. Such a predisposition would not necessarily be obvious as a family history of the disease: if several gene variants are implicated, each conferring only a modestly increased risk, only those people who happen to inherit a combination of several unfavourable variants – some from each parent – may have a markedly increased risk.

Most of the common genetic variants (polymorphisms) that predispose to cancer are unknown. However, research is beginning to implicate some genetic polymorphisms in cancer risk. For example, individuals who are homozygous for a deletion in the glutathione *S*-transferase M1 (*GSTM1*) gene, resulting in a lack of GSTM1 protein activity, are around 50% more likely to develop bladder cancer than are people with an active *GSTM1* gene. There is also evidence that the bladder cancer risk in people who lack GSTM1 activity is increased by smoking; that is, that there is a combined effect of genotype and an environmental factor.

Some complexities of the relationship between genes and disease

Penetrance

In many – but not all – Mendelian diseases, a person with a specific genotype is virtually certain to develop the associated disease, though its symptoms, age of onset and/or severity may vary. In Chapter 1 we introduced the concept of penetrance: the probability that a person carrying a disease-associated genotype will develop the disease. Penetrance is always associated with a time frame, for example 'lifetime penetrance', or 'penetrance by age 50'.

Both Huntington's disease and cystic fibrosis are virtually 100% penetrant. Cystic fibrosis is fully penetrant at birth, whereas Huntington's disease is fully penetrant by age 70 or so. The mutations in the *BRCA1* gene that are associated with breast cancer are highly penetrant, but not completely so; estimates of the lifetime penetrance of these mutations vary from about 60% to 85%. Most of the genetic variants associated with susceptibility to multifactorial disease are thought to be common in the population (so they are generally described as polymorphisms rather than mutations), but of low penetrance. Variations in penetrance are caused by the modifying effects of other genes and/or by environmental factors.

Inherited and new mutations

The mutations underlying some genetic disorders, for example cystic fibrosis, appear to have arisen many generations ago, with very few new mutations arising. In the case of these disorders, an affected individual will almost always have a parent who carries the same mutation. The birth prevalence of these diseases may vary in different populations; for example, cystic fibrosis is most common in populations originating from the north and west of Europe, whereas sickle-cell anaemia is more common in African or Afro-Caribbean populations and Tay Sachs disease is relatively more prevalent in Ashkenazi Jewish communities.

However, there are other diseases, for example neurofibromatosis type 1, for which new mutations appear to be more frequent, so an affected individual may carry a mutation that is not present in either parent. If this is the case, the parents usually have a low risk of having another child with the same disease, but the child itself is at risk of passing on the disease-causing mutation to his or her children. This example makes it clear that a disease may be *heritable* but not necessarily *inherited.*

Genetic heterogeneity

Most Mendelian diseases were originally classified on the basis of the phenotype associated with them; that is, the clinical manifestations of the disease. As the genes associated with these diseases have been identified and characterised, it has sometimes turned out that what appears to be the same disease clinically may be caused by different mutations. An example is autosomal dominant polycystic kidney disease, which in most families is caused by mutation of a gene on chromosome 16 but can also arise from mutation of a gene on chromosome 4. Genetic heterogeneity resulting from disease-causing mutations at different genetic loci is called non-allelic or locus heterogeneity. When different mutations at the same locus cause the same disease, this is known as allelic heterogeneity. Allelic heterogeneity is very common; for example, hundreds of different pathogenic mutations have been discovered in the *BRCA1* and *BRCA2* genes, and in the *CFTR* gene associated with cystic fibrosis.

The cloning and characterisation of increasing numbers of 'disease genes' has also revealed that sometimes different mutations in the same gene can cause different diseases. For example some mutations in the *RET* gene cause the familial cancer syndrome multiple endocrine neoplasia type 2, while other *RET* mutations cause Hirschsprung disease, a congenital disorder affecting the intestine. The reason is that the cancer-causing mutations lead to production of a protein with a new, abnormal, function, while the mutations causing Hirschsprung disease lead to loss of protein function.

Variable expressivity

Even if a disease genotype is fully penetrant, the severity and symptoms of the disease can vary in different affected individuals, presumably because they are influenced by other genetic and environmental factors. An example of a disease showing such variable expressivity is Marfan syndrome, a disease affecting the skeletal system, the eyes and the heart, which can vary widely even among affected individuals from the same family. Variable expressivity can be considered the rule rather than the exception for virtually all genetic disease, suggesting that the concept of the 'single-gene disease' is in fact very much an oversimplification.

Genetic technology

The era of modern molecular genetics began with the development of technology that enabled DNA molecules to be manipulated. Specific pieces of DNA can, for example, be detected in a mixture, isolated, cut into smaller pieces, recombined with other pieces of DNA, copied and their base sequence determined. This technology, sometimes called recombinant DNA technology, has been at the heart of the project to map and sequence the entire human genome. It has also been central to the development of techniques for testing DNA to find mutations or polymorphisms associated with disease or other characteristics. The applications of DNA technology to genetic testing will be described in Chapter 4.

Cutting and joining pieces of DNA

Some applications in molecular genetics and biotechnology begin with cutting DNA into smaller pieces so that it can be worked with more easily, and so that individual genes and other sequences can be isolated from it. DNA can be cut either by shearing it mechanically or by using enzymes, isolated from bacteria, which cut the DNA at specific places, usually at characteristic sequences of four or six base pairs. The enzymes used to cut DNA are called restriction enzymes. There are many different restriction enzymes, which recognise and cut the DNA at different sequence-specific sites.

Pieces of DNA can be joined together end-to-end to form a single longer piece, by use of enzymes called DNA ligases.

Separating pieces of DNA in a mixture

Pieces of DNA of different sizes can be separated from one another using the process of electrophoresis (Figure 2.15). The mixture of DNA is placed at one end of a gel (a slab of polysaccharide matrix) soaked in liquid, and an electric field is applied across the slab. Because DNA has a net negative electric charge, it will start to move through the gel towards the positive electrode. However, the particles that make up the gel impede the movement of the DNA molecules and so the smaller molecules, which can more easily pass through the gel, move faster than the larger pieces and the result is a ladder of DNA bands representing pieces of different sizes. The bands of DNA can be visualised in various ways, for example by staining with a chemical that binds to the DNA molecule and glows when viewed under ultraviolet light.

Detecting specific sequences: hybridisation

Often, a particular piece of DNA (or RNA) of interest needs to be detected in a mixture containing many pieces with different sequences. One way to do this,

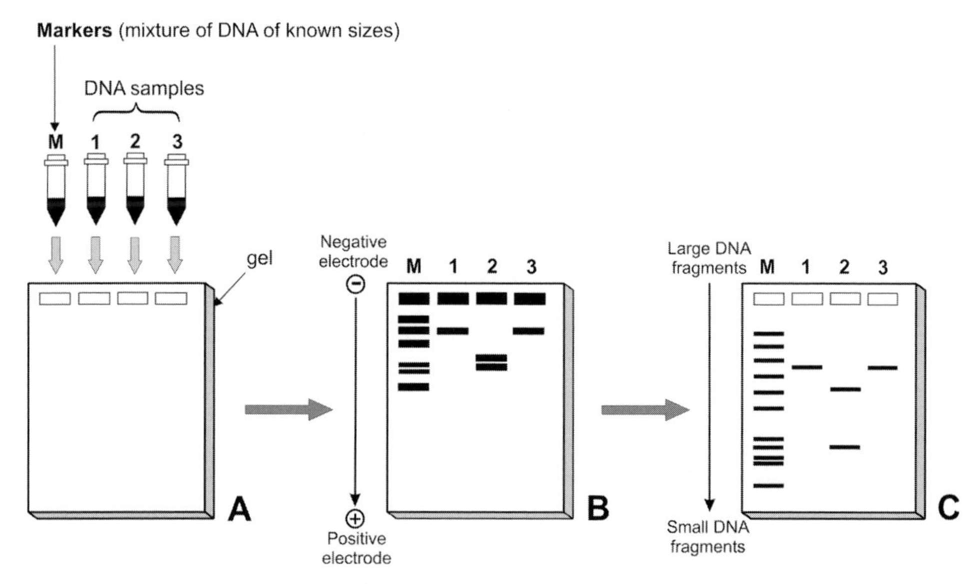

Figure 2.15 Gel electrophoresis. **A** DNA mixed with dye is loaded into wells in a gel; **B** an electric field is applied and the DNA fragments begin to move through the gel at different speeds according to their size; **C** different DNA fragments are separated by size, with the smallest fragments having moved the furthest along the gel

provided a purified sample of the sequence of interest is available, is by hybridisation. Hybridisation refers to the process in which two single-stranded pieces of DNA (or a piece of DNA and a piece of RNA) with complementary sequences will stick – or 'anneal' – together to form a double-stranded molecule. The piece of DNA or RNA used to detect complementary sequences in this way is often called a probe. If the probe is 'labelled' in some way, for example by making it radioactive or fluorescent, then any pieces of DNA or RNA that it hybridises to will also be labelled and can be detected.

Before it can be used for hybridisation, a double-stranded DNA molecule must first be denatured, so that the two strands separate. Denaturing is usually achieved by heating the sample; when it is cooled again, the single-stranded molecules will hybridise to any complementary molecules in the mixture, including those of the labelled probe.

Fluorescent in situ hybridisation (FISH)

An important technique that relies on hybridisation of complementary nucleic acid sequences is fluorescent in situ hybridisation (FISH; Figure 2.16). This technique makes use of fluorescent probes to detect and locate specific DNA sequences '*in situ*' in cells and tissues. In human genetics, FISH is commonly used to analyse the chromosomal content of cells and to detect mutational changes

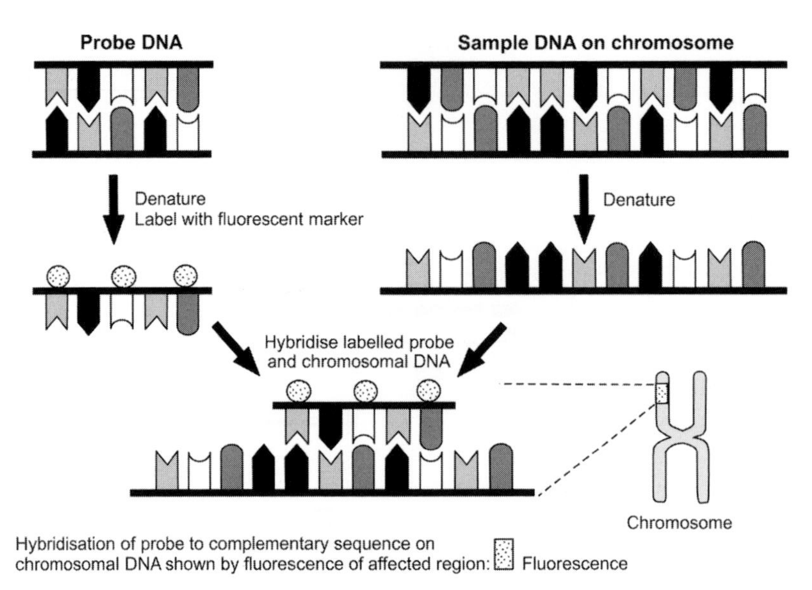

Figure 2.16 Fluorescent in situ hybridisation (FISH). Labelled probe DNA sequences hybridise to the complementary sequences of interest, if present; binding is detected by the presence of fluorescence

in chromosomes (see Chapter 4). FISH is so sensitive that it can detect single copies of specific genes in individual cells.

DNA cloning and clone libraries

The amount of any specific sequence of DNA in a typical biological sample is very small. Many applications in genetic medicine and biotechnology depend on being able to make many more copies of a sequence of interest. There are two main ways of copying DNA. The first, called molecular cloning (not to be confused with the cloning of a whole organism, such as Dolly the sheep), involves inserting a piece of DNA into the cells of a host organism, usually a single-celled organism such as yeast or a bacterium, and using the natural processes of DNA replication and cell division in the host organism to make multiple copies of the additional piece.

In order to ensure that the piece of interest will be replicated within the host, it has to be manipulated by joining it to a vector – a piece of DNA that includes all the additional sequence information necessary to make the host cells copy the DNA and pass it on as they divide and multiply. Cloning vectors come in various types and sizes. The smallest are plasmids, which are circular pieces of DNA that survive in bacteria. Plasmids can only take relatively small pieces of DNA into the bacteria (up to several thousand bases). If larger pieces of DNA need to be used then other vectors are needed. Cosmids allow pieces of DNA up to about 45 000 bases (45 kilobases [kb]) to be cloned in bacteria. BACs (bacterial artificial chromosomes) and YACs (yeast artificial chromosomes) are so called because they can accept very large pieces of DNA (100–400 kb) and contain sequences that allow them to behave like whole chromosomes in the host cells.

Many projects in genomics (the study of genomes and their functions) involve the construction of 'libraries' of clones that together contain a set of sequences of interest. There are different sorts of libraries. Genomic libraries contain, in a set of clones, all the sequences in the original genome. cDNA libraries are constructed by taking the messenger RNA produced by a particular type of cell or tissue and copying it 'backwards' (using a special enzyme) to produce DNA. A library produced from this 'copy DNA' (cDNA) will represent all the genes that are expressed in that particular cell type.

The polymerase chain reaction

The second way of copying DNA, the polymerase chain reaction (PCR), is a particularly powerful technique because it amplifies a specific DNA sequence exponentially, does not require the use of a living organism to propagate the DNA, and needs only a tiny amount of starting DNA that does not have to be pure. Like cloning, PCR relies on the natural process of DNA replication, but uses a purified enzyme called DNA polymerase and a supply of all the nucleotides needed to make new DNA. PCR is a cyclic process controlled by the temperature of the reaction mixture: in each cycle, the two strands of the piece of DNA are separated, copied and the daughter strands re-annealed (Figure 2.17A). With each cycle, the amount of the target sequence (the amplicon) increases exponentially (Figure 2.17B).

One other essential feature of the process is that in order for the DNA polymerase to start copying DNA, there must be a short 'primer' piece of DNA bound by hybridisation to each strand of the template at opposite ends of the sequence to be amplified. The polymerase reaction then extends these primers so that two new double-stranded copies of the template are made. As well as giving the DNA polymerase a starting platform, the primers ensure that the process is specific: using primers to the ends of a particular sequence will make sure that only that sequence is amplified, even if it is part of a mixture of DNA containing many different sequences.

Originally devised as a way of amplifying DNA, PCR has been adapted in recent years to enable its use to detect mutational changes in DNA. Examples of some PCR-based techniques for mutation detection are described in Chapter 4.

DNA sequencing

Once a piece of DNA has been purified and amplified sufficiently, for example by cloning, it can be sequenced. Once again, the process used in sequencing relies on

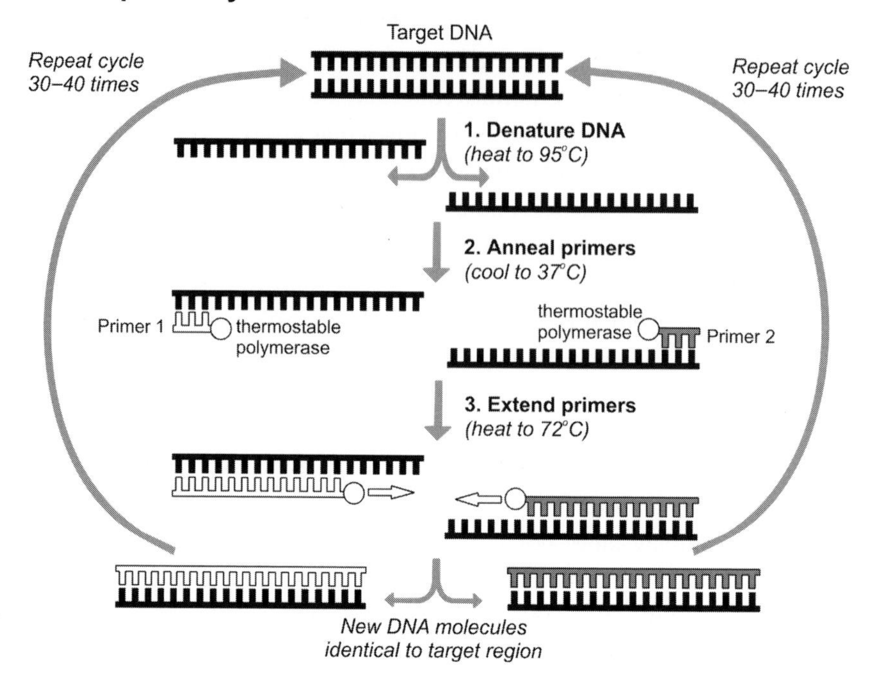

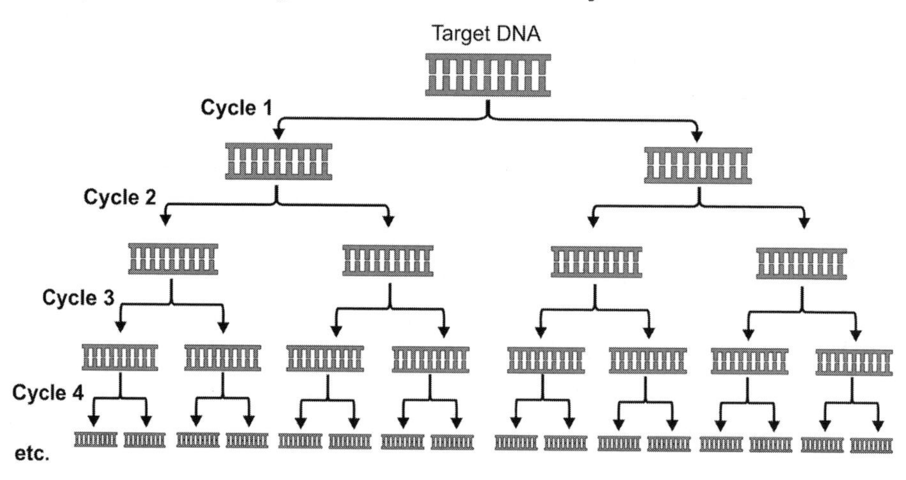

Figure 2.17 **A, B** **A** Polymerase chain reaction (PCR). **B** Exponential increase in DNA product during PCR

DNA polymerase to copy the template. Four reaction mixtures are set up, each including the DNA to be sequenced, the enzymes needed for replication and a supply of nucleotides. However, in each reaction mixture, the supply of nucleotides is 'spiked' with a small amount of a variant of one of the usual bases (A, C, G or T), which stops the chain elongation whenever it is incorporated into the growing chain. The result is, for each reaction, a nested series of DNA chains of different lengths, each stopping at a position in the sequence corresponding to that base. The products of the four reaction mixtures are run side-by-side in four lanes on an electrophoresis gel. In each lane a ladder of bands corresponding to DNA chains of different lengths is produced, and the sequence can be deduced by reading from the smallest to the largest piece. If different fluorescent labels are used for the four different bases, it can all be done in one single reaction, the bands can be detected and the sequence read out automatically. The entire process of DNA sample preparation and sequencing is now highly automated, a development that has been essential for the timely and cost-effective completion of the human genome project.

DNA microarrays

New techniques are being developed that enable many different analyses to be carried out simultaneously on a single sample. One of these is DNA 'chip' or microarray technology. A DNA microarray is prepared on an inert surface (glass, for example) that is divided into a grid of tiny squares. In each square is placed a spot of cloned DNA corresponding to a particular gene. DNA spots corresponding to thousands of different genes, or even the whole genome, can be accommodated on a single array no bigger than a microscope slide. In an alternative approach, short DNA sequences (known as oligonucleotides) that can act as probes for specific genes are synthesised directly onto a silicon support by the process of photolithography.

For both types of microarray, a DNA or RNA sample of interest is applied to the chip. Any sequence in the sample that matches a sequence on the chip will hybridise to it and, if the sample is suitably labelled, usually with a fluorescent tag, the pattern of matches can be visualised and analysed by computer, giving a read-out of the presence or expression level, in the sample, of thousands of different genes simultaneously.

DNA chips have many potential applications in biology and medicine. For example, they can be used to look for mutations in a gene (see Chapter 4), to measure how active a set of genes is in a particular cell or tissue type, to analyse how gene activity changes over time, or to compare the genotypes or gene expression profiles of different samples, for example the genotypes of people who do or do not respond to a particular drug, or the gene expression patterns of tumours compared to normal tissue (Figure 2.18).

Markers and maps

Studies aimed at finding genes associated with diseases or other characteristics rely on the use of genetic 'markers': identifiable DNA sequences whose location on a

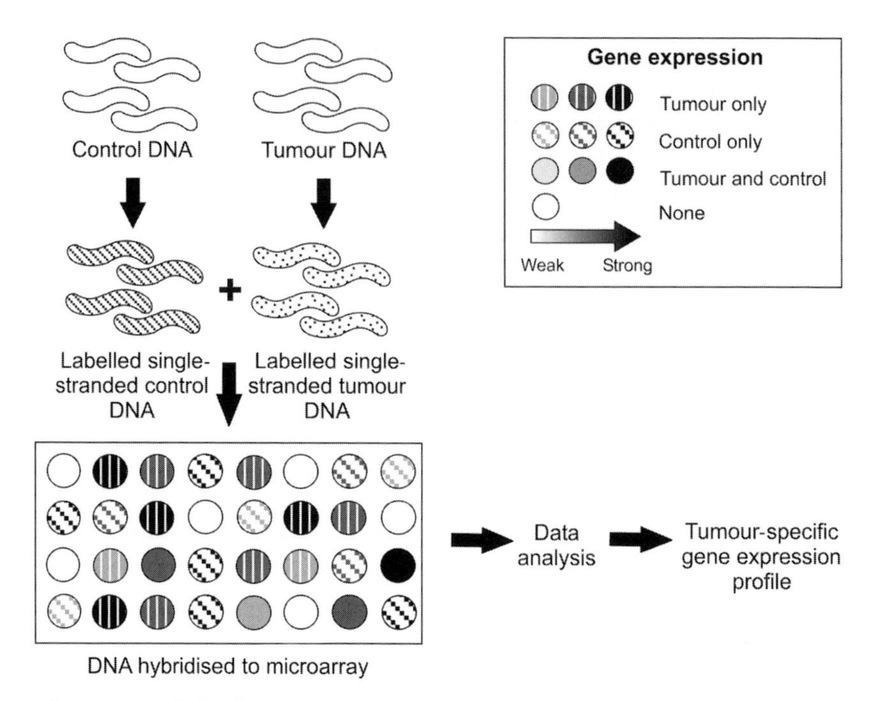

Figure 2.18 Microarray analysis of tumour gene expression patterns

specific chromosome is known. Genetic 'maps' of the chromosomes have been drawn up by ordering pairs of markers on the basis of how frequently they are inherited together in families. The markers used must be polymorphic; in other words they must exist in two or more slightly different, distinguishable versions in the population so that the inheritance of different alleles can be tracked. To be useful in practical terms, each allele needs to be found at a frequency of at least 1–2% in the population. The use of polymorphic genetic markers in linkage analysis – where 'disease genes' are located by comparing the inheritance of a disease through a family with the inheritance of genetic markers – is discussed in detail in Chapter 3.

Several types of polymorphic markers have been used for genetic mapping and linkage analysis. In the early days of recombinant DNA technology the most commonly used marker was the restriction fragment length polymorphism. If a piece of DNA is cut with a restriction enzyme and the pattern of fragments is analysed, the same sequence will always produce the same pattern, whereas a difference in the sequence may lead to the enzyme cutting in a different place, yielding a different pattern. Such a difference is called a restriction fragment length polymorphism (RFLP).

Other more recent types of polymorphic markers include microsatellite markers and single nucleotide polymorphisms (SNPs). Microsatellites, which are usually within the non-coding DNA, are segments of DNA consisting of repeated, short sequence motifs. Microsatellites are abundant within the genome and, because the number of repeated units at each site can vary, are often highly polymorphic. SNPs, bi-allelic polymorphic sequences that differ at just a single base pair, are useful markers because they are small, easily identified, and frequent within the genome, occurring about once every 300 bases.

The human genome project

Nowhere is the power of recombinant DNA technology more evident than in the human genome project – the international effort to sequence all three billion base pairs of the haploid human genome – which reached completion in time for the 50th anniversary of Watson and Crick's discovery of the structure of DNA.

Each human chromosome is far too large to be analysed or sequenced intact, so the overall strategy of the project had to involve breaking the chromosomes into pieces small enough to be sequenced, and then working out how the pieces fit together to form the complete sequence. A publicly funded international human genome consortium approached the task chromosome by chromosome, first preparing libraries of DNA cloned in YACs and BACs and using the marker content of these pieces to relate them back to detailed maps of the chromosomes. Sets of clones that covered the chromosomes with minimal overlap were chosen and the DNA within them was broken down into pieces small enough to be sequenced. Computer analysis was used to reassemble these sequenced fragments in the right order.

A private company, Celera, competed with the public consortium but took a different approach, called 'shotgun' sequencing, which involved breaking the whole genome into a huge number of small pieces, sequencing these pieces, and using powerful computing techniques to put the entire sequence together by analysing the overlaps between pieces. The difficulty of this approach is that the many stretches of repeated DNA in the genome make the task of reassembly very complex, and there is some controversy over whether Celera would have been able to complete the task without the availability of the publicly funded maps and sequence data for reference. Nevertheless, the shotgun approach has been extremely successful for sequencing the genomes of a large number of microbial pathogens, and has also been used for larger genomes such as those of the fruit fly (*Drosophila*) and the mouse.

The 'reference sequence' that has resulted from the human genome project does not relate to any single individual. The DNA that was used was extracted from sperm and blood samples taken from a small number (about six) volunteers who are all anonymous except for Craig Venter, who announced that his own DNA was used in the Celera project.

Mapping human genetic variation: SNPs and haplotypes

Linkage analysis in families has proved invaluable in identifying scores of genetic loci associated with rare single-gene diseases such as cystic fibrosis and Huntington's disease (see Chapter 3). However, in searching for the genetic variants associated with susceptibility to common diseases, attention has turned increasingly to association studies in populations. These studies, also explained more comprehensively in Chapter 3, compare the frequency of specific alleles in 'cases' (people with the disease) and unrelated 'controls' (unaffected individuals).

SNPs have emerged as the most promising type of genetic marker for use in association studies. An international project has focused on identifying and mapping millions of SNPs in the human genome, with the aim of systematically testing these variants for association with disease. If an association is found, it could indicate that the SNP itself is a functional variant associated with the disease, or that a disease-susceptibility gene lies nearby on the chromosome.

It is an enormous task to type every one of many thousands of SNPs in the large numbers of cases and controls that need to be studied in order to identify a statistically robust association between a genotype and a disease phenotype in a population. In the last few years, attention has turned to a possible way of simplifying the analysis. This relies on the phenomenon of linkage disequilibrium. Within a large population the chromosomes will have been extensively shuffled by recombination over the many generations through which the population has evolved. Eventually, after an infinite number of generations, all possible combinations of alleles at two nearby loci would be equally probable in the population. Over a large but still finite number of generations, however, particular combinations of alleles at nearby loci may persist; this is known as linkage disequilibrium. For example, within given populations, certain combinations of alleles such as SNPs have tended to stay together so that most of the corresponding chromosomes of individuals in the population carry one of just a few specific sets, or haplotypes, of these alleles (see Chapter 3, Figure 3.2). (A haplotype is a set of alleles found together on the same chromosome.) The blocks of linkage disequilibrium observed in populations are much smaller than the blocks of linked alleles shared by members of a single family, simply because they reflect a much larger number of recombination events.

The observation of linkage disequilibrium offers the hope that, instead of needing to type millions of SNPs in association studies, it might be possible to achieve the same result by typing a smaller number of SNPs that would be representative of specific haplotype blocks, thus greatly simplifying the task of finding gene–disease correlations. To this end, an international project, the HapMap project, has mapped common haplotype blocks within several different populations and identified representative SNPs for use in association studies.

The advantages, criteria and pitfalls of the haplotype mapping approach are discussed in more detail in Chapter 3.

The post-genome challenge

The human genome project represents not the end, but the beginning of the challenge of genomics. With the reference sequence as the starting point, researchers are now identifying and characterising not just all the genes and other functional sequences, but also the myriad products of the genome. Ways are being devised to study the functions of genomic sequences and their products, and how these components work together in biological systems. Such is the scale and complexity of this task that it is demanding the development of new computational tools.

Identifying genes and studying gene function

There are various methods for identifying sequences that are likely to be genes. For example, the sequence database can be searched by computer for characteristic sequences found in known genes – both human genes and genes discovered first in other organisms. Another method is to look for sequences that are expressed as mRNAs in various tissues and relate these expressed sequences back to their origins in the genome. The expressed sequences of the genome are those of greatest interest in the search for novel genes, and Expressed Sequence Tags (ESTs) are an important tool in genomic analysis. ESTs are short DNA sequences (200–500 base pairs) corresponding to part of the sequence of an expressed gene, and are used as tags to identify genes within genomic DNA.

Now that virtually all the genes have been identified, the focus is shifting to attempts to understand what they do, both in normal physiological processes and when disease develops. In order to grapple with the complexities of gene function and expression, technologies (such as DNA microarrays) are being developed that attempt to analyse the activity of many genes simultaneously.

Proteomics

For the most part it is proteins, rather than DNA or RNA, that perform the work of the cell, and relative levels of gene expression inferred from RNA measurements or microarray experiments often do not correlate with the levels of the corresponding proteins. For this reason, attention has also turned to analysing the types and amounts of all the proteins present in different tissues or organs, and attempting to relate these patterns to characteristics of interest such as disease status or progression. Because these approaches involve the analysis of thousands of proteins simultaneously, the term 'proteomics' has been coined to describe them.

It is technically much more difficult to work with proteins than with DNA or RNA. Proteins have three-dimensional structures that must often be maintained during analysis (if function is required) yet which are more easily disrupted than the simple helical forms of DNA and RNA. Protein structure can be destroyed by a variety of factors including heat, physical disruption or enzymes. Moreover, it is not possible to amplify samples of protein (unlike DNA), so proteins produced at low levels are harder to detect than more abundant proteins.

There are several key techniques used in proteomics. Two-dimensional polyacrylamide gel electrophoresis (2-D PAGE) is used for the separation of proteins from each other based on differences in charge in one dimension and mass in the second dimension. Up to 10 000 different proteins can be resolved as separate spots on a single high-resolution gel. These spots can then be identified by mass spectrometry, a technique that separates protein fragments based on their mass-to-charge ratio and can be used to calculate the precise mass (and hence composition) of proteins and peptides. Post-translational modification of proteins such as the addition of phosphate groups or sugars is an important feature in determining protein function; modifications can be detected using enzymes that remove the additional groups, or alternatively using antibodies that bind to them.

Proteomic analysis is expected to find many clinical applications in areas including oncology, toxicology and drug testing. In oncology, for example, proteomic patterns in body fluids such as serum or urine may provide an early, non-invasive indicator that a tumour is developing in the body, enabling therapy or preventive treatment to start at earlier stages than is possible at present. If cancer has already developed, proteomic analysis of tumour biopsy samples may be used to determine tumour stage or prognosis, to guide choice of treatment and to monitor treatment response.

Research is also underway on the use of proteomic approaches as an aid to drug development: the protein profiles of target tissues and organs before and during drug administration can indicate biochemical pathways involved in drug metabolism, adverse reactions, or development of drug resistance, for example.

Protein arrays, analogous to the gene expression arrays discussed above, are also being developed. Once again, the technical difficulties are much greater than for DNA arrays, mainly because each protein only has biological activity when it is in a specific three-dimensional conformation that is easily denatured under the conditions used for biochemical analysis. These difficulties are being overcome, however, and several potential applications are being developed for protein arrays. Arrays of antibodies, for example, could be used to screen simultaneously for the presence of many different molecules in body fluids, as an aid to disease diagnosis. Some researchers predict the development of 'protein chips' that will be used routinely by primary care practitioners as diagnostic tools and may eventually even be available over the counter.

Comparative genomics

Comparative genomics, the comparison of the human genome with that of other organisms using powerful computational tools to align and analyse different genome sequences, is an area of ongoing research. Studying similarities and differences between the sequence and architecture of different genomes provides insight into the structure and function of genes and non-coding regions, as well as the evolution of the human genome. Genomic regions that are strongly conserved across different species are likely to include critical components such as key genes for common features (such as proteins involved in fundamental metabolic processes), genes encoding functional RNAs (for example, tRNAs and ribosomal RNAs), and elements involved in the control of gene expression. Determining the degree of similarity between genomes helps identify such functional regions; for example, if a region of the mouse genome known to encode a particular gene is found to align with and show strong sequence similarity to a coding region of the human genome of unknown function, then that region may be predicted to encode a similar gene product. This can then be verified experimentally.

Information from comparative genomic studies can often be of great value in understanding aspects of disease, including pathogenesis, susceptibility and resistance. It can allow the identification of disease-related genes, or help researchers to select which gene products to target for therapeutic effect. The identification or creation of human disease models is another useful output; for example, if the functional equivalent of a key gene involved in a human genetic disease is identified in another organism, targeted disruption of that gene may create a physiological model of that disease.

Recently completed and ongoing genome sequencing projects include several species of insect, fungus, yeast and worm, along with a range of animals including mouse, rat, guinea pig, rabbit, dog, cat, cow, chicken, armadillo, elephant, chimpanzee, orang-utan and rhesus macaque. In addition, multiple microbial genomes have been sequenced, and the comparison of sequences from closely related pathogenic and non-pathogenic strains provides valuable data on genes that encode key pathogenic features of the disease-causing varieties, which in turn may be used to develop treatments to combat the disease.

Bioinformatics

In order for biologists to make use of the vast amount of data emerging from genome projects, it has been essential to develop ways of collecting, storing, organising, inter-relating, searching and analysing these data. The discipline of bioinformatics developed in response to this need. Bioinformatics is an interdisciplinary field merging knowledge and expertise from computer science, mathematics, physics and biology.

Organisations such as the European Bioinformatics Institute and the US National Center for Biotechnology Information have cooperated to assemble a variety of different genomic and proteomic databases used by the research community. As well as databases cataloguing genes and other DNA sequences, there are, for example, databases of sequence variation (for example, SNP and haplotype databases), repositories of microarray data, databases of protein structure and research literature databases. New computational methods are constantly being devised for 'mining' information from these databases, and for linking information from different databases.

Systems biology

Genomics promises to provide information that will help us to understand, at the molecular level, how the human body functions in health and disease. For this purpose it is not enough to have lists of genes and proteins; we must also know how these elements interact with each other in functioning biological systems: at the level of molecular pathways, in cells, tissues, organs and ultimately whole organisms (see Figure 2.5). Scientists are increasingly turning their attention to the challenges posed by 'systems biology'; it is clear that the sheer complexity of biological systems will require computing power considerably beyond that of the most powerful computers currently available, and will demand imaginative new approaches.

Epidemiological and biomedical informatics

Enthusiasts foresee a time when salient features of an individual's genetic make-up, perhaps even their entire genetic code, will be a part of their electronic health record, providing information that will guide not only diagnosis and treatment of disease, but also preventive health care decisions. Development of the evidence base for genomic medicine will involve amassing and analysing information, at the population level, about how genetic variation is related to disease (genotype–phenotype correlations) and how interactions between genes and environmental factors influence the onset and progression of disease. A substantial investment is needed in population-level bioinformatics and knowledge management to marshal and make sense of this information. Population-based projects such as UK Biobank (discussed in Chapters 3 and 6), requiring storage, analysis and correlation of genetic, medical and lifestyle information, will also be a spur to the development of new bioinformatics approaches.

A new discipline of biomedical informatics, bridging the gap between bioinformatics and clinical informatics, is emerging to address the issues raised by the incorporation of biomolecular data into electronic health records. Initiatives are underway to develop agreed standards for the description, transfer and storage of genetic data. Biomedical informatics systems need to be able to cope with the complexity and variability of DNA information such as that obtained from gene expression and microarray analysis. Genetic data will have to be stored and retrievable in a way that is comprehensible to clinicians and compatible with standard medical coding systems. Genetic test information will need to be linked with other clinical information including results from other types of medical tests and information about the patient's condition at the time the sample was taken. Pharmacogenetics may provide the first impetus in this direction.

Further reading and resources

Basic genetics

Strachan and Read's *Human Molecular Genetics* (2003) is an excellent in-depth reference, covering genetics, gene expression and genetic technology. For further information on the basics of genetics, there is a wealth of useful online resources: the Genetic Science Learning Center website from the University of Utah in the US includes a section called *The basics and beyond*, with animated and interactive units covering DNA, genes and proteins, as well as cloning, stem cells, gene therapy and other topics. The DNA Learning Centre in Cold Spring Harbor, US has a website called *DNA From the Beginning* which is an animated tutorial that outlines the basics of classical and molecular genetics, genetic regulation and control with a historical perspective, including references to experiments that revealed key concepts in genetics.

For a discussion of the role of DNA in the developmental programme of cells and organisms, see Chapter 1 of *Molecular Principles of Animal Development* by Martinez Arias and Stewart (2002). Evelyn Fox Keller discusses the changing concept of the gene and stresses the complexities of genetic systems in her 2000 book *The Century of the Gene*.

Genes and disease

For a classic clinical textbook, the latest edition of *Emery's Elements of Medical Genetics* (Turnpenny and Ellard 2005) provides an extremely useful reference, with sections on principles of human genetics, genetics in medicine and clinical genetics. *Human Molecular Genetics* (Strachan and Read 2003) also includes a relevant section on mapping and identifying disease genes and mutations, as well as chapters on post-genomic technologies. *Blazing a Genetic Trail*, available online from the Howard Hughes Medical Institute, is an engaging introduction to the search for disease genes that provides scientific and historical information along with examples.

General information on genes and genetic disease is available from a number of online resources, including the National Coalition for Health Professional Education in Genetics (NHGRI) health site, which also links to the *Genetics Home Reference*, a searchable guide to genetic conditions hosted by the National Library of Medicine. The US National Center for Biotechnology Information *Genes and Disease* website provides a collection of articles that discuss genes and associated diseases. The UK Wellcome Trust Human Genome website includes both general and specific information about genetic disorders, as well as news and special feature articles on selected topics related to genes and disease. The National Library for Health's specialist library for clinical genetics (GenePool) contains basic genetics information with a practical clinical focus.

For information on specific human genes and related genetic disorders, the GeneTests website is an invaluable, regularly updated US-based medical genetics information resource that includes GeneReviews, comprehensive genetic disease profiles covering clinical features, diagnosis, inheritance, genetic testing and counselling and other features, as well as an on-screen glossary of all technical and scientific terms. Online Mendelian Inheritance in Man (OMIM) is a useful searchable database of human disease-related genes, with extensive information on gene cloning, mapping and function, disease phenotypes, allelic variants, animal disease models and such like. GeneCards™ is a similar database of human gene functions, products and related disorders; this site provides more technical data and links to OMIM entries, as well as to related medical news items and scientific publications. Firth and Hurst's 2005 book *Clinical Genetics*, in the *Oxford Desk Reference* series, is a superb compendium of information. Written from a clinical standpoint, it takes the clinical consultation as its starting point and covers diagnosis, investigation, management and counselling for patients.

Also written for clinicians, *The Genetic Basis of Common Diseases* (edited by King and colleagues in 2002), is a useful starting point for information about genetic factors implicated in a range of common conditions, but for a fully up-to-date picture it needs to be supplemented by more recent reviews in the major medical journals. The book contains a useful introductory section on methods and approaches in the study of the genetics of common complex diseases.

The review 'Epigenetics: regulation through repression', published in *Science* in 1999 by Wolffe and Matzke, may be of interest to those wanting to know more about epigenetic phenomena and their role in human disease. For a recent discussion of the potential importance of epigenetic changes in cancer, see the 2006 review by Feinberg and colleagues in *Nature Reviews Genetics*. The website of the Human Epigenome Consortium contains information about a public/private collaboration to identify, catalogue and interpret genome-wide DNA methylation patterns in different cell and tissue types.

Genomics and the human genome project

Matt Ridley's 1999 book *Genome* is a highly readable introduction to the human genome, written for a general audience. John Sulston's *The Common Thread*, written with Georgina Ferry in 2002, is a personal account of the 'race' to the human genome sequence. In his 2003 book *Nature via Nurture*, Ridley develops in an accessible way the concept that human characteristics arise from interactions between the individual's genetic endowment and his or her environment.

The Genome News Network is an online magazine with special focus on news relevant to genomics and human medicine; the *Genes and Genomes* section includes collected articles on chromosomes, the human genome, biobanks, proteomics, RNA interference and other topics.

The National Human Genome Research Institute (NHGRI) website contains information about the human genome project and links to other useful resources, including a glossary of genetics terms and fact sheets aimed at a non-scientific audience and covering topics such as DNA sequencing, PCR, FISH and DNA microarray technology. Excellent information is also available on the web pages of the Human Genome Program of the US Department of Energy. A free-access article published in 2003 in *Nature* by Francis Collins and colleagues from NHGRI outlines their vision of how the human genome project can provide a starting point for new initiatives to improve human health, transform biology and benefit society. The website of the Human Genome Organisation (HUGO) contains links to resources including powerpoint presentations, meetings and lectures, the *Genome Digest* newsletter and the work of HUGO's committees.

For further reading in genetics and genomics at a more advanced level, the online version of the scientific journal *Nature* hosts the Nature Genome Gateway, a site that provides free access to collected articles on genomics (original papers plus news and commentaries), including special sections on the human genome and post-genomic technologies. The website of the Wellcome Trust Sanger Institute, the home of the human genome project in the UK, also provides information for a more specialist audience.

The post-genome challenge

Bayat's 2002 article on Bioinformatics in the *British Medical Journal* provides a clinical review including discussion of basic tools, applications and future prospects. See also the 2003 paper by Kanehisa and Bork, which reviews the development and current and future applications of bioinformatics. Mount and Pandey (2005) review, at a more specialised level, applications of bioinformatics in cancer research and the search for new therapeutic interventions. The European Bioinformatics Institute website is a portal to world-wide bioinformatics resources.

A now slightly dated but nevertheless useful article outlining the basis and biomedical applications of proteomics is 'Proteomics: new perspectives, new biomedical opportunities' by Banks and colleagues (2000). For a more recent review, 'Proteomics: the first decade and beyond', by Patterson and Aebersold (2003), looks at the evolving field of proteomics over the last 10 years, including the range of technologies used to analyse proteins and future prospects for integrated systems to allow an improved understanding of biological function. Calvo, Liotta and Petricoin, in a 2005 review on clinical proteomics in the journal *Bioscience Reports*, predict an era in which analysis of disease-specific biomarkers will lead to individualised therapies tailored to the specific molecular pathology of a patient's disease. The website of the Human Proteome Organisation sets out the aims and work of an international consortium of research associations and industry partners.

'Searching for the genome's second code', by Elizabeth Pennisi (2004), is an interesting article on the hunt for non-coding DNA sequences that control gene expression. Web pages developed by the Human Genome Program of the US Department of Energy contain a brief guide to functional and comparative genomics, with links to sources of further information on genome projects for other organisms and research goals in this field.

An optimistic overview of systems biology and its application to medicine can be found in the review 'Systems biology and new technologies enable predictive and preventive medicine', published in 2004 by Hood *et al.* in *Science* magazine. As part of a series on systems biology published in the journal *Cell* in May 2005, a commentary by Aderem outlines some of the scientific and organisational challenges facing this new field.

A 2004 paper by Sanchez-Martin and colleagues outlines the challenges of developing biomedical informatics systems to support genomic medicine.

3

Fundamentals of genetic epidemiology

An understanding of genetic science does not, on its own, provide a sufficient basis for identifying or developing clinically useful applications of genetics. Epidemiological information is also essential. We must, for example, know the frequencies of potentially relevant genetic variants in different populations, assess the strength of proposed associations between genetic variants and disease risk, and understand the quantitative contribution of genetic factors to the incidence and prevalence of diseases in populations.

Epidemiology can be defined as 'the study of the distribution and determinants of disease frequency' or more simply, 'the study of the occurrence of illness'. In this chapter, we present a brief overview of relevant general epidemiology before concentrating on the details of genetic epidemiology. We are using the term 'genetic epidemiology' not in the narrow sense of statistical genetics, but to describe the study of genes and disease in populations, the design of epidemiological studies, and assessment of the impact of random variation, bias and confounding on their results. This first section focuses on concepts of causation and association, measuring the occurrence of illness, the design of cohort and case–control studies, and an introduction to the concept of interaction.

An overview of classical epidemiology

Causation and association

Studying and measuring the effect of exposures is a primary goal of epidemiology. An exposure can be any factor that may be related to disease risk; for example, the family history of disease or a lifestyle factor such as cigarette smoking. In epidemiology, an *effect* is defined as the change in a population's disease frequency caused by an exposure. However, there is a fundamental problem with this conceptual approach: it is impossible to measure causal effects directly in observational studies of human populations or in individuals. There is very little scope for experimental studies of exposures and outcomes in human populations; for example, a study investigating lung cancer that randomised people to smoke or not would be unethical. This means that epidemiologists can only measure association, which is defined as the statistical dependence between two or more events, characteristics or variables. Ideally, the association measured should equal the causal effect we are interested in but this may not be the case: exposed people may develop the outcome of interest in the absence of a true causal relationship. Observed associations may therefore also be the result of:

- Random variation: this occurs because we are inferring the experience of a population from only a sample of that population; the smaller the sample, the greater the role of chance.
- Bias: this is any systematic error in a study that distorts an assessment of the true relationship between exposure and outcome. Common sources of bias are problems in the selection of subjects or from factors related to the measurement of exposure and outcome.
- Confounding: the observed association is due to the mixing of effects between exposure, outcome and other factors independently associated with both exposure and disease; these may be known or unknown.

It is the task of the epidemiologist to obtain a valid measure of association, one that is free from bias and confounding. Nevertheless, an understanding of the principles of causation is essential in grasping the epidemiological approach. Rothman has outlined a number of helpful principles to better understand causality. The most important principle is that every causal mechanism (or 'sufficient cause') involves the joint action of multiple component causes; no single component cause acts alone (Figure 3.1). For example, whilst cigarette smoking causes lung

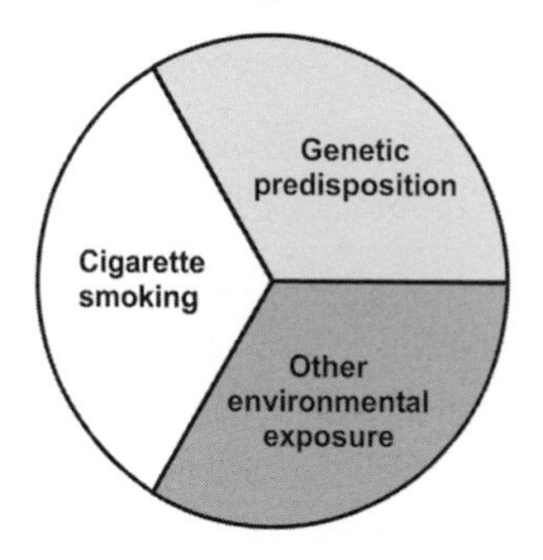

Figure 3.1 Component causes of lung cancer

cancer, not every person who smokes develops the disease. This is because other component causes are required before lung cancer develops, such as certain genetic traits or exposure to other non-genetic (or environmental) factors.

The next principle is that an effect can have more than one cause. Thus every disease can be conceptualised as having both genetic and environmental causes. This means that from one perspective, all disease is inherited (in the sense that all diseases will have some genetic cause). Similarly, all disease is environmental, even for those conditions that are usually defined as 'genetic diseases'. For example, phenylketonuria (PKU) is considered by many to be a purely genetic disorder. However, as discussed in Chapter 1, if we consider the outcome of PKU (learning disability), we can prevent it by restricting dietary phenylalanine. Thus this 'genetic disease' also has environmental causes; without the environmental exposure learning disability does not occur. Even conditions that are considered as purely 'environmental' (such as trauma) may have genetic factors that influence risk-taking behaviour or that impair sensory functions, such as eyesight, balance, or hearing.

Measuring the occurrence of illness

Classical epidemiology recognises a distinction between descriptive and analytical epidemiology. Descriptive studies measure the frequency of diseases and exposures in order to generate hypotheses about the causes of disease. Analytical studies measure associations between exposures and outcomes in order to test hypotheses about possible causal relationships. In both types of approach the key step is obtaining a valid measure of the relevant study variables. Epidemiologists generally use four basic measures of disease frequency in descriptive epidemiology: risk, cumulative incidence, the incidence rate and the prevalence proportion (see Box 3.1).

Risk is the probability of an individual developing disease during a specified time period and is a readily understood concept but is usually calculated as an average in a population; this is known as the cumulative incidence (or incidence proportion). It is vital that risk values are related to a specified time period to be meaningful.

However, risk has an important drawback as a tool for measuring the occurrence of disease: it is impossible to measure individual risk directly in most studies. This is because subjects will be lost from the study from causes other than the outcome of interest (known as competing risks) or from loss to follow-up. It is therefore sensible to consider risk as hypothetical. Other measures of disease occurrence are therefore required; the most commonly used measure is the incidence rate, which can be used to estimate risk indirectly. Incidence is the number of new cases occurring in a population; the incidence rate measures the number

Box 3.1 Epidemiological measures of disease frequency

- **Risk**: the probability of an individual developing disease during a specified time period
- **Cumulative incidence**: the average risk for a population during a specified time period
  Cumulative incidence = number of new cases of disease / number of people at risk (during a specified time period)
- **Incidence rate**: the number of new cases of disease occurring in a population during a specified time period
  Incidence rate = number of new events / total time experienced for subjects followed (known as the person-time at risk)
- **Prevalence proportion**: the proportion of a population that has disease at a given moment in time
  Prevalence proportion = number of people with disease / total number of people in the population (at a specified time)

of new cases of disease occurring in a population during a specified time period. It is a rate because of the time dimension.

Person-time at risk is determined by the size of the study population, the time contributed by each study member and whether the event of interest can recur or not (for example, death can only occur once). All units of person-time are treated equally, whether or not they come from the same individual or from different individuals. So a total of 30 person-years could be derived from one person contributing 30 years of time at risk or from 30 people contributing one year's time at risk. The key point is that only the time at risk of the disease occurring is counted, so even people leaving the study from competing causes can still contribute time at risk to the investigation.

What relevance does this have for genetic epidemiology? Genetic exposures are fixed at conception, so theoretically person-time at risk should be calculated from conception. However, different genes may act at different stages of a causal pathway and may influence factors related to aetiology, survival or response to treatment. It is also impossible to define the time of conception so date of birth is often used as a proxy. Thus, different time points for calculating person-time at risk may be adopted that fit with the particular hypothesis being investigated.

The prevalence proportion (usually shortened to prevalence) measures the burden or status of disease or risk factors in a population. It is the proportion of people with a disease in a defined population at a given time (sometimes called the point prevalence), although the terminology is not always consistently used. Prevalence is influenced by two main factors: the incidence rate of disease and the duration of disease. The average duration of disease is determined by factors such as the condition's severity, natural history and available interventions.

The inter-relationship between prevalence and incidence can be expressed mathematically as:

Prevalence = incidence rate × average duration of disease

Prevalence is less useful than incidence for describing causation because it mixes factors influencing aetiology and disease duration. However, prevalence is often used in the study of the aetiology of congenital malformations because it is impossible to measure incidence. This is because it is extremely difficult to determine the size of the population at risk (embryos), or to ascertain factors such as the timing of a malformation or the proportion of affected fetuses that die before birth. Prevalence is also a vitally important measure for public health practitioners because it can be used in the planning, organisation and delivery of health care.

Measuring associations in analytical epidemiology

To measure an association, the disease experience of exposed people is compared with the disease experience of unexposed people. There are three main groups of effect measures: relative, absolute and attributable fractions (Box 3.2).

Relative measures

These are presented as ratios of risks, incidence rates or prevalence proportions in exposed and unexposed groups. The general term 'relative risk' is often used but more precise definitions are preferable. Relative measures reflect the amount by

Box 3.2 Measures of association in analytical epidemiology

1. **Relative risk**
   - **Risk ratio** = ratio of risks or cumulative incidences (incidence proportions)
   - **Rate ratio** = ratio of incidence rates
   - **Odds ratio** = ratio of odds of exposure in cases versus odds of exposure in controls

   If the risks are sufficiently small, the risk ratio and rate ratio are approximately equal
2. **Absolute measures**
   - **Risk difference, attributable risk, excess risk** = difference between risks or incidence proportions
   - **Incidence rate difference** = difference between incidence rates
3. **Attributable fractions**
   - **Attributable fraction** = amount of disease associated with exposure in the exposed study group
   - **Population attributable fraction** = amount of disease associated with exposure in the total population

which an exposure multiplies the baseline risk. A relative risk of 1.0 indicates no effect; a relative risk greater than 1.0 indicates an increased risk and a relative risk of less than 1.0 indicates a decreased risk. Relative measures are often used in studies of aetiology because of their empirical and logical properties. Empirically, they provide a stable summary measure of effect in a variety of human populations. Logically, they facilitate the judgement of the extent to which an effect is causal or not (for more information, see Breslow and Day, cited in Further reading).

Another commonly used relative effect measure is the odds ratio, which estimates the incidence rate ratio in case–control studies. It is interpreted in the same way as a relative risk.

Absolute measures

The absolute effect of an exposure is the observed difference between risks, incidence rates, prevalence proportions, or survival in exposed and unexposed groups. Some of the commonly used terms and their synonyms are presented in Box 3.2. Absolute measures reflect the additional risk of disease in exposed versus unexposed groups. These measures are often used to estimate the public health impact of an exposure in a population. Nevertheless, a degree of caution should be exercised about this interpretation because it assumes that there is a true causal relationship between exposure and disease.

Attributable fraction and population attributable fraction

These measures (Box 3.2) estimate the amount of disease associated with a particular exposure, expressed as a proportion or percentage. They can be calculated from risks or, in certain circumstances, from rates. Again, it must be assumed that there is a true causal relationship between exposure and disease. The attributable fraction for a population is calculated from the attributable fraction in the exposed group multiplied by the proportion of all exposed cases of disease in the entire population. These measures, along with the risk difference, are very useful from a public health perspective and can be used to estimate the burden of disease from an exposure and the possible impact of preventive measures.

Cohort and case–control studies

Experimental designs are not used in studies of human genetics for ethical reasons, so non-experimental (observational) designs take precedence. Cohort and case–control designs have been widely used in genetic epidemiology: the cohort design in population DNA collections (such as the UK Biobank; see Box 3.3) and the case–control design in population-based gene–disease association studies. Although observational studies have their limitations, studying genetic variation as an exposure has three important advantages: the exposure does not change over time; the

Box 3.3 UK Biobank

The UK Biobank project is a collection of DNA samples, medical and lifestyle information from 500 000 men and women aged 40–69 from the general population of the UK. Its aim is to build a resource for studies on the combined effects of genetic variants and environmental factors on the development and progression of disease.

At enrolment, baseline information about health and lifestyle factors (such as smoking status) is collected by questionnaire, interview and medical examination. Information from the Office of National Statistics, cancer registries, hospitalisation data and medical records held by general practitioners are used to track endpoints (disease onset or death) occurring over a period of several decades.

Case–control studies nested within the cohort (that is, studies comparing disease cases from within the cohort with suitable controls also from within the cohort) will be the main means by which the combined effects of genes and environment will be studied. For example, the risk of disease associated with a particular environmental exposure can be compared in people with and without a genotype of interest. Similarly, the risk of disease associated with a particular genotype can be compared in people with and without an exposure of interest. The data will also be analysed for evidence of formal statistical interaction between genotype and exposure.

Calculations in the study protocol indicate that for conditions where the expected number of events is greater than 5000 (for example, diabetes, breast cancer, colorectal cancer and myocardial infarction), the study will have power to detect a relative risk of 1.5 for exposure within the genotype of interest, and an interaction ratio of 1.4 for exposures and genotypes present in 20–80% of the population (at 95% power and 0.1% significance). (The theoretical basis of studies on the combined effects of genes and environment is discussed later in this chapter.)

For conditions where the expected number of events is in the range 1000–2000 (for example, rheumatoid arthritis, Parkinson's disease or bladder cancer), the corresponding detectable relative risk is 1.8–2.0 and interaction ratio 1.7–2.0.

For further details on UK Biobank, see www.ukbiobank.ac.uk

exposure can be measured with considerable accuracy and precision (compared to many non-genetic factors such as diet or physical activity); and DNA-containing samples may often only need to be obtained once and can be stored for long periods of time, allowing the potential for re-analysis at a later date.

Cohort studies

The cohort study involves tracing a defined group of people over time and measuring the occurrence of outcomes in exposed and unexposed sub-groups. They are useful for studying the relationship of an exposure with a number of outcomes, and for the direct measurement of incidence rates. Cohort studies can be prospective, when the exposure is determined before the outcome, or retrospective, when the cohort is defined by the occurrence of the outcome; assessment of exposure status is made from past records (or in genetic studies by measuring the genetic variant of interest). A number of factors are important when designing cohort studies.

The first qualification for cohort membership is that members must be at risk of developing the outcome(s) of interest; members are then categorised with respect to the exposure of interest. Whether a study can measure risks or rates depends on whether the cohort is closed (members can be lost but no new members can be added) or open (members can be lost from and added to the study group). Risk can be measured in a closed cohort but not in open cohorts, where rates are measured. The calculation of time at risk is determined by the specific hypothesis being investigated with respect to the induction period (time until disease occurrence after exposure), the latent period (time until diagnosis from disease occurrence) and whether the outcome of interest can recur or not (myocardial infarction can occur more than once; death from myocardial infarction cannot). Careful consideration must be given to these factors to ensure that the outcome is not wrongly attributed to the exposure.

Exposure must be accurately measured to ensure the validity of later comparisons. Similarly, standardised case definitions are required for the outcome(s) of interest. Misclassification of exposure or outcome can be random (non-differential) or systematic (differential), each having its own impact on the validity of the results. Random measurement error often biases results towards the no-effect value, whilst systematic error can bias the results in any direction depending on its source and its relationship to the exposure or outcome. Retrospective cohort studies depend on determining outcomes from existing records, and they are particularly vulnerable to information bias concerning the exposure of interest; this is not a problem for studying genetic variants, although it will be for other exposures that require information from study subjects.

One of the main causes of bias in cohort studies is inability to trace some members of the cohort as the study progresses. Bias may arise if the probability of loss from the study is linked to the exposure or outcome of interest (or both). The problem can affect measurement of the outcome (numerator error) or calculation of the time at risk (denominator error) or both. Tracing cohort members in long-term prospective studies is therefore challenging and resource-intensive.

Case–control studies

The essence of the case–control study design is assembling a group of cases (people with the outcome of interest) and comparing them with a group of controls (people without the disease or outcome of interest) sampled from the source population for cases. This source population can be considered to be the hypothetical cohort that would be defined if a cohort study were being designed instead. Exposure is measured in the two groups and relative risks can be estimated by the odds ratio. There are a number of variants of the case–control study including nested designs, case–cohort variants and case-only studies which have been used in genetic epidemiology. There are several key factors in designing case–control studies.

First, the source population must be carefully defined so that people who develop the disease of interest are included as cases in the study. Thus, the source population (also known as the study base) is determined by the criteria for including cases in the study.

Careful selection of controls is also vital. The purpose of the control group is to provide an estimate of the exposure distribution in the source population that gives rise to the cases. This means that sampling of controls must be independent of the exposure. A number of sources for controls can be used, including general population registers, close contacts (neighbours, relatives or friends), random-digit dialling, hospital-based controls or even dead controls. Each has its own set of problems and potential biases, but carefully designed studies should be able to mitigate these problems in advance.

A common misconception is that cases and controls should be as similar as possible; this is incorrect because the primary function of the control group is to provide a valid estimate of the exposure distribution in the study base. The utility of matching as a means of controlling confounding has often been overstated because there are circumstances when matching can actually introduce confounding and selection bias into studies. There is also the problem that one cannot study factors that are used for matching.

As in cohort studies, definition and measurement of exposures and outcomes is vital to ensure valid results. The impact of misclassification has already been discussed above. Ascertainment of exposure is generally considered to be less of a problem in genetic epidemiology because the exposure (genotype) can be objectively measured. However, genotyping error is not uncommon and it is important that investigators maintain high technical standards. Other information about non-genetic factors obtained directly from the study subjects may be less complete and correct and may be subject to information biases, such as recall bias. This is of particular importance in studies attempting to investigate interaction between genes and non-genetic factors.

Interaction

The concept of interaction is extremely important in both classical and genetic epidemiology. The term interaction can be used to describe statistical, epidemiological or biological phenomena. In statistics, interaction is used to refer to any departure from the underlying form of a statistical model. In classical epidemiology, interaction occurs when the effect of one risk factor is dependent on the level of others. Biological interaction refers to the joint effect of two or more factors in a causal mechanism for development of disease. In genetic epidemiology, the two key interactions are between different genes and between genetic and non-genetic (environmental) factors.

The concept of statistical interaction has been criticised because it ignores biological interaction, it is model-dependent and it depends critically on the type or scale of an effect measure. So, if the measure of effect for an exposure and outcome is the relative risk, combined independent risk factors act multiplicatively; statistical interaction is said to occur if the joint effect of independent risk factors is not multiplicative. However, if an absolute measure is used, such as the risk difference, the effect of independent combined risk factors is additive; statistical interaction is said to occur if the joint effect is not additive. Statistical interaction between small numbers of variables can be assessed using model-based approaches, such as regression analysis.

However, as the number of potentially interacting variables increases, major limitations in these methods become apparent. Where data are multi-dimensional, and many interactions are modelled, there will be many contingency table cells that contain zero observations, resulting in large coefficient estimates and standard errors. In these situations, model-free methods have greater power for identifying interactions in relatively small samples. The implications of these concepts for genetic epidemiology will be explored later in the chapter.

Genetic epidemiology and human disease

The goal of genetic epidemiology is to identify and characterise variants in the human genome that are associated with specific disease phenotypes. In order to achieve this, three related questions must be answered:

- Is genetic variation between individuals important in the variation of disease susceptibility?
- Which genetic variants confer altered disease susceptibility?
- What are the characteristics of these variants?

Genetic variation and disease susceptibility

Evidence that many normal traits and diseases have an inherited component was obtained many years before the molecular basis of inheritance was discovered. This means it is possible to determine whether or not genetic factors alter disease risk using methods that do not require the measurement of specific genes.

The key tasks in determining whether genetic variation plays an important role in disease susceptibility are to assess whether diseases cluster in families; to assess the relative contributions of genetic and non-genetic factors; and to identify the mode of inheritance.

Clustering in families and the familial relative risk

The first step in determining the contribution of genetic variation to the aetiology of disease is to assess whether there is clustering of the disease in families. The second step is to quantify its extent. The observation that a disease 'runs in families' is insufficient by itself to establish a genetic contribution because familial aggregation may occur for several reasons and, in particular, because of a shared environment.

The degree of familial clustering can be expressed as the familial relative risk (known as λ_R). This is the ratio of disease risk in different types of biological relatives of affected individuals, compared with disease risk in the general population. Separate values can be calculated for each type of relative, for example the familial relative risk for siblings (λ_s). In general, the higher the familial relative risk (FRR) the stronger the genetic effect. The FRR for first-degree relatives of a dominant Mendelian trait such as Huntington's disease is approximately 5000. The sibling FRR for the Mendelian recessive disorder cystic fibrosis is about 500; familial risks for common complex disorders tend to be considerably lower (see Table 3.1). However, the absolute value of the FRR is not the whole story, because a strong genetic effect in a common disease will have a smaller value than the same strength of effect in a rare disease.

The FRR also provides information on how potential disease-related genes are interacting. For example, the FRR for siblings due to a gene acting in a recessive manner will be greater than the FRR for offspring, even though both risks relate to first-degree relatives; this reflects the increased likelihood of siblings sharing the

Table 3.1. Sibling familial relative risk (λ_s) for a number of diseases

Disease	λ_S	Lifetime risk %[a]
Coeliac disease	60	3
Multiple sclerosis	25	1
Insulin-dependent diabetes mellitus	15	6
Testicular cancer	8	2
Alzheimer disease	4	35
Breast cancer	2	14

[a] Cumulative risk of disease by age 80.

disease, compared with a parent and offspring. The change in FRR for different relationships may also be informative depending on the number of loci involved and how they interact, specifically whether they add to the disease risk or whether they multiply the disease risk.

The family history of a disease may be treated as an exposure for investigation, so that standard epidemiological study designs can be used to measure the FRR. Many early studies of common complex diseases used the retrospective cohort design. Detailed family information is obtained from a series of individuals with the outcome of interest (cases). Their relatives are then treated as a cohort of exposed individuals (individuals with a positive family history) followed from birth. The observed incidence of disease in these relatives is compared with the expected incidence of disease, using disease incidence in the general population to estimate the risk in unexposed individuals; that is, individuals with no family history of disease.

This most widely used design for estimating the FRR is the case–control study, in which cases and suitably selected controls are interviewed to ascertain whether their biological relatives have the disease of interest. Presence of a positive family history is again treated like any other exposure and the relative risk is estimated (using the odds ratio). The first problem with this design is the possibility of recall bias caused by differential recall of family history in cases and controls, leading to an overestimate of the true risk. The second problem is that reliable information is often only available from first-degree relatives; comparison of the FRR for first-degree relatives and more distant relatives is therefore difficult.

The prospective cohort study design avoids the problem of recall bias but the relative rarity of exposures and outcomes, even for common conditions such as the major cancers, has generally limited its usefulness.

Using heritability to assess genetic and environmental contributions

Disentangling the relative contribution of genetic variation and environmental factors to disease susceptibility is extremely challenging. This is where the concept of heritability becomes extremely useful. Heritability is the proportion of phenotypic variance attributable to genetic factors. It was first developed from the demonstration that many normally distributed quantitative traits (such as height and weight) can arise from the action of multiple genes (called polygenes), each with relatively small effects. In statistical terms, the range of such continuously distributed traits in the population is described by its variance (or standard deviation). Variances have the useful statistical property that they can be added when they are due to independent causes. Thus, the total variance in a phenotype (*V*p) is the sum of the variances due to genetic variance (*V*g) and environmental variance (*V*e); see Box 3.4.

Box 3.4 Heritability and partitioning of variance

Total phenotypic variance Vp = Genetic variance (Vg) + Environmental variance (Ve)

Genetic variance Vg = Variance due to additive genetic effects (Va) + Variance due to dominant effects (Vd)

Thus: $Vp = Va + Vd + Ve$

Heritability (broad) = Vg / Vp, the proportion of variance due to all genetic factors

Heritability (narrow) = Va / Vp, the proportion of variance due to genetic factors that can be passed from parents to offspring

Notes

Heritability (h^2) is often expressed as a percentage.

The heritability is frequently incorrectly interpreted as the proportion of *disease* due to genetic variation; it is in fact the proportion of the *variance* in disease risk attributable to genetic factors.

Interpreting heritability

In the context of a dichotomous disease trait (disease present or absent), the concept of phenotypic variance (and so heritability) has little meaning. However, if the risk of disease is viewed as having a continuous distribution in a population, the heritability for that disease is the proportion of variance in population disease risk attributable to genetic variation among individuals. The interpretation of heritability is dependent on assuming that there are no interactions between genes or between genes and environmental factors. However, genetic and environmental factors may be correlated; for example, genetic and social disadvantage may go together. It is important to recognise that estimates of heritability are population specific and therefore cannot necessarily be generalised to other populations. Two approaches are commonly used to measure heritability: twin studies and adoption studies.

Twin studies

Twin studies involve comparing the phenotype of different types of twins reared under different circumstances. They allow researchers to examine what proportion of the total phenotypic variance is explained by genetic factors, shared environmental factors, and non-shared environmental factors.

Monozygotic (MZ) twins come from the same fertilised egg and are genetically identical, having 100% of their alleles in common. Non-identical or di-zygotic (DZ) twins share on average 50% of their alleles, as with other siblings. If both twins of a pair have the same disease trait, they are said to be concordant. A greater similarity or degree of concordance between MZ twins and DZ twins indicates a genetic influence.

A concordance rate of 100% in MZ twins would indicate that a disease is entirely genetically determined. Under these circumstances, concordance in DZ twins would be expected to be 50% for a dominant genetic effect and 25% for a recessive genetic effect. Twin studies can be useful in providing basic information on what sorts of factors influence variation in a trait and in refining definitions of characteristics and are increasingly being used to assess the contribution of environmental factors. Criticisms of the twin study design include:

- Twin studies focus on populations not individuals, so that estimates of heritability refer only to the population studied and they may not generalise to other groups.
- In population-based twin studies, most participants do not show extreme phenotypic characteristics. Estimates of heritability and environmental variance may not necessarily apply to groups of extremely high or low scorers.
- The assumption that MZ and DZ twin pairs share very similar environments may not be true. Shared environment is often greater in MZ twins than in DZ twins; for example, they may be dressed identically.
- Twins, unlike other siblings, have shared the same prenatal environment at the same time even if they are subsequently separated.
- Findings in twins may not be easily extrapolated to non-twins. Twins experience greater intrauterine and perinatal adversity; the experience of being brought up as a twin is often very different from that of non-twins.
- Despite the fact that MZ twins share the same genome, they are never truly identical. Although we make the assumption that MZ twins are genetically identical, there are biological mechanisms that lead to genetic differences between them.

Although these are valid criticisms of the twin study design, they are not sufficiently strong to cast doubt about the usefulness of this approach. Nevertheless, there are clearly good reasons to use a variety of research strategies in examining the contribution of genetic and environmental influences before drawing firm conclusions.

Adoption studies

Adoption studies involve examining the biological and adopted relatives of people who have been adopted. They provide a powerful means of examining genetic and environmental influences and gene–environment interaction. If genetically related individuals (biological relatives) are more similar for a particular characteristic than genetically unrelated adoptive relatives, this suggests that genetic factors influence that trait. If genetically unrelated relatives are more similar for that trait, this is suggestive of a contribution from shared environmental factors.

However, adoption studies have two main problems. First, they are extremely difficult to conduct because information about biological parents often cannot be obtained; it may be considered unhelpful to approach them at all. Second, adoption is not a random process, meaning that children are placed in families resembling their biological family or in families that provide low-risk environments. Adoption is also an unusual event in itself.

Nevertheless, adoption studies have added to twin study evidence in demonstrating a genetic contribution to a number of conditions, including schizophrenia. Adoption studies have also shown that genes and environment can have an interactive influence: the effects of environmental adversity are much more marked when there is also genetic susceptibility.

Determining the genetic model of inheritance: segregation analysis

Segregation analysis compares the patterns of observed disease transmission in families with those expected from different genetic models. Its purpose is to determine the type of genetic model that best explains the observed familial clustering; for example, a single major gene, a combination of many genes (polygenic) or a combination of both (mixed model). Environmental factors can also be included in the modelling process.

Where a single major gene is predicted to be the cause of a trait, segregation analysis attempts to identify the Mendelian model that best describes transmission: dominant, recessive, co-dominant, dominant with reduced penetrance, etc. Segregation analysis is usually performed using maximum likelihood methods in powerful software packages (such as PAP or MENDEL), which examine the competing genetic models. These models require many parameters to be specified, including the anticipated number of major gene alleles, allele frequencies in the general population and the age-specific penetrance of each genotype.

Several assumptions are needed to model the effects of multiple genes, and especially how these genes interact. In most cases, the trait is assumed to be the result of many genes that have small additive effects, following a normal distribution with a mean and variance that can be estimated. For a discrete trait, the normal distribution is the distribution of disease risk.

Problems with segregation analysis

Segregation analysis requires large datasets and is very sensitive to subtle biases in the way information is collected. The main problem is ascertainment bias, when information about relatives is identified through families with affected children.

Families in which the gene is segregating but the disease is not expressed will not be identified. For example, if a disease were inherited in a recessive manner, the expected segregation ratio would be 1 in 4. However, biased ascertainment results in a ratio higher than expected, because only families with affected children will be identified. It is possible to statistically correct for this problem but caution should be exercised when interpreting the results of segregation analysis.

Identifying specific genetic determinants related to disease susceptibility

Once it has been established that genetic variation plays an important role in disease susceptibility, the next task is to identify the specific gene variants responsible. Initial successes in finding variants were confined to diseases with clear patterns of Mendelian inheritance, such as cystic fibrosis (autosomal recessive), familial hypercholesterolaemia (autosomal dominant) and Duchenne muscular dystrophy (X-linked recessive). In recent years, greater attention has been paid to unravelling the genetic basis of complex diseases that cannot be described by such simple genetic models. Gene-finding approaches can be grouped into two broad categories: linkage analysis and association analysis.

Both types of analysis involve the use of genetic markers. Introduced briefly in Chapter 2, genetic markers are variable DNA or protein sequence variants, derived from a single location on a chromosome, that are used in gene mapping. Ideally, these markers should be numerous, spaced out across the entire human genome, sufficiently polymorphic so that a randomly selected person has a good chance of being heterozygous, and easy to type and score. Genetic markers are not usually the disease susceptibility variant; in most instances, they simply provide a 'tag' to identify a DNA segment for further analysis.

Early markers were the blood groups, followed by the HLA antigens. More recently used markers are restriction length fragment polymorphisms (RLFPs), variable number of tandem repeat markers (VNTRs), and tri- and tetra-nucleotide repeats. Single nucleotide polymorphisms (SNPs) are the newest generation of markers and are now being widely used in genetic epidemiology. They are very numerous and can be easily typed using high-throughput genotyping methods. They are also thought to be responsible for about 80% of the genetic variation between individuals. However, they are bi-allelic and so are less informative than other types of polymorphic markers that have more alleles, such as VNTRs.

Linkage and linkage analysis

Linkage, also introduced in Chapter 2, is defined as the tendency of genes (or other DNA sequence variants) at specific loci to be inherited together as a consequence of their close physical proximity on a single chromosome. The concept of linkage is based on understanding the process of recombination.

Recombination is the exchange of DNA between homologous chromosomes that occurs during meiosis (see Chapter 2, Figure 2.8). These exchanges are also known as crossovers. The probability of recombination increases with the distance between loci on a chromosome. Thus, recombination is a function of the genetic distance between loci, so that the recombination fraction can be used to calculate the genetic distance between them.

Two loci with a recombination fraction of 0.01 are defined as being one centiMorgan (cM) apart on a genetic map. For two loci, *A* and *B*, the recombination fraction is the probability that an offspring will be a recombinant between those loci. If loci *A* and *B* are on different chromosomes, they cannot be linked and the recombination fraction is 0.5 (recombination fractions never exceed 0.5). Completely linked loci – with no recombination between them – have a recombination fraction of 0. Loci are linked if the recombination fraction is < 0.5. The relationship between genetic distance and physical distance is not linear and is not the same across the human genome. Also, the fact that loci are linked does not imply any functional relationship between them.

Recombination will only rarely separate very tightly linked loci. As a result, sets of alleles on small chromosomal segments tend to be transmitted as a block through a family pedigree; as mentioned in Chapter 2, these blocks of alleles are called haplotypes. A haplotype is the physical arrangement of multiple alleles along a chromosome or segment of chromosome. For example, take three loci *A*, *B* and *C* with alleles *Aa*, *Bb* and *Cc*. These alleles can be arranged on one chromosome in eight different combinations: *–A–B–C–*, *–A–B–c–*, etc to *–a–b–c–* (the number of haplotypes is calculated by the formula 2^n). Haplotypes are useful in genetic epidemiology because they identify chromosomal segments that can be tracked through pedigrees or populations. We will describe their use later in the chapter.

There are two main groups of linkage analysis methods: those that require the specification of a genetic model of inheritance (model-based linkage analysis) and those that do not (model-free linkage analysis).

Model-based linkage analysis

Model-based linkage analysis tests for the co-segregation of alleles at two or more loci within family pedigrees, based on a specified genetic model of inheritance. It determines the genetic distance between loci by estimating the recombination fraction.

The key to the power of linkage analysis is being able to distinguish recombinants from non-recombinants. This is not easy because humans are diploid organisms, family sizes are often small, and reduced penetrance can act as a confounding variable. Information is therefore usually required from parents and multiple pedigrees. An informative mating in linkage analysis is one where the offspring can be scored as recombinant or non-recombinant. Such individuals must be heterozygous at both loci under consideration, so that the combination of alleles passed on to their offspring can be determined. This is known as determining the phase of linked loci. Phase can often be inferred with certainty from parental genotypes, and with a high probability of certainty from multiple offspring. However, in practice, recombination fractions must be calculated for all possibilities consistent with the observed data, especially when multiple loci are being investigated.

When analysing linkage data, the null hypothesis is that there is no linkage (recombination fraction $= 0.5$) and the alternative hypothesis is that there is linkage (recombination fraction < 0.5). A ratio is computed of the odds of the observed pedigree assuming linkage, divided by the odds of the observed pedigree assuming no linkage, which is then converted to a logarithm. This quantity is called the 'logarithm of the odds score', and is known as the LOD score (see Box 3.5 for details). A LOD score of 3 or more is generally accepted as being good evidence of linkage (odds of 1000:1) and a LOD score of –2 as evidence against linkage. Because a large number of loci can be tested in a study, a conservative value of $\gg 3$ is often used to guard against false-positive results.

Box 3.5 The LOD score

The likelihood of a particular combination of genotypes can be determined for a given value of the recombination fraction, θ. For a sibship where phase is known and there are N individuals of whom R are recombinant, the likelihood is given by:

$$L = \theta^R (1-\theta)^{N-R}$$

Where phase is not known the number of recombinants under one phase is calculated and the likelihood is then given by:

$$L = \left[\frac{\theta}{2}\right]^R \left[\frac{(1-\theta)}{2}\right]^{N-R}$$

The likelihood of observing a given configuration of genotypes in a pedigree at a recombination fraction $0 \le x < 0.5$ is then compared with the likelihood of observing that pedigree under the assumption of no linkage ($\theta = 0.5$). The LOD score is the $\log_{10}$ of the ratio of these likelihoods. Thus, it is the logarithm of the odds in favour of linkage at a given recombination fraction.

$$Z(x) = \mathrm{Log}_{10}\left[\frac{L(\text{pedigree given } \theta = x)}{L(\text{pedigree given } \theta = 0.5)}\right]$$

$Z(x)$ is referred to as the two-point LOD score as it involves linkage between two loci. Where multiple families are used, the LOD scores at $\theta = x$ can be summed because they are logarithms. The value of x at which θ takes its maximum value is the maximum likelihood estimate of θ.

Using linkage to find disease loci

In practice, finding a disease locus is usually done by genotyping family pedigrees for a set of 300–400 markers at known locations evenly spaced across the genome. Strong evidence of linkage to a marker suggests that the disease gene/allele is in the same region. Further closely spaced markers in the region may then be genotyped in order to 'home in' on the disease locus. Once a small region has been identified, positional cloning can be used to identify the gene and the disease susceptibility variant(s). Positional cloning was an extremely laborious process before the human genome had been sequenced, but the availability of the complete sequence, with details of the locations of possible genes within that sequence, has simplified the process considerably.

The main problem for any model-based approach is specifying the correct model. Incorrect model specification may lead to true linkages being missed or false ones accepted. Model-based linkage analysis has therefore been most successful in mapping single-gene disorders inherited in a Mendelian manner. Multiple testing is also an issue, with implications for the significance level used to declare linkage. Complex traits are hard to analyse using linkage analysis.

The other major problem is that the calculations require powerful statistical packages (such as LINKAGE) to conduct the analyses. However, results from these programmes are highly dependent on the underlying algorithms used to estimate probabilities in the branching trees of family histories; they may also be unable to analyse certain types of family history. Linkage analysis can also be undermined by locus heterogeneity (also known as non-allelic heterogeneity, see Chapter 2), where the same clinical phenotype can be caused by genes at other loci, and also by problems in determining phase (see above). Despite these problems, model-based linkage analysis remains one of the most powerful tools in genetic epidemiology.

Model-free linkage analysis

When the underlying genetic model cannot be specified, model-based linkage analysis may be misleading. The solution is to use model-free (or non-parametric) methods that are based on identifying chromosomal segments (alleles or haplotypes) shared by relatives with the phenotype of interest (unaffected relatives are usually not analysed). The principle is that affected relatives should inherit identical alleles or haplotypes more often than would be expected by chance.

Because genetic model specification is not required, these methods tend to be more robust: affected relatives should show excess allele sharing even in the presence of incomplete penetrance, phenocopies and genetic heterogeneity. The analysis of affected sibling pairs is one example of the approach. Model-free methods can be broadly divided into two groups: those based on identifying genetic markers shared identical by state and those based on identifying genetic markers shared identical by descent.

Two alleles are said to be identical by state (IBS) if they are the same variant of a given polymorphism but are not derived from a known common ancestor. Thus, the simplest test is to compare the proportion of sibling pairs sharing zero, one or two alleles IBS with that expected under the hypothesis of free recombination between the disease locus and the marker locus. The expected proportions for IBS allele sharing will depend on the number of alleles at the marker locus and the allele frequencies.

Two alleles are said to be identical by descent (IBD) if they are IBS *and* have been inherited from the same common ancestor. In order to determine whether a sibling pair shares alleles IBD it is necessary to have genotype information from parents. Even then, unambiguous determination of IBD may not be possible. As with an IBS analysis, the simplest test is to compare the proportion of sibling pairs sharing zero, one or two alleles IBD with that expected under the hypothesis of free recombination between the disease locus and the marker locus. Where parents are genotyped and are fully informative, the proportions of pairs sharing zero, one and two alleles are expected to be ¼, ½ and ¼.

These methods can be extended to include genotype information for multiple affected and unaffected family members in large, extended pedigrees and for quantitative traits. As with model-based linkage analysis, powerful software programmes are used to analyse the data (such as MAPMAKER/SIBS and GENEHUNTER).

Association analysis

An alternative approach to identifying disease susceptibility gene variants is based on the concept of association. Whilst linkage deals with a specific genetic relationship between loci on a chromosome, association describes a statistical relationship between alleles and phenotypes. Association studies are a model-free approach to gene finding, because a specified genetic model is not required for their analysis.

The theoretical basis for most genetic association studies is the 'common variant: common disease' hypothesis. This states that spontaneous mutations during meiosis constantly give rise to genetic variants. The genetic material of offspring will therefore differ from that of their parents wherever such a mutation has occurred. These mutations will then be transmitted to subsequent generations and some of these will become common in the population, as a result of factors including selective advantage (people with the gene variant are more likely to survive and reproduce) and population bottlenecks or expansions. Some of these variants may predispose to common diseases; combinations of variants underlie differences in disease susceptibility within the population.

The principle of association studies is based on identifying disease susceptibility gene variants by comparing allele or genotype frequencies between people with and without the phenotype of interest. For quantitative traits, they aim to estimate the proportion of phenotypic variation associated with genetic variation. Association studies can be either population- or family-based. Population-based studies are case–control studies in which allele frequencies at a particular locus are compared in cases and unrelated controls (see Box 3.6 for a brief description of their analysis). In family-based studies, samples from an affected individual and his or her parents are needed; an 'internal control' group is constructed from the genotypes of family members. The frequency of alleles transmitted to affected offspring is then compared to the alleles not transmitted.

Box 3.6 Analysis of unrelated case–control association studies

The statistical analysis of an unrelated case–control study depends on the type of genetic variant studied.

The simplest case is for bi-allelic polymorphisms such as a SNP, which generates three genotypes (common allele homozygote, heterozygote and rare allele homozygote). The common allele is often referred to as the *wild-type* allele. Because it is not usually known whether the variant has a dominant, co-dominant, or recessive mode of action, the primary test of association is usually a χ^2 test based on odds ratios.

The results are often presented as the odds ratios for disease in individuals who carry one or two copies of the rare allele compared to the common homozygotes. Where the genetic model is expected to be dominant or recessive the appropriate genotypes can be combined and a χ^2 test carried out. A χ^2 test for trend can be used to test for allele dose effects (based on a co-dominant model).

The following example shows the genotype data from a breast cancer case–control study of a polymorphism that causes a change in the coding sequence of the *STK15* gene, which alters the amino acid at codon 31 from phenylalanine to isoleucine (F31I).

	Genotype			
	II	IF	FF	Total
Cases	192	262	66	520
Controls	256	214	50	520
Total	448	476	116	1040
Odds ratio	1.0 (reference)	0.61 (0.47 – 0.79)	0.57 (0.38 – 0.86)	

These data show a significant association between genotype and disease ($\chi^2 = 16.2$, 2d.f., $P = 0.0003$), with an apparently dominant protective effect for the rare allele.

Interpreting statistically significant results from gene–disease association studies

Associations can have a number of causes, not all of them genetic. There are four possible explanations for the finding of a positive association between alleles at a given locus and disease:

- Type 1 statistical error (false-positive results)
- The risk allele measured is a marker for another true biological variant (linkage disequilibrium)
- Confounding (population stratification)
- The allele has a true biological effect on disease risk.

Type I statistical error and false-positive results

Type I error is the probability of concluding that there is a true association when in fact there is not (a false-positive result); it is denoted as α, and it determines the critical level of significance (often taken as 0.05 in classical epidemiology). However, the appropriate significance level for use in genetic association studies is highly controversial. This is because the number of possible risk alleles is very large so that the prior probability that any one of them will be associated with disease is low.

The prior probability can be increased by carefully selecting variants to test (see 'the candidate gene approach' below). Even then, the expected number of loci, allele frequencies and risks are often not known before a study is conducted. Furthermore, alleles at different loci may be associated with each other (see 'linkage disequilibrium' below) so that tests at each locus are not independent. Many association studies test a large number of variants at different loci, which may result in generating spurious associations caused by random variation.

Consider a disease for which the familial relative risk to siblings (λ_S) is 2. A dominant allele with a population frequency of 30% that confers an increase in disease risk of 30% (RR = 1.3) would account for approximately 1% of the excess familial relative risk. Thus there would be a maximum of 100 such alleles to be found. If we assume that there are 10^5 candidate loci across the genome, the probability that a random candidate variant will be associated with disease is just 1 in 1000 (prior probability). If these loci are tested for disease association with 90% statistical power to detect a true association at the 0.01 significance level, the possible outcomes are shown in Table 3.2.

In the example shown in Table 3.2, the probability that an observed, statistically significant association is correct is just 8% (the positive predictive value; 90/1089). If the significance level is made more stringent the positive predictive value improves: 47% for a significance of 10^{-3}, 90% for a significance of 10^{-4} and 99% for a significance of 10^{-5}.

Therefore, some experts have suggested that much more stringent significance levels for genetic studies should be adopted ($10^{-4} - 10^{-6}$ have been proposed).

Table 3.2. Illustration of Type 1 statistical error

	Variant being tested		
Result of association study	True susceptibility allele	Not true susceptibility allele	Total
Positive	90	999	1 089
Negative	10	98 901	98 911
Total	100	99 900	100 000

The difficulty with this approach is that studies with a sample size of a few hundred to a thousand (as commonly carried out at present) will not yield very small significance levels. However, very large studies are difficult to conduct and expensive to analyse.

Techniques that correct for the effects of multiple testing have been devised, for example the Bonferroni method. However, some argue that because tests of several variants within a single gene cannot be assumed to be independent of one another, the basis for a multiple testing correction is not clear, and techniques such as the Bonferroni method are too conservative. The most satisfactory solution will probably be to set criteria for evaluation of a 'first pass' analysis which will provide the optimum retention of true positive results for further testing and confirmation, and rejection of true negatives. What these criteria should be will depend upon the properties of the genetic variants that are thought to be important; these will vary from study to study.

It is also worth mentioning here the related problem of Type II statistical error (denoted as β). This is the probability of concluding that there is no association when in fact one exists (a false-negative). This is related to the 'power' of a study, which is its ability to detect an effect where one truly exists ($1 - \beta$). For association studies investigating complex disorders, the likely effect of a single gene will be small. This means that many current studies are underpowered and that very large sample sizes will be needed to detect true effects (sample sizes of 1000 or more). Underpowered studies are also one of the reasons why the results of association studies are often not replicated by subsequent studies. Whilst non-replication may reflect true differences in the genetic epidemiology between different populations, the most common reason for non-replication is a false-positive result or a false-negative result.

Linkage disequilibrium

Linkage disequilibrium (also known as allelic association) is the non-random association of alleles at two genetic loci. In the context of a genetic association study, this means that the measured risk allele may be acting only as a marker for another nearby disease susceptibility locus. Whilst this may create problems it can be a very useful finding: it is not always necessary to measure a true functional variant because a marker allele in linkage disequilibrium with a functional variant can be used as a proxy (see Box 3.7). And because linkage disequilibrium is a short-range phenomenon, it can mark a segment of DNA as a candidate region for further investigation. This approach was used in studies identifying the disease susceptibility gene for cystic fibrosis.

The degree of linkage disequilibrium in a population reduces over time, because recombination separates linked loci (see 'Linkage and linkage analysis' above). The further apart two loci are, the more likely that recombination will remove any

Box 3.7 Linkage disequilibrium and its measurement

Consider a polymorphic genetic locus with two alleles (locus *A*). When a new mutation occurs during meiosis on the same chromosome as locus *A*, the new allele (mutation) will be associated with one or other of the two possible alleles at locus *A* – the marker allele – in the first generation offspring. The chromosome with the mutation will then be transmitted to the offspring of the individual. In the absence of recombination, the marker allele and the mutation will be transmitted together. Each generation provides an opportunity for recombination to occur, which rearranges the association between the mutation and the marker allele. Over an infinite number of generations, and thus infinite recombinations, the marker allele and the mutation would become randomly associated in the population (equilibrium). However, over a *finite* number of generations the association between marker and mutation will persist and so may be detected in genetic association studies.

The simplest measure of linkage disequilibrium is the linkage disequilibrium coefficient, *D*. Consider two loci, one with alleles *A* and *a*, and the other with alleles *B* and *b*. The common allele frequencies of *A* and *B* are denoted as P_A and P_B respectively. There are four possible haplotypes: *AB*, *Ab*, *aB* and *ab*. If they occur with frequencies P_{AB}, P_{ab}, P_{aB}, and P_{ab} then let

$$D = P_{AB} - (P_A)(P_B) = (P_{AB})(P_{ab}) - (P_{aB})(P_{ab}).$$

If $D =$ zero, then alleles *A* and *B* are independently distributed according to their allele frequencies. If *D* is not zero, then the population exhibits disequilibrium. The maximum value that *D* can take is 0.25. This occurs when the allele frequencies are 0.5 and the common alleles always occur together. The minimum value of *D* is –0.25 and occurs when the allele frequencies are both 0.5 and the common alleles never occur together. With allele frequencies of 0.5 one of the two alleles is arbitrarily defined as the common allele. Because *D* depends on allele frequencies as well as the degree of linkage disequilibrium, the coefficient *D′* is more commonly used, which corrects *D* for allele frequencies and has possible values $-1 \leq D' \leq +1$.

allelic association through the exchange of genetic material between chromosomes. On the other hand, if two loci are very closely linked, allelic association may persist for a considerable period of time, provided that the relevant chromosomes have been inherited from a common ancestor. Linkage disequilibrium is a complex phenomenon that varies both within and between populations and is affected by the population's history and structure. Interested readers should consult the texts listed in 'Further reading and resources' for more information.

Confounding in genetic association studies (population stratification)

A confounding factor is one that is associated with both the exposure and outcome of interest. In genetic association studies, confounding may arise from population stratification, which is also known as population admixture (see Box 3.8). Population stratification occurs when cases and controls are selected from genetically different subsets of a population, where the frequency of the disease and genetic variant are especially common in one of these subsets. These subsets may be different ethnic groups, for example. The choice of the study population and selection of controls is therefore crucial in the design of association studies.

There has been considerable debate about the impact of population stratification on the results of genetic association studies. Population stratification has been proposed as one reason for the non-replication of association studies. However, the existence of substantive population stratification, resulting in a false-positive genetic association, has never been empirically demonstrated. On the other hand, few published case–control studies have been formally evaluated for its presence.

One study that did this concluded that carefully matched, moderate-sized case–control samples in cosmopolitan North American and European populations

Box 3.8 Population stratification in a case–control study

Consider a heterogeneous population consisting of two sub-populations. In sub-population 1 the rare allele frequency is q_1 and in sub-population 2 is q_2. If there is no association between disease and locus then the allele frequency in cases from the two populations will also be q_1 and q_2.

Now assume that the disease incidence differs between the two populations ($i_1 > i_2$). If we select cases and controls at random from our mixed population, cases are more likely to be selected from population 1 and controls are more likely to be selected from population 2. The allele frequency in cases will then be weighted towards q_1, and in controls will be weighted towards q_2. Thus in our mixed population, the case and control allele frequencies will differ, generating an apparent gene–disease association where no true association exists.

are unlikely to contain levels of population stratification that would result in inflated numbers of false-positive associations. Nevertheless, in order to minimise the possibility of population stratification, cases and controls should be as similar as possible in genetic background (selected from the same source population). A test for spurious association using genetically unlinked markers within studies can be used to check for the presence of these effects.

Another approach is to use family-based association studies.

Family-based association studies and the transmission disequilibrium test

The principal advantage of family-based association studies is that they can circumvent the problem of population stratification. Essentially, they are genetic association studies using internal controls, usually the affected individual and both of their parents. The transmission disequilibrium test (TDT) is the most popular method. It is based on the principle that a disease susceptibility allele (or a marker allele in linkage disequilibrium with the disease susceptibility allele) should be transmitted to affected offspring more often than an allele that is not associated with the disease. Homozygous parents are discarded from the analysis because they are uninformative. Although the TDT is a powerful approach, it may be impossible to obtain parental data, especially for late-onset conditions. In this situation, unaffected siblings can be used instead.

Haplotype analysis in association studies

Allele frequencies defined by multiple loci (haplotypes) can be compared in the same way as single alleles in association studies. If there is a block of N independent bi-allelic SNPs in close physical proximity to one another on a chromosome, they could in theory generate 2^N different haplotypes. However, the observed haplotype structure of the human genome is much less complex, because alleles at adjacent loci tend to group together because of linkage disequilibrium (Figure 3.2). This results in chromosome segments (known as haplotype blocks) where relatively few haplotypes are found. It is therefore not necessary to genotype all of the polymorphisms in these haplotype blocks to capture all the relevant information for that block. Indeed, haplotype blocks containing 10–30 polymorphisms can be identified by genotyping as few as 3–8 SNPs.

Although the haplotype architecture of the complete human genome has not yet been defined, empirical studies have revealed substantial diversity in local haplotype structure. The relative contributions of mutation, recombination, selection and population history have resulted in some haplotype blocks that extend for only a few kilobases (kb) and others that may be 100 kb or more. However, estimating haplotype frequencies in a population is complicated by the fact that haplotypes are not usually directly observable (see the concept of phase above).

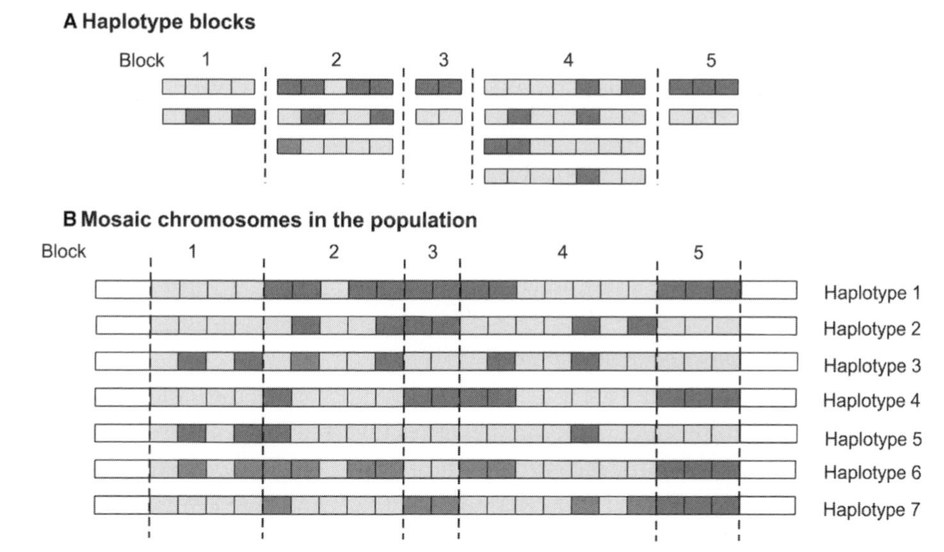

Figure 3.2 Haplotype blocks. Chromosomal regions with a commonly occurring characteristic pattern of alleles are known as haplotype blocks; different individuals within a population will have different combinations of these alternative blocks. Adapted from Cardon, L. R. and Abecasis, G. R. (2003). *Trends Genet.* **19**, 135–40. Figure 1. Copyright (2003), with permission from Elsevier

This problem can be minimised by using parental genotype data or by using other statistical estimation techniques.

Genome-wide association and the candidate gene approach

Theoretically, disease susceptibility genes could be identified by looking for linkage disequilibrium between genes and markers spaced out across the entire genome, as happens in genome-wide linkage studies. However, linkage studies in families have the advantage of only requiring markers spaced at intervals of several million base pairs, whereas population-based association studies need markers at much closer intervals.

The reason for this is that there will have been only a few recombinants (even in multi-generation families) so that family members share large sections of DNA. On the other hand, there are likely to have been many recombination events between unrelated individuals in a population, with much greater variation in their DNA sequences. The International HapMap is a catalogue of common genetic variants that occur in human beings. It describes what these variants are, where they occur in our DNA, and how they are distributed among people within populations and among populations in different parts of the world. The project has recently released data on over four million polymorphisms for four populations with African, Asian and European ancestry. These data suggest that approximately 500 000 markers would need to be genotyped to capture all the common genetic variation. Until recently, genotyping on such a scale was prohibitively expensive, but the rapid development of genotyping technologies has made genome-wide association studies possible. Several such studies are currently in progress for a variety of disease phenotypes. The results of these studies are likely to provide important insights into genetic susceptibility to common, complex disease and will inform future study design.

The candidate gene approach

Candidate genes are usually selected on the basis of the biological function of their protein product (for example, genes involved in cholesterol metabolism may be good candidates for coronary heart disease). An association study is relatively straightforward if there is a variant of the candidate gene known to have a functional effect or be directly responsible for predisposition to the disease. However, this is not usually the case: several variants in the gene may be known, but there is often no evidence that any one of them has a functional effect or is directly responsible for the disease. In this situation, several variants must be tested in the hope that one will prove to be a functional variant or that one or more of them will be in linkage disequilibrium with an unidentified functional variant.

Whether or not a given variant will act as an adequate marker depends upon several factors, not all of which can be predicted when the study is carried out. The main problems are:

- The marker will only perfectly reflect the functional variant if they are in complete linkage disequilibrium. However, this is unlikely unless they are physically extremely close; incomplete linkage disequilibrium will result in the loss of some statistical power.
- The association will be weakened if the functional variant has arisen independently on more than one occasion in the history of the population, because it is likely to be associated with markers on two or more different versions of the chromosome in the population.
- Even if the marker and functional variant have each only occurred once in the population, if they arose at very different times, their frequencies are likely to be very different. In general, recent variants will have a low frequency because they are present in a smaller segment of the population. This can very considerably weaken the power of the statistical analysis to detect associations, with a requirement for larger sample sizes.

Each of these problems disappears if a known functional variant is used; for example, it does not matter how many times a variant has arisen in the population, so long as it is the same variant.

Otherwise, the problems are not so easily solved. Information about the extent of linkage disequilibrium across genes and their regulatory regions (where important variants might well lie) is still fragmentary; what there is suggests that it is different for different genes. There is, in principle, no way of knowing whether presumed functional variants have arisen once or many times, and at what point they occurred in the history of the population. If the common variant: common disease hypothesis is wrong and most polygenic susceptibility is based on a large number of recently arisen, individually rare variants, the association study design will fail. A coherent strategy for assessing a candidate gene would be as follows:

1. Identify the full set of 'common' (say greater than 1% or 5% frequency) variants in the gene to be investigated.
2. Genotype a small number of samples for those variants, to define the linkage equilibrium structure across the gene, and to identify the set of SNPs that efficiently captures all the common genetic variation.
3. Genotype these 'SNP tagging' SNPs in a large case–control study and compare genotype frequencies in cases and controls. Where a significant difference is found, the task of identifying the true causative variant then can begin.

The history of the search for disease genes suggests that guessing such candidates is not often successful. Alternative ways to identify candidates are available (see Box 3.9). Eventually, it may be possible to avoid the problems of guessing candidate genes and to use an empirical whole-genome approach.

Defining the phenotype in association studies

Association studies may fail to detect true associations if the phenotype is not precisely defined, with the result that the group defined as 'cases' is heterogeneous. The 'all or nothing' endpoint of occurrence (disease present or absent) is most

Box 3.9 Alternative ways of identifying candidate genes

- **Animal models**: loci associated with susceptibility or resistance to disease can be mapped empirically, and the genes from the corresponding genomic region in humans assessed as candidates.
- **Consistent somatic changes in tumour cells**: these may provide clues to cancer susceptibility genes.
- **Assayable phenotypes**: a search for inherited variation in phenotypes (such as radiation response, inflammation and growth factors) may be used as a basis for a subsequent gene search based on that phenotype.
- **Sensitised screen approach**: this method is derived from animal systems. Linkage methods are used to search for genetic modifiers of the phenotype in carriers of known, highly penetrant predisposing genes.

often used in association studies but other endpoints may have advantages. For example, breast cancer is almost certainly heterogeneous in its aetiology. Greater analytical power may be obtained by defining subsets of breast cancer – for example by age, by tumour molecular markers (such as oestrogen receptor status), or by histological type. Other aspects of the clinical phenotype may also be used as endpoints, such as survival.

Clinical disease represents the final result of many biological processes, and so might be regarded as the most distant read-out from the causative genetic variation. 'Intermediate phenotypes', such as serum markers of disease, may be more closely correlated with a given genetic variation; if the phenotype can be treated quantitatively as a continuous variable rather than dichotomously, there will also be additional gains in statistical power.

Conclusion: linkage and association are complementary approaches

Linkage analysis can scan the entire genome using only a few hundred markers and can be conducted relatively quickly. However, identified candidate regions may still be too large for positional cloning. One way of tackling this is to start with genome-wide linkage studies, probably in affected sib-pairs, followed by finer mapping of candidate regions using association studies. However, for susceptibility genes and their variants with weak effects and for complex diseases, association studies will take precedence because linkage studies would require unfeasibly large sample sizes. A combined approach using both family-based studies and association studies in unrelated cases and controls is being adopted by the Generation Scotland project (for further details, see www.generationscotland.org and Chapter 6, Table 6.1).

Systematic review and meta-analysis of genetic association studies

The literature of genetic epidemiology is littered with reported gene–disease associations that have not stood up to further scrutiny; that is, the association has not been replicated by subsequent, independent studies. Several recent reviews have identified the reasons for lack of replicability of gene–disease association studies, including varying extent of linkage disequilibrium, population stratification and limitations in study design, all discussed in this chapter. Many studies are simply too small to have the power to detect, with convincing statistical significance, odds ratios of the magnitude expected for the influence of a single genetic polymorphism on disease risk (that is, in the range 1.1–1.5). Furthermore, the possibility of false-positive findings due to chance is high when many associations are studied. These problems are exacerbated in the presence of reporting bias: the tendency for statistically significant findings to be published in preference to weak or less exciting findings.

The main reason for the continuing problem with replicability of gene–disease association studies is the enormous cost of studies large enough to have sufficient power to detect robust effects. One way of overcoming this problem has been the setting up of large, collaborative projects that can effectively share resources.

An additional strategy is to pool the results from several studies using the approaches of systematic review and/or meta-analysis. A systematic review attempts to identify all relevant studies fitting pre-defined criteria, and systematically summarise the validity and findings of these studies using explicit criteria that aim to minimise bias. An international collaboration, the HuGENet initiative (Box 3.10), has been established to encourage the preparation of systematic reviews on proposed gene–disease associations, and to develop methodologies for this application of the systematic review process.

A meta-analysis is a statistical synthesis of the results of multiple studies and is usually undertaken within the context of a systematic review. In a meta-analysis of gene–disease association studies, the estimated associations are combined across studies typically using a weighted average, with weights inversely proportional to the variances of the estimates. Thus, larger studies have more influence on the summary estimate than smaller ones (see Figure 3.3 for an example). Variation of results across studies, known as heterogeneity, may be addressed by performing a

Box 3.10 The HuGENet initiative

HuGENet was established in 1999 by the Office for Genomics and Disease Prevention (OGDP) at the US Centers for Disease Control and Prevention in Atlanta, USA. It has grown into an international network currently comprising hundreds of collaborators in several dozen countries. HuGENet's core activities are collation of evidence (through preparation of systematic reviews), information exchange (through its website at www.cdc.gov/genomics/hugenet/default.htm), training and technical assistance.

Over 40 HuGE systematic reviews have been published. Each review attempts to identify human genetic variations at one or more loci, describe what is known about the frequency of these variants in different populations, identify diseases that these variants are associated with, summarise the magnitude of risks and associated risk factors, and evaluate associated genetic tests. Reviews point to gaps in existing epidemiological and clinical knowledge, thus stimulating further research in these areas.

HuGENet is evolving into an organisation similar to the highly successful international Cochrane Collaboration. An international executive committee for the network has been established and additional coordinating centres are being designated around the world. The Public Health Genetics Unit (PHGU) in Cambridge became a second coordinating centre in 2005. Several international consortia are working together with HuGENet on specific diseases such as Parkinson's disease, cardiovascular disease, pancreatic cancer and oral cleft. HuGENet is becoming, in effect, a network of networks.

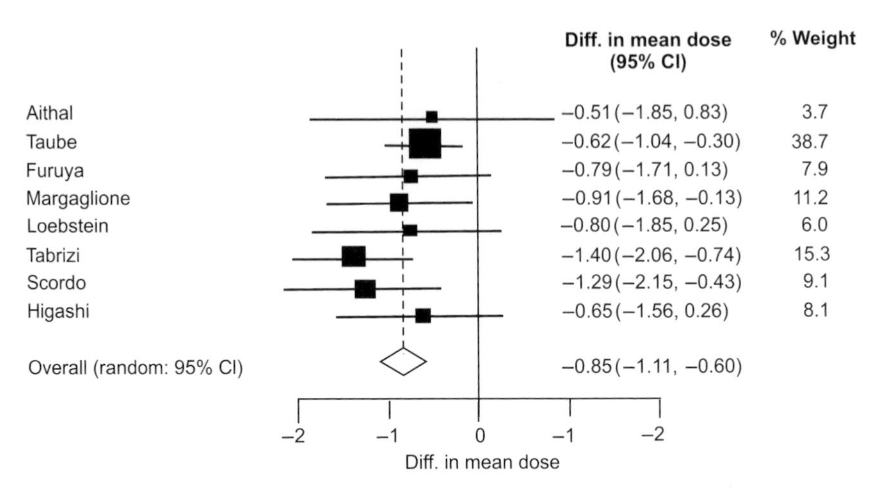

Figure 3.3 Meta-analysis. The meta-analysis provides firm evidence of a lower warfarin dose required by carriers of the CYP-2C9*3 allelic variant. From Sanderson, S., Emery, J. and Higgins, J. (2005a). *Genet. Med.* **7**, 97–104, Figure 1. With permission from Lippincott, Williams & Wilkins

random-effects meta-analysis (allowing the true associations to vary across studies) or by undertaking meta-regression (relating the sizes of association to characteristics of the studies). Meta-analysis is vulnerable to the effects of bias in the studies that are included in the analysis; research is underway to try to estimate the magnitude and effect of different sources of bias.

A robust bioinformatic structure is needed to support the meta-analysis and systematic review of genetic association studies, and indeed genetic epidemiology in general. Projects are underway at both OGDP in Atlanta and PHGU in Cambridge UK to develop new systems for capturing and storing the relevant data in an appropriate format.

Evaluating the characteristics of disease-susceptibility genetic variants

Once a disease-susceptibility gene variant has been identified, its precise role in disease aetiology needs to be established, which requires an understanding of the structure and function of genes. Although this is beyond the scope of standard genetic epidemiology, there are a number of important characteristics that need further discussion:

- Identifying whether gene variants are pathogenic variants
- Estimating disease-associated allele frequency in the population
- Estimating penetrance of disease-associated alleles
- Identifying and characterising gene–gene interactions
- Identifying and characterising gene–environment interactions.

Identifying whether gene variants are pathogenic variants

Many gene variants will not be causally related to disease because they do not affect the level of gene expression or the function of its protein product. In Chapter 2 (Box 2.1) we have described the main types of genetic variants (mutations and polymorphisms) that can be identified in the human genome. In practice, it is commonly assumed that protein-truncating variants (frameshift, nonsense and confirmed splice site or regulatory variants) are disease-causing unless there is evidence to the contrary. Other variants (intronic, missense, in-frame insertion/ deletion) are only classified as disease-causing if there are good supporting data. These include assessing whether:

- The variant is polymorphic in the population
- The variant segregates with disease in families
- The variant significantly alters gene expression or protein function in functional studies.

It is difficult to ascertain whether relatively rare variants are polymorphic in human populations because large samples are required. Although the presence of polymorphism does not always imply that a variant is not associated with disease, the risks associated with such alleles are likely to be modest, and they are therefore not usually relevant.

In order to test whether a new variant segregates with disease in a family, it may be possible to test multiple family members for the variant. However, if the number of affected individuals in the family is low or some affected family members are phenocopies (not carrying the variant allele), then this approach may not be definitive. Incomplete penetrance can also reduce the information available from testing (apparently) unaffected family members.

Other methods may be used to assess the disease risk of specific variants. For example, population-based studies may be used to compare if the frequency of a specific variant is increased in cases compared to controls. However, many variants will be very rare in the population and formally demonstrating that any one carries an increased risk of disease is rarely feasible.

Supportive evidence that a specific variant is disease-causing may be provided by functional studies, which demonstrate that the variant affects protein expression or its function. Thus, when a new variant is detected, it is important to determine its phenotypic significance particularly if a test for the variant will be used in clinical practice, where it may have important therapeutic consequences.

Estimating disease allele frequency

Where a single disease-associated allele has been identified, it is relatively straightforward to estimate its frequency in the population. In an association study, the allele frequency in controls provides a direct estimate of its frequency in the population. However, as discussed in Chapter 2, for many disease-associated gene variants, multiple alleles of the gene can give rise to disease susceptibility (this is known as allelic heterogeneity).

For example, protein-truncating mutations in the *BRCA1* gene are associated with a very high risk of breast and ovarian cancer in women. The gene is large, spanning over 80 kb of genomic DNA, comprising 22 coding exons with a total of 3400 base pairs. Over 250 different disease-associated variants have been described, many of which have been identified in only one family. These variants occur throughout the length of the gene with no apparent 'hotspots', so testing an individual for an unspecified variant involves scanning the whole gene – a laborious and expensive process, as outlined in Chapter 4. (In some populations, specific variants, known as founder mutations, are more common. For example, ~1% of the Ashkenazi Jewish population carry the 185delAG mutation; 5382insC is common in the Ashkenazim and parts of eastern Europe and the missense mutation C61G is also common in eastern Europe.)

Reliable, empirical estimation of the combined frequency of all disease-associated variants in a population would require a very large sample size, which is not feasible given currently available technology. Consequently, the population disease allele frequency is often estimated indirectly using empirical data for disease allele frequency in cases, combined with data on penetrance.

Estimating penetrance

As discussed in Chapters 1 and 2, the penetrance of a specific genotype is the probability that an individual with that genotype will express the phenotype of interest. For a disease phenotype, it is the probability that an individual will be affected by disease. The proportion of carriers of the susceptibility genotype that are affected will vary with age; therefore, age must also be specified when describing penetrance.

The ideal study design for estimating penetrance would be to identify all individuals with a specific genotype from a random sample of the population at birth and follow them up for the outcome of interest. This method would provide an unbiased estimate of the average penetrance for all those with the susceptibility genotype. However, such an approach is not usually feasible for a variety of reasons, including:

- Identifying individuals with the susceptibility genotype may be difficult both practically and ethically, especially for complex genes with multiple disease-associated alleles which make molecular genetic testing difficult.
- The time to develop the phenotype of interest in adult-onset disorders limits the possibility of truly prospective studies.

Thus, most studies of penetrance rely on identifying gene carriers ascertained in other ways. Multiple-case families with disease-associated mutations are often used for this purpose. Family members are treated as a retrospective cohort so that the disease incidence in family members with and without the mutation can be compared and penetrance computed. Some form of correction is normally applied to account for the different methods of family ascertainment. These approaches give consistent estimates of penetrance provided that the same penetrance function applies to all carriers. Differences occur if penetrance is modified by other risk factors (genetic or environmental) that also cluster in families or if penetrance is mutation-specific. Either of these phenomena would lead to the actual penetrance of mutations segregating in multiple-case families being higher than that of mutations segregating in the population as a whole.

Gene–gene interactions

One of the major challenges facing genetic epidemiologists is unravelling the complexity of polygenic disease susceptibility. This requires an understanding of how these genes interact to cause disease. The general issues around the meaning and interpretation of the term 'interaction' have been described above.

Box 3.11 provides an example of the difficulties facing genetic epidemiologists when exploring interactions between genes using model-based methods, such as

Box 3.11 Gene–gene interaction and model-based statistical methods

Two statistical terms are needed to model the main effect of a simple bi-allelic locus when using logistic regression in the analysis of a case–control study; two dummy variables are needed to generate three genotypes. Twenty terms would be needed to model ten such loci. The number of terms needed to describe the statistical interactions among a subset k of n bi-allelic loci is $[(n \text{ choose } k) \times 2^k]$.[†] So, as each additional main effect is included in a model, the number of possible interaction terms grows exponentially. Thus, a model to include all possible 2- to 10-way interactions for 10 loci would need 59 048 terms in a logistic regression model.

This example clearly shows that where standard model-dependent approaches are used for multi-variate data analysis, a limit on the analytic model is required (for example, by limiting the number of possible interactions). It is clearly not possible to generate sufficiently large datasets to use this type of approach in an unstructured way. Much of the recent impetus for the development of new analytic tools in molecular biology has come from the analysis of gene expression array data, which provide data on a large number of genes simultaneously.

Notes

[†](n choose k) is the number of different ways of choosing k samples from a total sample of n.

logistic regression. Thus, rather than posing the question of whether or not there is statistical interaction (according to some arbitrary, pre-defined model of interaction), it may be more pertinent to try to define the nature of that interaction in a biological sense.

An example of gene–gene interaction (also known as epistasis) is provided by the renin-angiotensin system. This system is responsible for the regulation of blood pressure, renal function and fluid balance. People carrying particular variants of the *ACE* gene and of the *AGTR1* gene are at much greater risk of myocardial infarction than those who do not have both variants.

Gene–environment interactions

If unravelling gene–gene interactions is a challenge, then identifying how genes interact with environmental factors adds even more complexity. Factors such as age, gender and diet influence the relationships between genetic variation and disease susceptibility. These factors are important because they may help to identify individuals at a greater risk of disease and provide opportunities for disease prevention. In this section, we consider some of the relevant study designs for evaluating gene–environment interaction and introduce the concept of Mendelian randomisation.

Study designs for gene–environment interactions

Twin, adoption studies and segregation analysis (outlined earlier in this chapter) can be used to investigate gene–environment interaction. However, when genetic markers are available, case–control studies and case-only designs have important advantages. Case–control studies are particularly useful when the exposure and genetic variants are common. Both the exposure and the susceptibility genotype can be designated as either present or absent. Using unexposed subjects without the susceptibility genotype as the reference group, odds ratios can be calculated using a 2-by-4 contingency table. For example, an interaction has been shown between the *Taq1* polymorphism and maternal cigarette smoking, increasing the risk of cleft palate in their infants (see Table 3.3). This shows there is a much greater risk of cleft palate in the infants of mothers who both smoke and have the *Taq1* polymorphism.

However, a major problem with case–control studies is information bias, which occurs when there are systematic differences in the way exposure data are obtained from cases and controls.

This has led to the development of an alternative approach, known as the case-only design. In this method, investigators use only case subjects to assess associations between environmental exposures and susceptibility genotypes. It provides

Table 3.3. Interaction between *Taq1* polymorphism and maternal cigarette smoking on risk of cleft palate

Smoking	*Taq1* polymorphism	Odds ratio cleft palate (95% CI)
No	No	1.0 (Reference category)
No	Yes	1.0 (0.3–2.4)
Yes	No	0.9 (0.4–1.8)
Yes	Yes	5.5 (2.1–14.6)

a simple tool to screen for gene–environment interaction. Cases are defined as those with the susceptibility genotype; pseudo-controls are defined as those without the susceptibility genotype.

If the genotype and exposure are independent in the source population from which cases arose, the odds ratio (designated as ORca) measures the joint effect of the genotype and exposure (assuming a multiplicative model). If there is no interaction, the ORca is expected to be 1; if the joint effect is more than multiplicative, ORca is greater than 1; and if the joint effect is less than multiplicative (for example, an additive effect), ORca is less than 1. This method can be used in the analysis of 2-by-2 contingency tables or in logistic regression models.

There are a number of important methodological issues involved in the case-only approach. First, the choice of cases is subject to the usual rules of case selection for any case–control study; for example, the use of population-based incident cases allows researchers to generalise their findings.

Second, researchers must assume independence between exposure and genotype in order to apply this method. This may seem reasonable for many genes and exposures but there are some genes whose presence may lead to a higher or lower likelihood of an exposure on the basis of some biological mechanism; for example, some gene variants may cause people to drink more or less alcohol.

Third, it is not possible to evaluate the effects of the exposure alone or the genotype alone, but only departure from multiplicative joint effects; however, additive effects may also be of interest. Usually, extreme departures from multiplicative effects will also reflect even greater departure from additive effects.

Finally, observed associations may be due to chance or linkage disequilibrium between the genetic marker and the true susceptibility allele(s) at a neighbouring locus.

Gene–environment interactions and Mendelian randomisation

Mendelian randomisation (MR) describes the random assortment of alleles from parents to children that occurs during formation of the gametes at meiosis (see

Chapter 2). Theoretically, this should result in genetic variants being distributed in the population in a way that is independent of behavioural or environmental factors that may confound the relationship between certain genetic variants and disease. Indeed, some have suggested that the term 'Mendelian deconfounding' may be more appropriate in this context.

This process of random assortment may provide a study design similar to a randomised trial in certain circumstances, for investigating functional variants and environmental exposures. Davey Smith (2003) has suggested that MR may help with solving a number of problems in observational epidemiology, particularly control of confounding and ruling out reverse causation (where the presence of the outcome influences the putative exposure). The principles of MR can be applied to the study of gene–environment interactions and confounding in a number of ways:

- Genetic variants may influence intermediate phenotypes, such as levels of serum cholesterol or the enzyme paraoxonase, which are known risk factors for coronary heart disease. The causal nature of associations between the genetic variants, the intermediate phenotype and the outcome can be assessed, as well as the impact of interventions modifying it (see Figure 3.4).
- Genetic variants that modify the biological response to an exposure, such as slow and fast drug-metabolising variants, or variants that predispose people to certain exposures, may be used as indirect indicators of different exposure levels (such as lower milk consumption in people with lactose intolerance, or lower alcohol consumption in people with particular *ALDH2* gene variants).
- Genetic variants may be used as a proxy for exposures that are difficult to measure, for example where total lifetime exposures are the relevant measure.

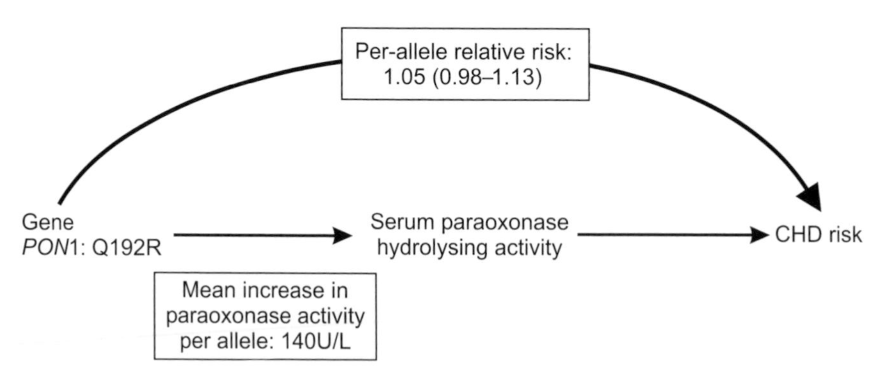

Figure 3.4 Mendelian randomisation. Mendelian randomisation in action: the relationship between genotype, intermediate phenotype and outcome for paraoxonase and coronary heart disease. Reprinted from Wheeler, J.G. *et al.* (2005). *Lancet* **363**, 689–95, Figure 3. Copyright (2005), with permission from Elsevier

For example, serum cholesterol levels influence coronary heart disease risk; certain genetic variants resulting in different levels of serum cholesterol may be used instead of single measurements of cholesterol at given time intervals. This can also mitigate the effect of regression dilution bias.
- Genetic variants should not be affected by factors that create selection or information bias.

However, the usefulness of MR in practice is limited by the lack of reliable gene–disease and gene–intermediate phenotype associations. Many genes have multiple effects, such as *APOE* gene variants. Different *APOE* gene variants are known to be associated with longevity, Alzheimer's disease, changes in serum cholesterol levels, gallstones and osteoporosis. This means that it can become very difficult to understand relationships between different *APOE* variants and specific outcomes because they may be confounded by the other effects of the variant being studied. There is also the phenomenon of canalisation, where the body develops compensatory mechanisms that can reduce the impact of specific genetic or developmental problems. Finally, the relationships between genetic variants, intermediate phenotypes and diseases may also be confounded by population stratification or by linkage disequilibrium. Despite these problems, MR is proving to be a very useful concept for genetic epidemiologists.

Further reading and resources

Classical epidemiology

Rothman's *Epidemiology: An Introduction* (2002) provides an excellent starting point for general epidemiology and would be suitable for those who are relatively new to epidemiology. This book is based on Rothman and Greenland's seminal 1998 text, *Modern Epidemiology*, which is superb. Definitions are crucial in epidemiology and Last's *A Dictionary of Epidemiology* (2001) is an excellent source of knowledge, succinctly expressed. Specific information on fundamental measures of disease and association is especially well described in Breslow and Day's *Statistical Methods in Cancer Research* (1980).

Genetic epidemiology

For those wanting an overall introduction to the human genome and its epidemiological implications, the recently published volume *Human Genome Epidemiology* (edited by Khoury, Little and Burke 2004a) is very readable. It includes sections on genetic epidemiology and genetic testing, and has a section devoted to specific case studies.

Burton, Tobin and Hopper have recently reviewed key concepts in genetic epidemiology. Their article is the first in a series of seven *Lancet* reviews, published in late 2005, that provide an authoritative and up-to-date compendium on modern genetic epidemiology. The concluding article in the series, by Davey Smith *et al.*, sums up the achievements and prospects of the field and its potential to contribute to public health improvement.

The *Lancet* series includes a review by Teare and Barrett on genetic linkage studies (article 2 in the series). Reviews by Cordell and Clayton (article 3), and Hattersley and McCarthy (article 5) tackle genetic association studies. Other recent reviews on genetic association studies include a 2002 paper by Romero and colleagues that is very well written and provides some good practical examples. Campbell and Rudan (2002) comprehensively review the background to interpreting association studies and deal with the application of traditional criteria for causality and their limitations in this particular context. Although we have discussed some of the problems posed by population stratification, a seminal paper by Wacholder and colleagues (2000) provides some empirical evidence that it may not be as big a problem as first thought.

Palmer and Cardon (article 4 in the 2005 *Lancet* series) discuss whole genome association, scanning using SNPs. Other recent reviews on the HapMap resource and the potential of genome-wide association studies have been published by McVean *et al.*, (2005), by Farrall and Morris (2005), and by Hirschhorn and Daly (2005).

Hopper, Bishop and Easton (article 6 in the 2005 *Lancet* series) discuss the advantages offered by population-based family studies for investigating the contributions of both genetic and environmental factors, separately or together, to disease risk. (Their discussion also includes studies of twin pairs; a thorough description of the use of classical twin studies may be found in a seminal paper by Martin and colleagues published in 1978 in the journal *Heredity*.)

A 2005 review by Hunter outlines the available models for describing gene–environment interactions and discusses how the analysis and interpretation of interactions are influenced by factors including study design, sample size and genotyping technology.

A paper by Clayton and McKeigue (2001) also provides an overview of some of the key epidemiological issues for studying interactions. It also (controversially) opposes the use of large, population-based cohort projects such as UK Biobank, instead advocating case–control studies as a more cost-effective approach. In response, several researchers have argued in favour of the value of such projects: see replies to the Clayton and McKeigue paper by Wacholder and colleagues (2002), Burton and colleagues (2002), and Banks and Meade (2002). The protocol for the UK Biobank project may be found on the project's website.

A detailed exposition of the concept of Mendelian randomisation and its applications in genetics research may be found in Davey Smith and Ebrahim's 2003 paper "'Mendelian randomization': can genetic epidemiology contribute to understanding environmental determinants of disease". Additional commentary on this approach and its limitations is provided in a 2003 paper by Little and Khoury.

Systematic review and meta-analysis

One of the main problems for epidemiological research is the lack of consistency in reporting study results. This has implications for those seeking to perform systematic reviews and meta-analyses, as well as those looking to assess susceptibility to bias. A proposal for the standardised reporting of genetic association studies is made by Little *et al.* in their 2002 paper 'Reporting, appraising, and integrating data on genotype prevalence and gene–disease associations'.

A recent review on systematic reviews in genetic association studies has been published by Salanti, Sanderson and Higgins (2005). The authors discuss a number of the key problems for those undertaking meta-analysis of the published literature and set out some of the issues that will need to be addressed in the future. Khoury has outlined the rationale for the HuGENet approach in a 2004 paper in the journal *Nature Genetics*. A strong case is made for an international endeavour to coordinate knowledge generation and synthesis to maximise the potential benefits of post-genomic research and its application. A commentary by Ioannidis and colleagues (2006) in *Nature Genetics* sets out a 'road map' for achieving this coordinated approach.

4

Genetics in medicine

In Chapters 2 and 3 we have discussed the relationship between genes and disease. We have also outlined the approaches that are being used to discover and quantify associations between specific genetic variants and disease risk, and to understand how genetic risk is modulated by environmental and lifestyle factors.

Although our knowledge of the genetic determinants of disease is incomplete, applications of genetics in medical practice are already in existence or are being developed. Within the specialist service of medical genetics in the UK, consultant clinical geneticists and genetic counsellors see individuals and families who are affected by, or at high risk of, conditions that may have a genetic basis. Genetics professionals attempt to assess whether the condition is, for example, a known disease caused by a single-gene lesion or chromosomal abnormality. They may suggest tests to aid diagnosis. In addition, they may give advice about a variety of issues including genetic risk to other family members, and reproductive options. Specialist genetic services, and related services within the healthcare system, are discussed in more detail in Chapter 5.

Many applications of genetics in health care, both actual and potential, rely on technology designed to test for the presence of specific genetic variants. We begin this chapter with a discussion of genetic testing and its uses in the diagnosis of disease and estimation of disease risk. We then move on to consider broader applications of genetics in the two major component areas of health care: disease prevention and disease management. Some of these applications are close to being adopted in routine clinical service, while others remain so far in the research sphere.

Genetic testing

The concept of a genetic test is rather more problematic than might appear at first sight. This is because the term can have two different meanings. It may mean a test for a genetic, that is an inherited or heritable, disorder, where the adjective 'genetic' qualifies the noun 'disorder'; or alternatively it may mean a test that is applicable to any disorder, with the word 'genetic' qualifying not the disorder but the nature of, or the technology used for, the test.

A test for a genetic disorder may use technologies that directly analyse DNA or chromosomes; or it may include non-DNA-based tests from which one is able to deduce genetic changes, for example biochemical tests or tests that rely on radiological or clinical manifestations. An ultrasound examination of the kidney is an example of a radiological test that may (at least in certain contexts) be considered a genetic test, since it may indicate the presence of the genetic variation responsible for adult polycystic kidney disease.

Most current clinical uses of genetic testing concern testing in relation to inherited or heritable disorders. Increasingly, such tests involve direct examination of the genetic material but in some cases biochemical or other types of tests are used. In the future, DNA-based tests that reveal genetic susceptibility to common (multifactorial) disease may enter the clinical arena.

Diagnostic genetic testing

The aim of diagnostic genetic testing is to establish the presence of a specific genetic disease, often in infants or young children, and ideally so that appropriate treatment may be undertaken. For example, in an infant with wasted muscles and difficulty in walking – symptoms consistent with muscular dystrophy but which might also have another cause – a genetic test could be used to provide, first, a definitive diagnosis of muscular dystrophy as distinct, for example, from a spinal muscular atrophy; and, second, a more accurate categorisation of the exact type of muscular dystrophy in that particular child.

Diagnostic testing may also be used antenatally to test for a genetic disease in a fetus; in this case, the aim is to provide the parents with information that they may choose to act on, for example by preparing for the birth of a disabled child, or by electing to terminate the pregnancy. The material used for testing is fetal cells, usually obtained by chorionic villus sampling or amniocentesis. A couple who have previously given birth to a child with a recessive single-gene disorder may decide to undergo antenatal diagnostic testing in subsequent pregnancies.

For some couples in this situation, termination of an affected pregnancy is unacceptable but they wish to avoid giving birth to another affected child. In some cases, the option of pre-implantation genetic diagnosis may be available. This procedure (Figure 4.1) involves the creation of an embryo by in vitro fertilisation. At a very early stage, one to two cells are removed from the embryo and tested for the disease-causing genotype. An embryo can compensate for the loss of these cells and develop to term. Only embryos that are unaffected by the genetic disease are used to establish a pregnancy.

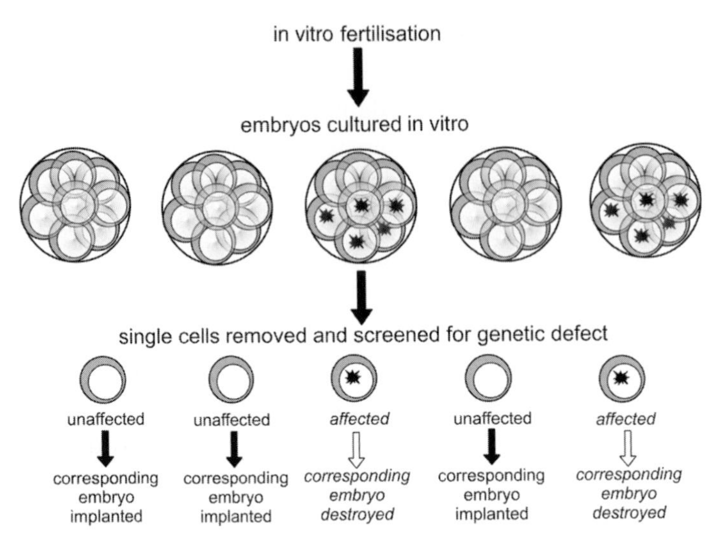

Figure 4.1 Pre-implantation genetic diagnosis (PGD). Embryos are grown for three days to the eight-cell stage before removal of one to two cells for genetic testing; embryos found to be free from the disease in question may be implanted

Carrier testing

Carrier testing identifies individuals who are themselves usually unaffected but are carriers of a recessive disease-causing mutation. Testing may be offered to individuals who have a relation affected by a recessive genetic disease. The reason for testing is to enable reproductive choice. If a couple knows that one of them is a carrier, they may decide that the other member of the couple should also be tested for carrier status. If both members of the couple prove to be carriers, various options are possible. They may choose not to act on the information, they may decide not to have children, or they may opt for antenatal genetic testing to determine whether the unborn child will be affected by the disease. If the fetus is found to be affected, again they may decide to take no action or they may wish to terminate the pregnancy.

In the case of X-linked recessive disease all carriers are female. Here, female relations of an affected male may wish to know their carrier status if they want to have children, so that they can choose to have antenatal testing or possibly pre-implantation genetic diagnosis to avoid the birth of an affected male child.

Predictive genetic testing

Predictive genetic testing (also known as pre-symptomatic testing) is the use of genetic testing to predict whether an individual will develop a genetic disease at a later stage of their life. The term is only applicable where the disease-associated mutation is known and is highly penetrant. A classical – but rare – example is predictive genetic testing for Huntington's disease. The gene associated with Huntington's disease was identified in 1993. The disease is associated with alterations in a specific part of the sequence, which can be detected by DNA analysis. As Huntington's disease is a late-onset disease, a person with a parent affected by the disease will not generally know whether they inherited it until they reach middle age. However, DNA testing at any age, even antenatally, will reveal whether the mutation is present, changing that person's individual risk from 50% to virtually 100% or zero.

Ideally, predictive genetic testing is used in association with prophylactic treatment for individuals who test positive. In families at risk of the highly penetrant familial form of bowel cancer called familial adenomatous polyposis, genetic testing can be used to identify family members who carry the disease-causing mutation, and prophylactic treatment is offered to prevent the onset of symptoms. The use of genetic testing in this context, and in particular the issues surrounding the testing of children, are discussed further in Chapters 5 and 6.

In contrast, Huntington's disease is untreatable and fatal, so careful counselling is essential for any person from an affected family who is contemplating undergoing genetic testing.

Testing for genetic susceptibility

As genetic research advances, genetic variants are being identified that appear to be associated with an increased risk of disease but which, because of incomplete penetrance, cannot be used with certainty to predict the development of disease. Tests to determine such changes are called susceptibility or predisposition tests. An allele of a gene encoding the blood protein apolipoprotein E is an example of a susceptibility allele: the *APOE4* allele of this gene has been shown to be associated with an increased risk of Alzheimer's disease. Specifically, someone with late-onset Alzheimer's disease (onset after the age of 65) is about 10 times more likely to carry two copies of *APOE4* than they are to have two copies of a different allele, *APOE3*. However, the presence of an *APOE4* allele is neither necessary nor sufficient for a person to develop Alzheimer's. Other factors, both genetic and environmental, are involved in determining whether disease will develop.

The boundary between 'predictive' and 'susceptibility' tests is not always a distinct one. Tests for *BRCA1* and *BRCA2* mutations, for example, can reveal a 60%–85% lifetime risk of developing breast cancer; whether this risk is stronger than a 'susceptibility' is essentially a personal judgement.

Testing for weakly penetrant alleles associated with susceptibility to common disease is rarely considered worthwhile at present, because of the limited predictive value of such tests. For diseases such as Alzheimer's, there is the added disincentive that there is as yet no effective treatment or prophylaxis for the disease. However, this situation may change in the future if it proves possible to identify sets of genetic variants that together substantially increase disease risk, and if interventions can be found that can effectively reduce this risk. Genetic susceptibility testing may then find a place in mainstream clinical medicine; the potential for using genetics in disease prevention is discussed later in this chapter.

Population screening

The term 'genetic screening' is often used as a synonym for genetic testing. Strictly speaking, the term should be reserved for the explicit and systematic application of a diagnostic genetic test across a whole population of asymptomatic people, or a subset of a population such as pregnant women or newborn infants. A further important characteristic of a screening test is that it is usually offered by the State or by physicians who approach the individual with the suggestion that they should take up the offer of the test. This differs from the usual clinical situation where the patient approaches the physician, and the test is used as a means of resolving the patient's problem. Screening therefore gives rise to certain ethical issues not found in clinical testing; hence, as we discuss further in this chapter and in Chapter 5, there is a need for such programmes to meet certain defined criteria.

Screening for genetic disease at present falls into three main categories: neonatal screening, antenatal screening and carrier screening (Box 4.1). In many cases

Box 4.1 Types of population screening programmes for genetic conditions

- **Neonatal screening**: A test is carried out on infants soon after birth to detect symptoms or markers of disease. The rationale for neonatal screening is that early identification of the disease enables specific management measures such as prophylactic treatment or special diets to be put in place to minimise harm. Screening for phenylketonuria and sickle-cell disease are examples.
- **Antenatal screening**: A screening test is offered to pregnant women to identify fetuses at risk of a condition associated with serious health problems, such as Down syndrome. Screening is carried out in order to offer parents the choice of whether to proceed with the pregnancy or opt for termination.
- **Carrier screening**: The aim of carrier screening programmes is to identify people who carry one copy of the harmful mutation in a recessive condition such as cystic fibrosis or Tay Sachs disease. Screening may be offered in communities or ethnic groups that have an elevated frequency of a disease-causing mutation. Screening may be available in early pregnancy, to couples who are contemplating starting a family, or even earlier to young people who might have children at some time in the future. Subsequent testing of the partner of carrier individuals can identify couples whose offspring might be at risk of the condition.

(antenatal Down syndrome screening is an example) an initial screening test gives an indication of risk, and those who are identified as being at higher risk are offered a definitive diagnostic test.

Population screening programmes for genetic conditions should in general terms conform to the criteria for population screening set out by Wilson and Jungner (1968). These include requirements (among others) that:

- The epidemiology and natural history of the condition should be understood.
- There should be a detectable risk factor or disease marker that can be measured by a simple, safe, precise and validated screening test that is acceptable to the population.
- The distribution of test values in the target population should be known and a suitable cut-off level for a positive test defined and agreed.
- There should be an effective treatment or intervention for those who test positive.

The National Screening Committee in the UK have developed their own set of criteria based on those set out by Wilson and Jungner.

Some additions and modifications to the Wilson and Jungner criteria have been suggested in order to cover features considered specific either to genetic conditions themselves or to genetic tests. For example, in some cases the aim of genetic screening is not to prevent or treat a disease in the person screened but, as in carrier screening, to provide information used for reproductive choices. Where single-gene diseases are under consideration, the consequences for other family members (who may not themselves have taken part in the screening programme) must also be considered. In the case of carrier testing, or where carriers of a recessive condition are identified as a 'by-product' of a programme to detect affected individuals, the natural history of people with carrier status should be understood, including any psychological effects.

Methods of genetic testing

As mentioned earlier in this chapter, tests used in the diagnosis of genetic diseases do not always involve analysing DNA or chromosomes. They may, instead, be designed to detect specific effects of a genetic mutation in the body, using methods such as biochemical analysis, neurological tests or physical examination. In the case of phenylketonuria, for example, the diagnostic test is based on the detection of elevated concentrations of the amino acid phenylalanine in a blood sample.

Those genetic tests that do involve analysis of the genetic material are generally classified as cytogenetic tests, which look for physical changes in chromosomes, or DNA tests, which look for specific changes in DNA sequence. However, the boundaries between these two categories are blurring, particularly as cytogeneticists make use of increasingly sophisticated molecular techniques for chromosomal analysis.

Cytogenetic testing

Until the last decade or so, cytogenetic tests were limited to examination of the number and gross structure of the chromosomes – the karyotype. A sample of cells had to be grown in culture, as their chromosomes could only be visualised by applying special stains to the condensed chromosomes in dividing cells and examining them under a microscope (see Chapter 2, Figure 2.2). Under these conditions each chromosome appears as a structure with a characteristic size, shape and pattern of transverse bands. The cytogeneticist is trained to spot any differences from the normal karyotype. Although slow (because of the time taken to culture cells) and of low resolution (the smallest differences that can be detected are equivalent to 4–5 million base pairs of DNA), this technique is still widely used in the diagnosis of chromosomal abnormalities such as trisomy 21(Down syndrome; see Figure 2.10).

The development of fluorescent in situ hybridisation (FISH; see Chapter 2, Figure 2.16) has revolutionised the potential of cytogenetics by enabling the detection of much smaller genetic changes, even down to the level of single genes. This increase in sensitivity and resolution has also made it possible to carry out cytogenetic analysis on non-dividing cells (interphase FISH), so that results can be obtained much more rapidly. Cytogeneticists are also increasingly adopting new molecular techniques such as quantitative fluorescent PCR (QF-PCR), described later in this chapter. QF-PCR, which can be used to detect changes in gene dosage, is finding application as a rapid method for detecting the presence of extra chromosomes. It is increasingly used in antenatal testing for chromosomal disorders such as the three most common trisomies.

A major difference between the new cytogenetic approaches and traditional cytogenetic analysis is that they are targeted: whereas traditional cytogenetics asks 'Is there any discernible difference between this karyotype and the normal karyotype?', the new techniques ask 'Do the chromosomes of this individual carry the specific alteration(s) I am testing for?'

DNA testing

Early approaches to DNA-based genetic testing, when some disease-associated genes had been mapped to chromosomal locations but the specific genes and pathogenic mutations had not yet been identified, relied on the use of closely linked polymorphic markers such as restriction fragment length polymorphisms (RFLPs, see Chapter 2). Inheritance of these markers through a family could be used as a surrogate for inheritance of the disease-causing gene variant. There are still some situations in clinical genetics where linkage analysis is the only option available, but they are becoming increasingly rare. The feasibility of testing using linked markers depends on having an appropriate pedigree structure, and the accuracy depends on the distance between the DNA probe and the gene, as this affects the probability that the marker will be separated from the gene by recombination during meiosis.

Once a gene associated with a genetic disease has been identified and a pathogenic mutation(s) has been characterised, direct DNA testing can be used to look for that mutation(s).

In some circumstances, a DNA test can give a definitive answer to the question of whether an individual is carrying a mutation that causes a specific disease. For example, diagnostic testing is rapid and accurate in cases where all people with the disease carry the same, known mutation. This is so, for example, for Huntington's disease, and for the most common form of sickle-cell disease.

Many – probably most – genetic diseases, however, can be caused by any one of a large number of different mutations, either within the same gene or sometimes in different genes; that is, there may be substantial genetic heterogeneity and it may be difficult to determine whether a detected sequence change is pathogenic or simply a polymorphism that is unrelated to the disease. Sometimes, a subset of mutations can be identified that account for most cases of the disease (cystic fibrosis is an instructive example; see Box 4.2). However, a negative result from such a test, although it lowers the probability that the individual carries a disease-causing mutation in that gene, does not always eliminate it altogether.

The spectrum of disease-causing mutations in a gene, and their frequencies, may be different in different population groups. For example, the major mutations causing the haemoglobin disorder beta-thalassaemia vary between people of Mediterranean, Asian and Afro-Caribbean ancestry. In such cases, it is important to use a test that is appropriate for the population group from which the individual comes, in order to maximise its sensitivity.

There are many genetic diseases which show substantial genetic heterogeneity but where there are no particularly common mutations that account for the majority of cases; sometimes, a specific mutation may even be 'private' to just one family. A particularly cogent example is provided by the *BRCA1* gene, associated with familial breast cancer. More than 600 different sequence variations have been identified in this gene. In order to offer DNA testing to a woman who is a member of a high-risk family (based on family history), but is herself so far unaffected, it is usually essential first to identify a pathogenic mutation in an affected family member. The first affected family member to come to clinical attention is known in clinical genetics as the proband or index case. If a disease-causing mutation can be found in the proband, it is then possible to determine

Box 4.2 Genetic heterogeneity and DNA testing: cystic fibrosis carrier testing as an example

Testing for cystic fibrosis mutations is complicated by the fact that the disease can be caused by any one of more than 800 different mutations in the *CFTR* gene. Most genetics centres in the UK currently test for about 30 mutations that together account for over 90% of CF cases in people of northern European extraction (one mutation, a three-base deletion called ΔF508, accounts for around 70% of cases). If the test were to be used for carrier screening, this means that if a couple from this section of the population were both to test negative, there would still be a small residual risk (less than 1 in 100 000) that they could conceive an affected child. This residual risk has several components:

- The possibility of a mistake in the test itself (no test can be 100% accurate).
- The possibility that both parents contain mutations in the gene other than those tested for (allelic heterogeneity).
- The one-in-four chance that two carriers of a recessive mutation will conceive an affected child.
- The possibility that a new mutation(s) has occurred in the child that is not present in the parents. (In the case of cystic fibrosis this last possibility is very remote; virtually all individuals with cystic fibrosis have parents who are both carriers.)

accurately whether other family members carry the same mutation. If no disease-causing mutation is identified in the proband, there is nothing to be gained by attempting DNA testing in relatives. In this situation, family members will still know that they are at high risk, because of their family history, but it is not possible to pinpoint the specific cause of disease in their family, or to identify which family members have inherited any specific genetic factor(s) responsible for increasing the risk of disease.

Techniques for finding mutations

Various approaches have been developed to 'scan' a suspect gene for mutations in situations where the exact mutation in a family is not known. High throughput mutation scanning requires techniques that are both sensitive and amenable to automation. Many of these techniques depend on detecting subtle physicochemical differences in the behaviour of DNA molecules with slightly different sequences; the piece of DNA to be tested is compared with a piece of DNA that is known to have the normal, or wild-type, sequence. Complete sequencing of the entire gene can also be used as a mutation scanning technique but at present this is generally too expensive for routine service use.

Generally, PCR amplification of the DNA region of interest is used to generate enough DNA for analysis, followed by techniques to compare normal and test amplicons (PCR product DNA molecules). If the presence of a mutation is indicated by these techniques, sequencing or mutation analysis will be required to determine the exact nature, and in some cases position, of the mutation.

A particular difficulty in interpreting the results from mutation scanning is that it is not always easy to say whether a sequence difference that is detected is a disease-associated mutation or a normal polymorphism. Population data are needed to resolve this question. One type of mutation scanning test that does discriminate between normal and abnormal sequences is the protein truncation test, which relies on the fact that many disease-causing mutations result in production of a shortened protein product.

Electrophoresis-based methods

Single-stranded conformation polymorphism (SSCP) detection is a widely used method for identifying mutations; it uses PCR amplification of the region of interest followed by gel electrophoresis (see Chapter 2 for a description of these basic techniques). The technique relies on the fact that two single-stranded DNA molecules that differ by as little as a single base will adopt different three-dimensional structures, and these alternative conformations will move differently through a gel. Fluorescent PCR primers can be used to allow automated detection of mutated sequences. SSCP is most sensitive for short DNA fragments of 300 base pairs or less.

Conformation-sensitive gel electrophoresis (CSGE) is based on mismatch pairing between normal and mutated base pairs (Figure 4.2). Double-stranded DNA samples are amplified by PCR, denatured to separate the DNA strands, then reannealed. Samples that contain mutations will form some mismatched (heteroduplex) double-stranded DNA that adopts a different conformation from the matching (homoduplex) double-stranded DNA and moves at a different speed through the gel. Mildly denaturing gel electrophoresis conditions exacerbate the conformational changes and enhance separation of matched and mismatched DNA samples. The use of fluorescently tagged PCR products and automated analysis produces an output pattern of fluorescent peaks that alters if changes as small as a single base pair are present; this is a very sensitive technique used for mutation detection.

Capillary gel electrophoresis uses gels within tiny capillary tubes to resolve DNA molecules. This adaptation of basic electrophoresis is much more amenable to automation (for example, using arrays of multiple capillaries combined with fluorescence detection systems) and is used for high-throughput genotyping and mutation analysis.

Mismatch cleavage detection refers to a general technique for the identification of unknown mutations based on mismatch between test DNA and wild-type

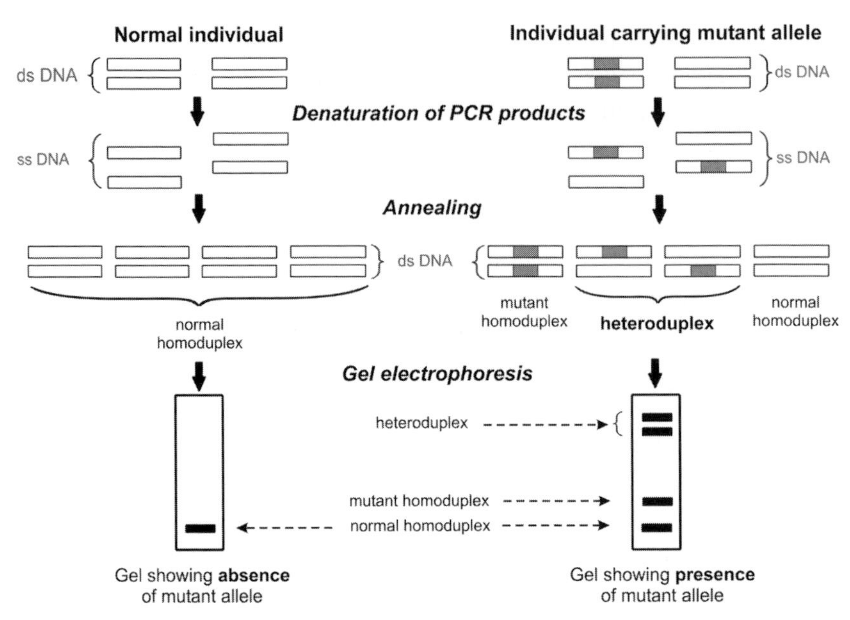

Figure 4.2 Conformation-sensitive gel electrophoresis (CSGE). CSGE can detect the presence of mutations because they create mismatched (heteroduplex) double-stranded DNA, which adopts a different conformation from homoduplex DNA and moves at a different speed through a gel

(labelled) probe DNA sequences when they form double-stranded DNA complexes. It can be used to both identify and position mutations in relatively large stretches of DNA.

Chemical mismatch cleavage (CMC) is based on the sensitivity of unmatched or mismatched C and T bases to modification by specific chemicals (hydroxylamine and osmium tetroxide). The hybridised DNA molecules are cleaved at the chemically modifed regions of mismatch by another chemical, piperidine, and the resulting fragments are separated by size to identify the location of the mismatches. Semi-automated fluorescent detection of the fragments is also possible. Enzyme mismatch cleavage (EMC) is a modification of the CMC technique using enzymatic digestion of mismatched DNA, which avoids the use of toxic chemicals. The enzymes used (such as T4 endonuclease VII) are resolvases, which recognise and cleave at sites of base mismatch in double-stranded DNA.

PCR-based detection

Information from PCR experiments is largely qualitative, but it is possible to obtain quantitative information using techniques known as quantitative or real-time PCR. Quantitative PCR relies on detection of a competitive reporter molecule that uses the same primers as the target DNA or RNA, but produces a different size

PCR product (amplicon). Target DNA is mixed with different (known) amounts of the reporter and the PCR products are analysed using gel electrophoresis. Equal amounts of the reporter and target amplicons will be produced when their respective template concentrations are equal; as the amount of reporter is known, the amount of target DNA can be estimated.

Real-time PCR uses fluorescent probes for the detection of PCR products and requires a machine that can monitor fluorescence during the reactions; fluorescence intensity is a measure of the amount of PCR product. This is a more accurate and sensitive technique than traditional PCR, which measures total DNA output at the endpoint of the reaction. It can detect as little as a twofold change in the total amount of DNA present. It is also much faster and can be fully automated. This technique has had a major impact on areas of genetics research such as gene expression analysis, and is also used in genetics laboratories for rapid antenatal testing and genotyping assays. Different types of fluorescent reporter molecules are used for real-time PCR; these include sequence-specific probes such as TaqMan®, and dyes that bind to double-stranded DNA amplicons, such as SYBR Green.

TaqMan® is a technique that relies on the ability of the Taq DNA polymerase enzyme to cleave fluorescently labelled probe molecules during PCR (Figure 4.3).

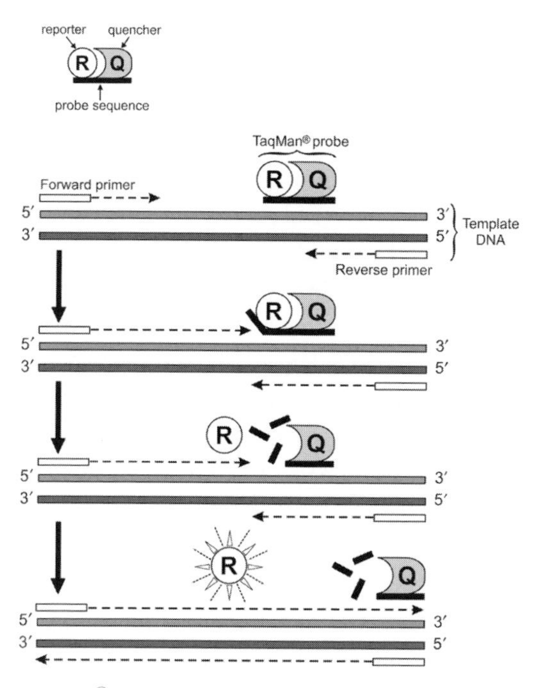

Figure 4.3 TaqMan®. Extension of PCR primers leads to cleavage of the TaqMan® probe and release of the fluorescent reporter component; levels of fluorescence are proportional to the levels of the DNA product

The TaqMan® probe is bound to target DNA, followed by binding of the two PCR primers either side; the TaqMan® probe binds at a lower temperature than the primers. It has two different fluorescent tags attached, one a 'reporter' tag and the other a 'quencher' tag that blocks fluorescence of the reporter label when adjacent to it. The reporter and quencher tags emit different wavelength fluorescence – typically green and red, respectively. During the PCR reaction, the Taq DNA polymerase cleaves the TaqMan® probe, releasing the reporter from the quencher and leading to an increase in reporter (green) fluorescence proportional to the amount of PCR product DNA. This fluorescence is detected and quantified to give a real-time record of the level of DNA produced by the reaction.

Molecular beacons also contain fluorescent reporter and quenching dyes, but in this instance the beacons comprise a short DNA sequence that forms a hairpin structure while free in solution, that keeps the quencher close to the reporter. When the beacons bind to target DNA during PCR, the reporter is separated from the quencher and fluoresces.

Multiplex ligation-dependent probe amplification (MLPA) is a technique to detect copy number variation in genomic sequences at high resolutions, which is increasingly used in genetic laboratories because it is sensitive, reasonably inexpensive and appropriate for high throughput of samples. MLPA allows relative quantification of multiple different nucleic acid sequences in a single reaction, and is typically used for the detection of duplications or deletions in the *BRCA1* gene and *MSH2* and *MLH1* genes involved in hereditary breast and colorectal cancer, respectively.

For MLPA, genomic DNA is hybridised to pairs of probes: one with a central target-specific sequence flanked by a universal primer sequence, and another with a target-specific sequence at one end and a universal primer sequence at the other, separated by a variable-length random fragment (Figure 4.4). The probe pairs are designed so that the target-specific sequences bind adjacently to the target DNA and can be joined by a ligase enzyme to create a single probe sequence flanked by primer binding sites that allow PCR-based amplification. The amount of ligated probe product produced is proportional to the target copy number; deletions or duplications of the target sequence can be identified by the relative peak heights/areas.

Comparative genomic hybridisation

Comparative genomic hybridisation (CGH) is a method for the identification of copy-number changes (amplifications and deletions) within the genome. It relies on the differential binding of reference (normal) and test DNA samples to a normal chromosome spread. The reference and test samples are labelled with different fluorescent dyes; say, red and green respectively. Changes in copy number

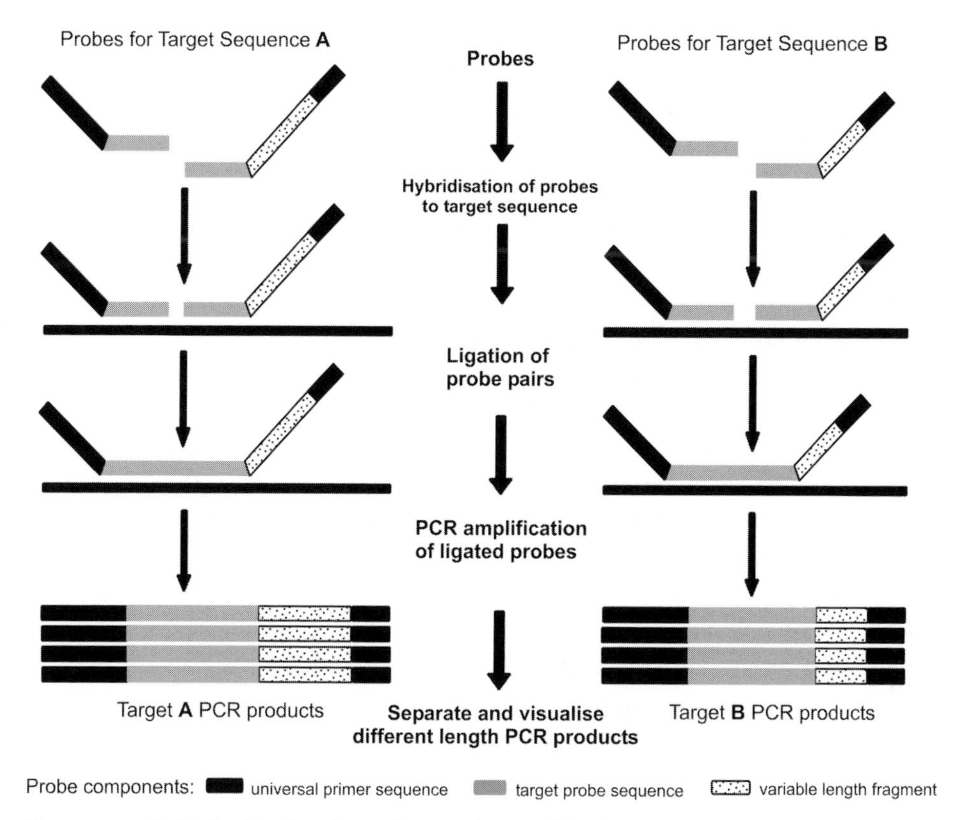

Figure 4.4 Multiplex ligation-dependent probe amplification (MLPA). MLPA can detect copy number variation in multiple different sequences simultaneously using fluorescently labelled target-specific probes of different lengths; the amount of ligated probe product for each sequence (detectable by the level of fluorescence) is proportional to the original copy number

in the test DNA can be identified by regions of red and green fluorescence, representing deletions and amplifications respectively. Where there has been no change, the fluorescence is yellow because equal amounts of red and green fluorescent material are present.

Microarray comparative genomic hybridisation, or array CGH, combines the principle of CGH with microarray technology. Microarray chips contain thousands of probe sequences representing the genome, and can provide much more precisely targeted identification of genetic abnormalities, comparable to performing multiple FISH experiments.

Denaturing high-performance liquid chromatography (DHPLC)

High-performance liquid chromatography (HPLC) is a widely used technique for the separation of different molecules. The molecules divide their time between a moving liquid and a static column; their relative affinities for the two determine the speed at which they move through the column. Molecules with different relative affinities move at different speeds through the column and will wash off (elute) at different times. DHPLC is used to detect the presence of mutations in double-stranded DNA, based on the fact that mismatch between wild-type and mutated DNA strands affects the conformation and ability of DNA complexes to bind to a column. Sequence variations alter the DNA molecule surface, making it bind less tightly to the column and elute earlier than wild-type DNA. Using conditions that cause partial denaturation of double-stranded DNA enhances the separation of wild-type and mutation-containing complexes. DHPLC can be fully automated, and permits rapid sample analysis. It can identify the presence of single base changes, small insertions and deletions, but not the nature or location of the mutations. In genetics laboratories, it is used to screen for the presence of *BRCA1/2* (breast cancer) mutations, and for mutations in the dystrophin gene associated with forms of muscular dystrophy. It is also used for high-throughput single nucleotide polymorphism (SNP) analysis in gene-association studies.

MALDI-TOF

MALDI-TOF MS (matrix assisted laser desorption / ionisation – time of flight mass spectrometry) is a technique used for the characterisation of biomolecules such as DNA or proteins. DNA molecules are mixed with a matrix and subjected to a laser pulse, which vaporises and ionises (electrically charges) them, before being accelerated through a flight tube to a detector at the far end. As they pass through the tube, the molecules separate out according to their size and charge, and so reach the detector at different times, generating different signals. Automated MALDI-TOF is widely used for genotyping and SNP analysis, but is also being developed for diagnostic mutation screening.

Future developments

In the future, microarray technology, already well developed in the technique of array CGH, is likely to have an increasing impact on the practice of DNA testing. The use of chips allows many sequence alterations to be tested for simultaneously, making it possible to test several samples for the same panel of mutations, or (as in the case of array CGH) to test a single sample simultaneously for a large number of possible sequence alterations. At present many uses of microarray technology are at the research and development stage; their application in a routine service setting will depend on further validation and probably reductions in cost.

Many future applications of genetic testing will require the use of methods for determining an individual's genotype at several different genetic loci. For example, a particular pattern of SNPs may indicate that an individual is likely to experience an adverse reaction to a particular drug, or to be particularly sensitive to the effects of an environmental chemical. High-throughput technology is being developed to enable this type of testing to be carried out rapidly on large numbers of samples. This is being applied at the research stage in large studies that aim to discover and validate associations between SNPs and characteristics of interest (see Chapter 3), and will also be necessary if routine application in health services becomes a reality.

Evaluation of genetic tests

Just like any other medical intervention or technology, genetic tests should be evaluated to assess the benefits of their use. Although genetic tests should not be singled out as uniquely problematic, there are a number of specific issues that need particular attention. The term 'genetic test' should be regarded as shorthand to describe a test to detect:

- a particular genetic variant (or set of variants)
- in relation to a particular disease
- in a particular population, and
- for a particular purpose.

All of these elements are important when evaluating genetic tests.

One important approach is the ACCE framework (Box 4.3), developed by the Office of Genomics and Disease Prevention at the Centers for Disease Control and Prevention in the USA. Although the ACCE framework is applicable to protein- or metabolite-based tests for genetic disorders, it has mostly been applied to DNA-based tests. A modified version of the ACCE approach, known as the 'Gene Dossier', has been adopted by the UK Genetic Testing Network to evaluate emerging DNA-based genetic tests in the NHS (also see Chapter 5).

Challenges for evaluating genetic tests

Rigorous evaluation of genetic tests is conceptually and methodologically difficult and the quality of many published evaluations is poor. A major problem for many new and emerging genetic tests is that the evidence base is very limited. In the case of new tests for rare disorders, for example, the very small numbers of available samples and test results may make it difficult to calculate the numerical indices used to evaluate test performance, such as specificity and predictive values.

Determining the genetic variants known to be associated with a disease entity, usually termed 'characterising the genotype of interest', is a key step but is not always straightforward. This genotype could be defined in three ways: as all known and unknown variants; all known variants; or specific selected variants.

One important problem concerns those tests where the genotype of interest cannot be easily specified, usually when there is extensive allelic and/or locus heterogeneity or when mutation-scanning methods are used. There are also

Box 4.3 The ACCE framework for evaluation of genetic tests

An ACCE evaluation begins with an introductory section that describes the relevant disorder and the setting in which the test will be used. It then moves on to an assessment of the **A**nalytical validity, **C**linical validity, **C**linical utility and the **E**thical, legal and social implications of the test in question.

- **Analytical validity** is essentially a measure of the technical accuracy of the test: in the case of DNA testing, it defines the laboratory test's ability to measure accurately and reliably the genotype of interest.
- **Clinical validity** defines the test's ability to detect or predict the presence or absence of the phenotype (disease). It includes assessment of the positive and negative predictive values of the test, which depend on the test's clinical sensitivity (the proportion of individuals with positive tests results who also have, or will develop, the disease); the clinical specificity (the proportion of individuals with negative test results who do not have, or will not develop, the disease); and the prevalence of the disease.
- **Clinical utility** refers to the likelihood that the test will lead to an improved health outcome. It encompasses, for example, the benefits and risks of positive and negative test results, the consequences of false positives and false negatives, the availability of effective interventions, and whether the test result contributes to decisions about patient management or alters clinical outcome. The clinical utility is not a fixed property of a test but will vary depending on the clinical and family circumstances of the person for whom testing is proposed.
- **Ethical, legal and social implications** include possible non-medical consequences such as stigmatisation or discrimination; these are included because they are acknowledged to be an important component of the test's impact on the individual undergoing it and, in some cases, his or her family.

considerable methodological issues to consider when evaluating techniques such as microarrays, where many genetic variants can be tested for simultaneously.

The classical techniques for evaluating clinical tests apply essentially to diagnostic tests. However, applying such techniques to the evaluation of tests indicating predisposition to future disease raises problems because of the need to incorporate the dimension of time. To detect genetic variants that confer an increased risk of developing the phenotype during a defined time period requires data from cohort studies; cross-sectional studies are generally inappropriate. Applying indices of diagnostic accuracy (such as sensitivity and specificity) is less meaningful, because the aim of susceptibility testing is to estimate absolute risks for individuals.

For some applications of genetic testing, the unit of analysis is the family and not simply individuals. The process involved in a 'genetic test' for an individual, unaffected family member may involve assessment of the likelihood that an inherited disease syndrome is segregating within the family, scanning the DNA of an affected family member(s) for a mutation that segregates with the disease and, depending on the outcome of these analyses, the offer of a direct gene test to the unaffected relative. Evaluation of the 'genetic test' in such situations must include evaluation of the whole assessment and test 'package', not just the final DNA test.

Some commentators have suggested that the assessment of clinical utility should be strengthened in the ACCE framework, particularly in recognising that genetic testing is a complex process and is one component of an overall complex intervention. A clear understanding of the relationships between clinical diagnosis, non-genetic diagnostics and genetic testing is required. This kind of analysis should include assessment of genetic testing instead of non-genetic testing or in addition to non-genetic testing, with estimation of the relevant benefits, harms and costs.

Genetics and disease prevention

A major aim of public health medicine is the prevention of disease. It follows, then, that public health genetics will be concerned with identifying ways in which advances in genetic science may be harnessed in the cause of disease prevention and the promotion of health.

Genotypic and phenotypic prevention

A popular scenario for the future involves using genetics to identify people who are at a significantly increased risk of disease, and offering them interventions that will reduce that risk. The rationale is that disease results from interactions between genes and environment, so it should be possible to modify risk by altering either the genotype (genotypic prevention), or the environment (phenotypic prevention), or both.

Genotypic prevention could in theory involve changing either the germ-line genome or the somatic genome of cells affected by the disease. Intervention at the level of the germ-line genome is fraught with many difficulties, both practical and ethical. Antenatal genetic testing followed by the offer of pregnancy termination if the fetus is affected by a genetic disease could be considered an example of this type of genotypic prevention but is viewed by most people as acceptable only if the disease in question causes severe disability (see Chapter 6 for further discussion).

Manipulation of the germ-line genome (the genome of the sperm or egg) to correct a genetic defect before disease becomes evident is not yet feasible in humans and raises many problems. Germ-line modification has been achieved in animal models but has not been attempted in humans and is illegal in many countries, including the UK, where genetic engineering even of non-human animals and plants has very low public acceptance. Alteration of the somatic genome (perhaps in the unborn fetus) with the aim of preventing disease would probably command more public support but would be affected by many of the same technical difficulties that have dogged attempts to develop gene therapy as a form of disease treatment. Gene therapy is discussed further later in this chapter.

Phentoypic prevention, at least in theory, avoids the practical and ethical problems associated with genotypic prevention. Here, there is no attempt to change an individual's genetic constitution; rather, disease development is slowed or prevented by a phenotypic intervention such as drug treatment, surgery or lifestyle change. In fact, the well-established public health messages concerning diet and lifestyle all rely on the idea of phenotypic prevention of common disease but they are applied indiscriminately, irrespective of genotype. As discussed in Chapter 1 there is an argument that this sort of advice might be more effective if it could be targeted at those groups or individuals who are at increased genetic risk.

Identifying individuals at high genetic risk: family tracing

Phenotypic prevention in the context of genetics relies on being able to identify those individuals who are at increased genetic risk. At present, the clearest examples of this approach come from the application of 'cascade' testing, also known as family tracing, in the families of individuals affected by certain adult-onset Mendelian diseases. In this approach, first-degree relatives of an individual affected by a treatable or preventable adult-onset genetic disease, but who are themselves so far asymptomatic, are actively sought out and offered a test to determine whether they also carry the causative mutation or perhaps other markers of the disease. Family tracing is considered an appropriate approach for conditions such as familial hypercholesterolaemia, which can be effectively treated by cholesterol-lowering drugs before its effects become life-threatening. Health-economic analysis suggests that it is more cost-effective than population screening for this condition. The approach is also being assessed for its suitability in families affected by hereditary haemochromatosis (Box 4.4).

Family history is already used in clinical practice as a form of triage to identify individuals at risk of highly penetrant familial forms of common cancers, particularly breast/ovarian cancer or bowel cancer. A strong family history of the disease in an affected person may prompt the offer of genetic investigation and perhaps testing for a mutation in one of the genes known to be associated with these conditions. If a mutation is found, at-risk relatives can be offered the option of testing and those who do not carry the mutation can be reassured that their risk is not significantly higher than the general population level.

For those who test positive, some preventive options are available. For example, prophylactic mastectomy and oophorectomy are effective, though drastic,

Box 4.4 Family tracing (cascade testing) for hereditary haemochromatosis
Hereditary haemochromatosis is an autosomal recessive condition leading to excessive iron accumulation that in some individuals can cause severe liver disease and other problems. An effective preventive intervention is available in the form of frequent phlebotomy. Ninety per cent of individuals of northern European origin who are affected by hereditary haemochromatosis are homozygotes for the C282Y mutation in the *HFE* gene. Some have advocated population screening for haemochromatosis but the disease is incompletely penetrant (estimates vary from 1% to 40%) so a population approach would identify many people who have the disease-associated genotype (approximately 1 person in 150 in northern European populations) but might never become unwell. As a compromise, it has been suggested that a family tracing approach might be a better way of identifying people who are likely to be at high risk of the disease and would stand to gain most from preventive measures. The reasoning is that first-degree relatives of clinically affected individuals may be more likely than unrelated people to share whatever other genetic and environmental factors are implicated in overall susceptibility to development of the disease.

preventive interventions for breast and ovarian cancer. Alternatively surveillance may be offered so that, if cancer does develop, it can be identified and treated as early as possible.

Susceptibility genetics

The examples in the previous section concern prevention of Mendelian diseases. The prospects for using genetics in the context of prevention of common, multifactorial disease are controversial.

In most cases, the increased risk conferred by individual disease-associated polymorphisms is likely to be very modest and not sufficiently predictive to warrant the use of genetic testing to identify susceptible individuals (see paper by van Rijn, van Duijn and Slooter 2005). The picture could change dramatically if several different disease-associated alleles were known that, acting together, had a much greater effect on risk, and some mathematical simulation studies support this view, suggesting that the power of genetic risk prediction rises rapidly as more genes are introduced (see the papers by Pharoah *et al.* 2002, and Yang *et al.* 2003, for examples).

However, the clinical usefulness of using 'multiplex' genetic testing to identify susceptible individuals in the general population has been questioned on the grounds that the sensitivity and specificity of a multiplex test are likely to be poor: accurate risk prediction may be possible only for the tiny proportion of people who have all (or nearly all) higher-risk variants, or all (or nearly all) lower-risk variants (see paper by Janssens *et al.* 2005). For the majority, with a mixture of higher- and lower-risk variants, no accurate prediction will be possible so use of the multiplex test could, it is argued, result in missing a large number of people who will develop the disease, while unnecessarily treating a large number who would not develop it.

In practice, we are a long way from knowing enough about the genetic factors associated with risk of common disease, or about how these genetic variants interact with specific environmental factors, to be able to use this information in disease prevention. It may be several decades before the scientific basis for the 'predict and prevent' scenario can be adequately evaluated. In the meantime, there is a need for substantial investment in social and behavioural research, to improve our understanding of how people perceive risk, and whether knowledge of genetic susceptibility would be likely to act as a motivator for preventive intervention or would induce counter-productive feelings of fatalism.

Early research in this field suggests that tests for genetic susceptibility do not necessarily induce undue worry but that risk information alone plays only a small part in people's ability to change their behaviour. The availability of an effective intervention is important, as is the individual's assessment of their ability to achieve behavioural change; this in turn is strongly dependent on their familial and social environment. One danger is that those identified as at lower genetic risk may be falsely reassured; there is already some evidence from behavioural science research that this can occur.

Family history as a tool in prevention of common disease

Family history information may provide a useful – and currently under-used – tool to identify individuals who are likely to be at increased risk of common disease. Family history (discussed from an epidemiological perspective in Chapter 3) is indicative not just of genetic risk but also of risk resulting from shared environmental/lifestyle factors.

We have already discussed the clinical use of family history to identify individuals who may be affected by highly penetrant Mendelian forms of some common diseases. Family history might also be clinically useful in situations where the familial risk is much lower. As a rule of thumb, having one first-degree relative affected by a common cancer approximately doubles an individual's risk of that disease. A stronger family history increases risk still further, with relative risks in the range of two to five. For some other common diseases, familial relative risks are substantial (see Table 3.1). It has been estimated that almost half of the population has a close relative with one or more common chronic diseases.

Enthusiasts for the use of family history to predict risk and prevent disease suggest that family doctors should prospectively elicit family history information from their patients and encourage those with family histories suggesting significant risk to adopt preventive measures such as dietary or lifestyle change. Caution is needed, however, as this approach has not yet been systematically evaluated. Research is underway in the US with the aim of establishing the accuracy of family history as a risk predictor, identifying interventions that are effective for individuals with a family history of a particular disease, and determining whether screening on the basis of family history leads to improved health outcomes. Ethical, legal and social implications are included in this analysis.

Ecogenetics

Often, the exact nature of the environmental factors that interact with genetic variants to influence disease risk is not known. However, there are some environmental exposures that we know, from long-standing epidemiological evidence, are likely to be implicated: these include, among others, dietary factors and certain environmental components such as toxic chemicals and radiation.

New areas of research are opening up that are attempting to elucidate these gene–environment interactions and their relevance for disease. These research areas are sometimes described by the general term 'ecogenetics', though terminology in the field varies. Ecogenetics has several different sub-branches including toxicogenetics and nutrigenetics.

Tobacco smoke is a known environmental toxin and differential genetic susceptibility to the carcinogenic effects of tobacco smoke has been investigated. An example is the relationship between genotype for the *N*-acetyltransferase genes *NAT1* and *NAT2*, smoking, and risk of bladder cancer. The *NAT1* and *NAT2* genes are involved in the metabolism and detoxification of aromatic monoamines, carcinogenic compounds found in tobacco smoke. Synthesis of evidence from several studies suggests that individuals carrying certain allelic combinations of the *NAT2* gene that confer a 'slow acetylator' phenotype are more susceptible to the carcinogenic effects of tobacco smoke than those with the 'fast acetylator' phenotype. Genetic effects on reactions to cigarette smoke are likely to be complex, involving interactions among variants of several genes including *NAT1* and *NAT2*, members of the cytochrome P450 family and the glutathione *S*-transferase M1 (*GSTM1*) gene.

Unravelling such complex interactions will be a difficult task, as discussed in Chapter 3. Additional difficulties arise if levels of exposure to a substance of interest are not known or cannot be measured accurately – this is likely to be the case for many, if not most, environmental exposures of interest.

From the standpoint of disease prevention, the contribution of an improved understanding of genetic susceptibility to environmental hazards is not yet clear. Differential genetic susceptibility to the effects of beryllium dust illustrates some of

Box 4.5 Ecogenetics: the example of beryllium sensitivity

Beryllium metal and ceramics are used in a wide range of machinery and processes in the nuclear industry. Inhalation of beryllium dust can cause sensitisation, leading to chronic lung disease that can be fatal. Genetic studies have shown that individuals with a specific polymorphism in the *DPB1* gene (part of the major histocompatibility complex, which encodes components of the immune system) have a risk of sensitisation to beryllium that is tenfold that of individuals without this polymorphism. However, although the relative risk conferred by the sensitising *DPB1* allele is high, the specificity of the *DPB1* marker is too low to justify its use. Beryllium sensitivity is a complex trait involving multiple factors including other genetic variants.

the problems of applying an 'ecogenetic test' in practice (Box 4.5). Any potential genetic tests used to assess susceptibility must be thoroughly evaluated by the criteria outlined earlier in this chapter.

The question of whether genetic testing should be used in the context of employment, to identify individuals at increased risk from occupational hazards, also has ethical, social and policy dimensions, which will be discussed in Chapters 6 and 7. There is obviously an argument for reducing everyone's exposure – regardless of genotype – to known toxins and carcinogens such as beryllium or the components of tobacco smoke. There is also a fear that those with lower genetic susceptibility might adopt a blasé attitude to exposure to such substances, misinterpreting 'lower risk' as 'no risk'. These arguments do not, however, undermine the value of studies on the interactions between environmental substances and the genome. A better understanding of the mechanisms of toxicity and the range of genetic susceptibility could lead to improved recognition of substances that are likely to have harmful effects, and to better definition of the maximum tolerable dose based on the most susceptible genotype.

In the US, the Environmental Genome Program has been established by the National Institute of Environmental Health Sciences (part of the National Institutes of Health) to investigate the relationships between environmental exposure, genetic susceptibility and human disease. The programme has identified a set of 'environmentally responsive genes' that are likely candidates for involvement in interaction with hazardous agents in the environment. The 554 genes currently under investigation include genes with roles in key cellular processes such as DNA repair, cell cycle, cell division or signal transduction, and genes encoding components of known pathways of metabolism for toxic substances.

In the first phase of the programme, these genes are being systematically searched for polymorphisms by resequencing in a set of DNA samples from 90 different individuals. Other aspects of the programme are concerned with functional analysis of the polymorphisms, population-based epidemiological studies, and the development of new technologies to support the programme.

Nutrigenetics and nutrigenomics

Nutrigenomics uses the new technologies developed in genomic research to investigate interactions between dietary constituents and the genome at the molecular, cellular and systems levels. An understanding of these interactions can help to identify key genes, variation in which may affect individual responses to diet. Nutrigenetics describes the use of knowledge about this variation to provide individually tailored dietary advice with the aim of preventing disease.

Both nutrigenomics and nutrigenetics are still in their infancy. Some interesting preliminary findings are emerging; for example, there is some evidence that an individual's *APOE* genotype influences the effectiveness of dietary modification in reducing blood lipid levels and therefore, presumably, the effectiveness of this type of intervention in reducing risk of cardiovascular disease. If this finding were confirmed, it might mean that genetic testing could be used to target lipid-lowering drug treatments at those most likely to benefit. There is also preliminary evidence that particular dietary interventions may have differential effects in people with different genotypes. Again, if confirmed, such findings could have important implications.

However, the complexity of this area, and the difficulties faced by researchers, must not be underestimated. Many reported research results have not been replicated and the literature is full of conflicting findings. There is evidence of selective reporting of 'positive' results.

Extremely large prospective studies (enrolling many thousands and perhaps up to half a million participants) are needed to obtain robust results and they must be prolonged (at least 10–15 years) to capture long-term effects. Attention must also be paid to other aspects of study design. For example, serious problems in the accuracy of dietary measurements must be overcome. In choosing what phenotypes to study, it may be helpful to use continuously distributed intermediate phenotypes such as body mass index or plasma hormone levels. Choice of genes to study is also important: the risk of chance findings may be minimised by focusing attention, at least initially, on genes for which there is a plausible biological hypothesis for involvement in a gene–diet interaction.

As well as observational studies seeking to correlate dietary factors and genetic variants with disease outcomes, large-scale and long-term interventional studies are needed to elucidate how specific dietary changes affect disease risk in people with different genotypes. For these studies it will probably be necessary to enrol participants on the basis of their genotype, introducing extra practical difficulties in cases where some of the relevant genotypes are rare. Pooling and meta-analysis of results from different studies will be needed to validate findings, and sophisticated bioinformatics tools will be required for the storage and analysis of vast volumes of data.

The science of nutrigenetics and nutrigenomics is exciting but the extent to which it can be translated into applications in mainstream health care, and how far in the future such applications may be, are unknown. In the meantime, it is important not to dilute or confuse the key public health messages concerning a healthy diet. These messages are unlikely ever to be superseded at a population level; genetic factors may, however, in the future identify some individuals or population subsets at very high risk for whom specific dietary advice will be appropriate.

Genetics and disease management

Increasing understanding of the genomic processes that occur during the onset and progression of disease, and of individual variation in these processes, will provide opportunities for new approaches to disease management.

Pharmacogenetics

It has been known for many years that individuals differ in their responses to therapeutic drugs. Many factors including age, sex, nutrition and physical activity can affect drug responses but a substantial proportion of inter-individual variation (around 20–95%, depending on the drug) appears to be genetic.

The study of individual genetic variation in drug response is known as pharmacogenetics. A related term, pharmacogenomics, is generally used to describe the use of genomic technologies to study the effects of drugs on the genetic programmes of cells and tissues, and to use this knowledge to identify potential new drug targets. These definitions are by no means universal, however, and many authors use 'pharmacogenetics' and 'pharmacogenomics' interchangeably.

In this section, we will discuss pharmacogenetics in the context of heritable variation in drug response. In the following section, we turn our attention to the use of molecular-genetic profiling in disease diagnosis and management; as part of this discussion, we will consider somatic genetic variation in tumours and its use to guide the choice of chemotherapy treatment.

Heritable pharmacogenetic variation

Heritable genetic variation can affect either the safety or the efficacy of a drug, or both (Figure 4.5). Variation in drug response is a serious clinical problem. It has been estimated that adverse drug reactions are responsible for around 1 in 15 hospital admissions in the UK, while in the US around 100 000 deaths each year

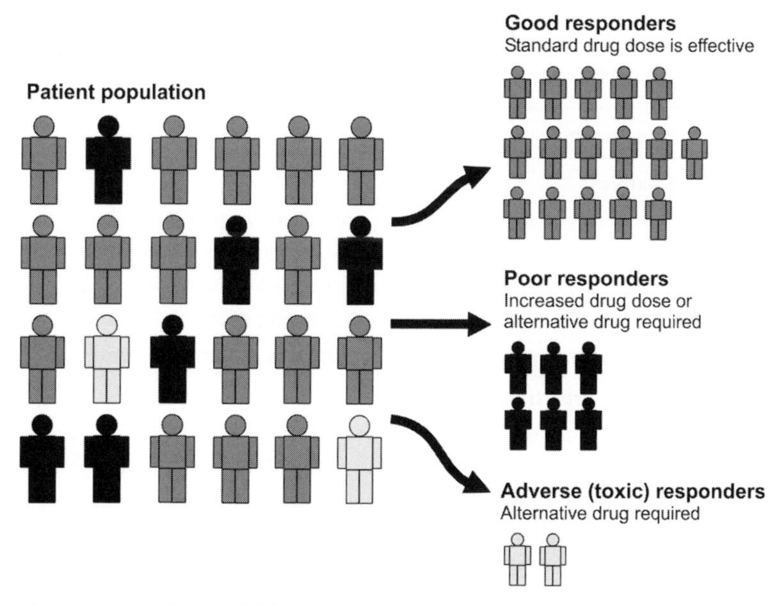

Figure 4.5 Pharmacogenetics. Individual genetic variation in drug response can affect safety or the efficacy

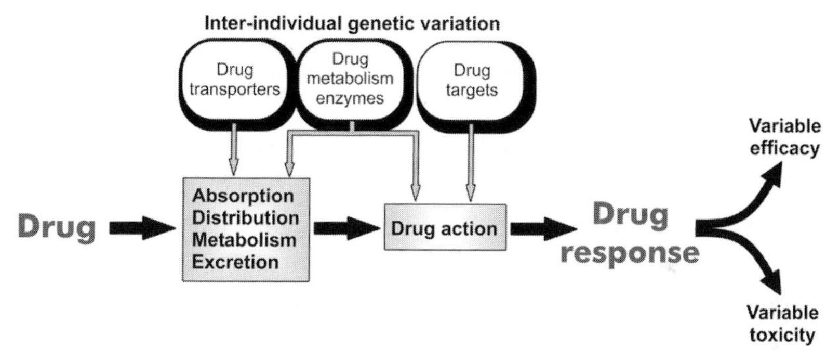

Figure 4.6 Drug response genes. Genes that influence drug response may be involved in various biological pathways that affect drug metabolism and action

have been attributed to this cause. Limited efficacy of drugs is commonplace: around 30% of patients who are prescribed a particular drug will obtain no clinical benefit from it. Most of the burden of morbidity and mortality from adverse drug reactions is due to poor prescribing, but some is due to genetic factors.

In pharmacological terms, there may be differences in any of a wide range of parameters including the absorption of the drug, its metabolism into a biologically active form, its distribution within the body and its excretion (Figure 4.6). The study of how drugs are metabolised and excreted in the body is known as pharmacokinetics. The mechanism by which they interact with target cells and

Table 4.1. Examples of genes that influence pharmacodynamic and pharmacokinetic aspects of drug response

Gene	Protein name	Phenotype/drug response
Pharmacodynamics		
ADRB1	Beta-1 adrenergic receptor	Increased response to salbutamol
COX	Cyclo-oxygenase	Responsiveness to aspirin and NSAIDs
CETP	Cholesterol ester transfer protein	Increased response to atorvastatin and pravastatin
HTR2A	Serotonin receptor 2A	Reduced response to clozapine
Pharmacokinetics: drug transporters		
ABCB1	Drug transporter MDR1	Resistance to anti-epileptic agents, e.g. phenytoin; increased immune recovery after starting anti-HIV drugs
Pharmacokinetics: metabolism		
CYP2C19	Cytochrome p450 2C19	Decreased response to omeprazole
CYP2D6	Cytochrome p450 2D6	Response to codeine
GSTM1	Glutathione *S*-transferase M1	Increased survival following chemotherapy for ovarian cancer

Reproduced from Brice, P. and Sanderson, S. (2006b). *Pharm. J.* **277**, 109–12, with permission from the Royal Pharmaceutical Society of Great Britain.

tissues is termed pharmacodynamics. Genetic factors can affect both pharmacokinetic and pharmacodynamic properties of drugs (Table 4.1).

Some genes have been implicated in several different examples of drug response variation. For example, a large family of enzymes, the cytochrome P450 (CYP) family, is involved in the metabolism and excretion of many of the drugs currently used in medical practice. These enzymes have evolved to play a role in the detoxification of harmful substances encountered in the environment. Variation in *CYP* genes has been implicated in differing responses to many drugs including warfarin, the analgesic codeine, and a large number of drugs used to treat psychiatric and neurological disease (e.g. clozapine, fluoxetine) and cardiovascular disease (e.g. timolol). 'Poor metabolisers' carry inactivating *CYP* gene mutations that may compromise drug metabolism and lead to toxic responses at normal doses. Conversely, rapid metabolisers may inactivate drugs so quickly that no therapeutic response is achieved.

The frequencies of the polymorphisms implicated in differing responses to drugs may vary in different populations. For example, the 'poor metaboliser' variant of *CYP2C9*, implicated in response to warfarin, is found in as many as 30– 40% of 'Whites' but fewer than 1% of Asians. Table 4.2 lists some common

Table 4.2. Common pharmacogenetic polymorphisms in human drug-metabolising enzymes

Gene	Phenotype	Frequency in different ethnic groups	Number of known drug substrates	Examples
Cytochrome P450 (drug oxidation)	Poor metaboliser	White 6%, African American 2%, Oriental 1%	>100	Codeine, nortriptyline, dextromethorphan
	Utra-rapid metaboliser	Ethiopian 20%, Spanish 7%, Scandinavian 1.5%		
CYP2C9	Reduced activity		>60	Tolbutamide, diazepam, ibuprofen, warfarin
CYP2C19	Poor metaboliser	Oriental 23%, White 4%	>50	Mephenytoin, omeprazole, proguanil, citalopram
N-Acetyl transferase (acetylation)	Poor metaboliser	White 60%, African American 60%, Oriental 20%, Inuit 5%	>15	Isoniazid, procainamide, sulphonamides, hydralazines
Thiopurine methyltransferase (*TPMT*) (*S*-methylation)	Poor metaboliser	Low in all populations	<10	6-mercaptopurine, 6-thioguanine, azathioprine

Reproduced from Wolf, C. R., Smith, G. and Smith, R. L. (2000). *BMJ* **320**, 987–90, Table 1, with permission from the BMJ Publishing Group.

Box 4.6 Pharmacogenetics of *TMPT* and the thiopurine drugs

Drugs such as 6-mercaptopurine, azathioprine and 6-thioguanine are widely used in oncology, dermatology and other specialist fields of medicine. These drugs have a number of potentially serious side-effects, including fatal myelosuppression. Metabolism of these drugs is performed primarily by the enzyme thiopurine *S*-methyltransferase (TPMT), although others are involved, including methylene tetrahydrofolate reductase (MTHFR). A number of common polymorphisms in the *TMPT* gene determine the level of enzyme activity; individuals with low or intermediate activity are at risk of drug toxicity unless the drug dose is reduced, usually to about 10% of standard doses. Pre-treatment genetic testing has been carried out in the US for around 10 years now, and there is evidence to suggest that it is cost-effective in certain healthcare settings. One of the difficulties of transferring testing to other countries is that there are around 13 known alleles associated with reduced TMPT activity, first identified in predominantly Caucasian patients. However, these variants have different frequencies in different population groups as well as variation in functional effects between heterozygous and homozygous individuals, suggesting that other genetic or environmental factors have a role in determining drug response to thiopurine drugs.

Reproduced from Brice, P. and Sanderson, S. (2006b). *Pharm. J.* **277**, 53–56 with permission from the Royal Pharmaceutical Society of Great Britain.

polymorphisms that are known to be involved in drug responses, and their frequencies in different populations.

Heritable pharmacogenetic variation has been known for over 40 years but tests for these variants have been slow to find a place in medical care. One test that is in clinical use in some oncology centres is a test for a polymorphism in the gene encoding the enzyme thiopurine methyltransferase (TPMT). TPMT is involved in the metabolism of thiopurine drugs used in cancer treatment. Individuals with polymorphisms that lower the activity of the enzyme experience severe toxic responses to normal doses of thiopurine drugs. For example, about 1% of White patients are homozygous for a polymorphism that lowers enzyme activity. However, genetic heterogeneity in different populations has prevented widespread adoption of *TPMT* testing in medical care (Box 4.6).

SNP profiling in pharmacogenetics

Some researchers are attempting to identify panels of polymorphisms (for example, SNPs and SNP haplotypes) that are associated with defined drug responses. The principle of this approach, and the problems that need to be overcome, have been discussed in detail in Chapter 3. In the context of pharmacogenetics, the most serious pitfall is likely to be errors in the choice of SNPs, leading to false associations. Such errors may be difficult to detect if the SNPs are simply anonymous variants not related to any known biological function. For this reason, some experts in the field suggest that the first line of attack should be to use carefully selected and validated sets of SNPs from candidate genes for which there is a plausible biological hypothesis for involvement in the drug response.

The first published example of the use of SNPs in a pharmacogenetic association study focused on an adverse hypersensitivity reaction to the drug abacavir, used to treat patients infected by human immunodeficiency virus (HIV). About 4% of patients treated with abacavir experience adverse symptoms including fever, rash and respiratory problems; such symptoms are characteristic of an immune system response. A set of SNPs in a panel of candidate genes known to be involved in immunological reactions was compared between hypersensitive patients and abacavir-treated controls. Polymorphisms were discovered in two genes that were associated with the hypersensitivity reaction and could be used to predict the response with an accuracy of 30–70% in White males. However, the predictive value of the markers varied in different populations and between men and women, limiting the clinical usefulness of the test.

Problems and prospects for pharmacogenetics

There are several reasons for the relatively slow pace of translation of pharmacogenetics from the research lab to the clinic. First, many pharmacogenetic association studies have used only small numbers of cases and controls, and have not been independently replicated by larger studies.

In addition, the predictive value of most pharmacogenetic tests is low, and clinical utility has often not been established. This is likely to be the case for most tests involving analysis of single genes. For example, the predictive value of testing for the *CYP2C9* polymorphism in relation to the warfarin reaction is not known with certainty but has been estimated at less than 20% and it is known that other genetic polymorphisms also influence warfarin response. It has been shown that a 'package' of known genetic and phenotypic factors can account for just over 50% of the observed variance in warfarin response but this may still be too low to be clinically useful. If predictive value is low, clinicians will often prefer to adopt a 'try it and see' approach, provided any adverse reaction is rare and not so severe as to be life-threatening. Box 4.7 summarises some of the factors that must be taken into account in decisions about the value of testing for *CYP2C9* polymorphisms in relation to warfarin response.

Before pharmacogenetic testing can be adopted by healthcare systems, demonstration of scientific and clinical validity will also need to be accompanied by health-economic analysis. It is likely that each test–drug combination will need to be assessed on a case-by-case basis. Pharmacogenetic testing may only be

Box 4.7 *CYP2C9* gene variants and warfarin response: to test or not to test?
Wide variation is observed in the dose required to achieve effective anticoagulation by the drug warfarin without excessive risk of bleeding. Part of this variation is due to variation in the enzyme cytochrome P450-2C9, encoded by the *CYP2C9* gene, which inactivates the drug in the liver: patients who require the lowest warfarin dose are homozygous for a *CYP2C9* variant that is ineffective in this function.

Warfarin prescription and therapy are now very carefully undertaken using clinical features, phenotypic tests and computerised decision support systems. Genetic testing for *CYP2C9* genotype may be advantageous in identifying patients who may be particularly vulnerable during treatment initiation. However, the predictive value of the genetic test for risk of bleeding is not known accurately and may be quite low, so it may not add much to standard management. New drugs, such as direct thrombin inhibitors which do not require intensive monitoring, will soon supersede warfarin and their use may be more cost-effective than a test-and-treat strategy for warfarin.

warranted in certain circumstances, for example for drugs that are very costly, or where the clinical procedure to establish an effective dose is expensive and time-consuming (see Chapter 7 for further discussion).

It seems likely that a modest number of pharmacogenetic tests will be ready for clinical application within a decade or so. In 2005, the US Food and Drug Administration approved the first two commercially available pharmacogenetic tests. The Roche CYP450 AmpliChip detects polymorphisms in two cytochrome P450 genes but is not being marketed in connection with any specific drug. The second test to be approved was the Invader UGT1A1 Molecular Assay (manufactured by Third Wave Technologies), which detects variants of the gene encoding UDP-glucuronosyltransferase. The enzyme is involved in breaking down drugs such as irinotecan, used in colorectal cancer treatment. The drug has been relabelled in the US to include dosing recommendations based on a patient's genetic profile for the UDP-glucuronosyltransferase gene.

Prescribing guidance in the US also now includes information on some genetic tests that may inform prescribing decisions. For example, the growth hormone somatropin is known to be unsuitable for individuals suffering from the genetic disease Prader–Willi syndrome. Reference to drug-metabolising enzyme genotypes is now provided for several drugs including theophylline, celecoxib and aripiprazole. However, prescribing decisions remain largely a matter for clinical judgement: although pharmacogenetic information may help, many other patient-specific factors need to be taken into account, including other conditions the patient may be suffering from, other medications they may be taking, age, nutritional status and likely compliance with treatment.

Molecular genetic profiling in diagnosis and disease management

The pharmacogenetic variants that we have discussed so far have been inherited genetic variants that affect an individual's response to drug treatment. However, the molecular-genetic characteristics of somatic cells – in other words, the way the genetic programme is played out in a particular cell type or tissue type, and how that programme is altered by the onset or progression of disease – may also provide information that can be used for diagnosis or treatment decisions.

Gene expression profiling in tumours illustrates the potential of this approach. A striking example of a successful targeted therapy is the drug imatinib (known as Glivec® in the UK and Gleevec® in the US), used in the treatment of a type of chronic myeloid leukaemia caused by a specific chromosomal rearrangement. The drug targets an abnormal tyrosine kinase enzyme produced by cells with the rearranged chromosome. Long-term efficacy of the drug has been demonstrated in more than 90% of patients receiving treatment.

A second example is the typing of *HER2* gene expression in breast tumours. Around 15% of breast tumours strongly over-express the *HER2* gene. In women with HER2-positive breast cancer, the risk of disease recurrence is markedly reduced if standard chemotherapy is supplemented with the drug Herceptin® (trastuzumab), an antibody drug that targets the HER2 protein. HER2-negative tumours do not respond to the drug.

New microarray approaches that enable simultaneous analysis of the expression levels of thousands of genes (see Chapter 2) are showing promise for improving cancer diagnosis, prognosis and management. For example, gene expression profiling has been used to identify different tumour subtypes from a set of malignant breast tumours, suggesting the existence of distinct disease entities (with different associated prognoses) in what was previously supposed to be a single class of tumour. Microarray analysis of gene expression patterns in diffuse large B-cell lymphomas has identified disease subgroups distinguished both by clinical outcome and by the recurrent presence of specific chromosomal abnormalities. Similarly, gene expression profiling has also been used to identify genetically distinct subgroups of acute myeloid leukaemias and prognostic sets of genes.

Prognosis is extremely important for any cancer patient; not only as a key element in selection of the most appropriate treatment, but also in predicting likely clinical outcome. Where prognosis is known to be good, it may be feasible to avoid unpleasant and debilitating adjuvant chemotherapy; even where the prognosis is poor some patients will prefer to have this information. Microarray studies are yielding information about outcome in many different types of cancer, and may allow the development of better prognostic tools than those currently available. In the future, microarray profiling could be of value not just in determining the likely prognosis for cancer patients, but also in dictating optimal treatment options from the array of available interventions, from surgery and radiotherapy to adjuvant chemotherapy and hormone treatment.

The use of microarray profiling in cancer has already reached the Phase III clinical trial stage. For example, in Europe a large-scale trial is underway to test the prognostic value of microarrays on lymph-node-negative breast cancer patients, who will be assessed according to conventional criteria and on the basis of their microarray profile. Where the microarray profile is inconsistent with the observed clinical/pathological findings, women will be randomly assigned to one of two groups and will receive adjuvant treatment based either on conventional criteria or on their microarray profile. There has been some criticism that this trial is premature, however, as the microarray signature has not been independently validated by other studies.

The same caveat applies to the first commercial test kits for breast cancer prognosis to appear on the market: Oncotype DX™ (from US-based company Genomic Health) and Mammaprint (from Agendia, a spin-out company from the Netherlands Cancer Institute), both launched in early 2004.

Despite the promise of gene expression profiling, many issues need to be addressed before mainstream clinical implementation can become a reality. These include the need for large-scale clinical trials and robust evaluation of the technology, the bioinformatics requirements for storing and analysing complex genomic data from large numbers of patients, the importance of assessing attitudes of patients and clinicians, health-economic implications, and potential ethical concerns.

Gene therapy

Gene therapy is the insertion of genetic material into cells with the aim of treating disease. Research on gene therapy has focused on two main applications: the correction of a genetic defect (usually a mutation causing a highly penetrant single-gene disease) in somatic cells by introduction of the corresponding normal gene, or the use of a gene to deliver a therapeutic drug or protein to a target tissue in the treatment of diseases such as cancer or heart disease.

Both types of gene therapy share some common features. For example, both require means of:

- getting the gene of interest into cells
- targeting specific cells or tissues involved in the disease
- maintaining adequate levels of expression in order to achieve a therapeutic effect
- avoiding undesirable responses such as immune rejection, inflammation or carcinogenesis; and
- achieving an acceptable level of bio-safety.

The only type of gene therapy that has been attempted in humans is somatic gene therapy; that is, altering the genetic make-up of normal somatic or body cells. Such genetic changes are not heritable. Germ-line gene therapy, which would involve a heritable change in the genome of sperm or egg cells or their precursors, has not been attempted and is prohibited in many countries, though some take the view that, if it were to prove possible, its use would be justified as a way of avoiding transmission of devastating genetic diseases to the next generation. There is a theoretical possibility that germ cells or their precursors might be inadvertently affected during somatic gene therapy; this risk has to be assessed separately for each potential application of gene therapy but is generally thought to be very low.

Most gene therapy trials to date have treated adults or adolescents, but in some cases where early treatment may be essential to prevent death or serious illness and disability (for example, X-linked severe combined immunodeficiency disease) trials have involved young children. The possibility of gene therapy in utero has also been considered as a treatment for genetic conditions, such as Type 2 Gaucher's disease or Hurler's disease, that have already caused substantial damage before the individual is born. However there are substantial questions concerning both the safety and the efficacy of gene therapy in utero, and there have been no clinical trials to date.

Gene therapy methods

Much gene therapy research to date has concentrated on developing effective ways of getting genes into cells (Figure 4.7) and achieving stable expression. Some gene therapy approaches (sometimes called in vivo approaches) involve direct introduction of the therapeutic gene into the patient's body, for example by injection at a target site such as muscle or a tumour, inhalation via a nebuliser for administration to the airways, or systemic injection. In others (ex vivo gene therapy), the gene is first introduced into target cells in culture, and then the treated cells are introduced into the body.

Cells can be induced to take up genes that are encapsulated within fatty particles known as liposomes, and even naked DNA can be inserted into cells treated by electroporation. Around 25% of gene therapy trials have used one of these methods, which tend to cause relatively few adverse responses such as inflammation. However, long-lasting gene expression has rarely been achieved because the therapeutic DNA tends to be lost from the target cells, making repeated treatment necessary.

Many trials, instead, have involved use of viral-based vectors (Figure 4.7). Viruses have evolved mechanisms for efficient entry into cells, where viral genes are expressed along with those of the host cell. Some viral vectors (for example, retroviral vectors) integrate permanently into the genome of the host cell, enabling

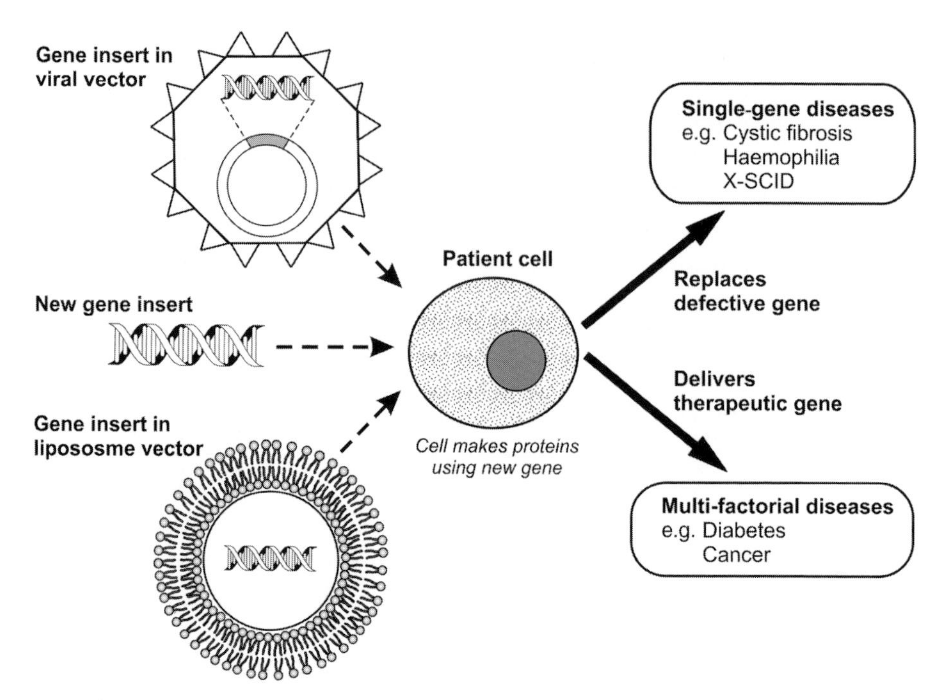

Figure 4.7 Gene therapy approaches. Genes that influence drug response may be involved in various biological pathways that affect drug metabolism and action

long-lasting expression to be achieved because the viral genome is replicated as the host cell divides, but with the risk that the insertion site into the genome cannot be controlled and may cause a mutation in the host genome. Integrating viral vectors are generally used in ex vivo gene therapy approaches and for target cells that are rapidly dividing. Viral vectors that do not integrate into the host cell genome (for example, adeno-associated virus vectors) may be appropriate for in vivo administration to slowly dividing or non-dividing target cells such as liver, brain or heart.

By January 2006 there had been over 1100 clinical trials of gene therapy worldwide; most of these have been Phase 1 trials, assessing the safety of the treatment in healthy volunteers. Around two-thirds of the trials have tested gene therapy treatments for cancer. Only 9% have been concerned with single-gene disease, and around the same percentage with vascular diseases. A small number of trials (about 7% of the total) have explored gene therapy treatments for infectious disease. So far, no gene therapy product has been approved for worldwide clinical use.

Gene therapy for single-gene disease

Single-gene diseases caused by deficiency of a specific gene/protein (generally autosomal or sex-linked recessive diseases) are good candidates for gene therapy, at least in theory. Several such diseases, including cystic fibrosis, haemophilia and

Box 4.8 Gene therapy treatment for X-SCID

X-linked severe combined immunodeficiency syndrome is a rare genetic disease caused by mutations in the gene encoding a common protein segment which forms part of five different cell-surface receptors that are essential for normal development of T cells and natural killer cells in the immune system. If untreated, the disease is fatal in early infancy, as affected babies die from multiple infections. The disease can be treated by bone marrow transplantation from a matched donor, but treatment is not always fully successful and sometimes no suitable donor can be found.

Gene therapy treatment involved removing bone marrow cells from affected baby boys and treating them with a viral vector containing a normal copy of the defective gene. The cells were then infused back into the patients. Out of 18 babies treated by early 2005, 17 had responded by showing long-term reconstitution of the immune system to near-normal levels. They were able to resist infections and it had been possible to discontinue conventional treatment.

Duchenne muscular dystrophy, have been the focus of gene therapy research over the last 10–15 years. Although results in animal models have in some cases been encouraging, clinical trials in humans have generally proved disappointing.

There has, however, been some success in gene therapy treatment for rare genetic immunodeficiency diseases. The first was announced in 2000, when French researchers reported the use of gene therapy to treat the disease X-linked severe combined immunodeficiency (X-SCID) (Box 4.8). Subsequently, other groups have reported success in treating X-SCID, and there have also been reports of successful treatment of two other genetic immunodeficiency diseases: adenosine deaminase deficiency (ADA-SCID), and X-linked chronic granulomatous disease.

Unexpectedly, however, three of the successfully treated X-SCID babies in France subsequently developed a leukaemia-like disease involving uncontrolled proliferation of T lymphocytes. In two of these cases, it was discovered that the gene therapy vector had integrated into the genome within the promoter of a gene that, when mutated in this way, can trigger cancer (that is, a proto-oncogene). The chances of such an event had been thought to be vanishingly small; the fact that it occurred in two children indicates that the integration site was not random, a possibility that will have to be taken into account in other applications of gene therapy that make use of viral vectors. The young age of the children treated and the nature of the target cells in X-SCID may also be relevant factors. These adverse events are a serious setback. However, it must be kept in mind that without gene therapy treatment the children would probably have died from X-SCID, as no matched bone marrow donors were available.

Gene therapy for cancer

As mentioned previously, most gene therapy research in the context of common disease has focused on finding new treatments for cancer. Two general approaches have been used: the use of gene therapy to deliver toxic agents to tumour cells, and its use to stimulate a host immune response to the tumour. An example of the first of these approaches is the use of the 'suicide gene' thymidine kinase (TK) from the herpes simplex virus to make tumour cells sensitive to the cytotoxic drug ganciclovir: the gene therapy construct is delivered directly to the tumour, for example by injection, and the patient is then treated with the drug. Tumour cells that contain the TK gene convert the pro-drug ganciclovir to its active cytotoxic form, ganciclovir triphosphate, while other body cells are spared. Other applications of this approach are also being investigated, for example in the treatment of cardiovascular disease by preventing re-occlusion of blood vessels after angioplasty.

Immunostimulatory gene therapy has been pursued in a variety of ways. For example, a gene encoding a known tumour antigen may be introduced into a patient with the aim of stimulating antibody production that will eliminate the tumour. In another approach, genes encoding key immunostimulatory proteins are introduced into tumour cells outside the body. These cells are then used as a 'vaccine' that stimulates the body to mount an immune response against the tumour.

Although approaches such as these have proved promising in pre-clinical research and in small-scale clinical trials, none has yet proved sufficiently effective and reproducible to enter mainstream clinical use.

Safety of gene therapy

The potential dangers of gene therapy were brought to public attention in 1999 with the death of a young man in a gene therapy trial in the United States. Jesse Gelsinger died from liver failure after treatment with a high dose of a viral vector engineered to treat the disease ornithine transcarbamylase deficiency. Other potential safety problems for patients include anaphylactic shock (an acute immune response), inflammation, infection or carcinogenesis (as occurred in two of the children treated for X-SCID).

There are also potential risks to the wider population, for example from the remote possibility that recombination between a viral gene therapy vector and a replication-competent virus might generate a new viral pathogen.

Recognition of the potential dangers of gene therapy has led most countries to strengthen procedures for regulating clinical trials of gene therapy and to work towards developing a robust regulatory framework for any gene therapy products. The regulation of gene therapy is discussed in Chapter 7.

RNA therapies

There has been much excitement in the last few years about the potential use of functional RNA molecules as therapeutic agents. These strategies attempt to modify the expression level of a specific gene by targeting its mRNA (see Chapter 2), and may be useful in treating diseases that are caused by over-expression of a protein or production of a harmful mutant protein.

One such approach, RNA interference (RNAi), uses small double-stranded RNA molecules containing a sequence complementary to part of a target gene. These 'short interfering RNAs' (siRNAs) activate an intracellular processing mechanism that results in the release of a targeted RNA-silencing complex which selectively destroys the mRNAs produced by the target gene, or blocks their translation (Figure 4.8). This mechanism is thought to have arisen during evolution as a defence against viral infection. RNAi may still have a role in defence against viruses but has also been found to function in the regulation of normal gene expression.

RNAi has rapidly gained a place in biomedical research, providing a valuable tool for investigating gene function both in normal physiological processes and in disease. Both human and animal RNAi libraries have been constructed, enabling

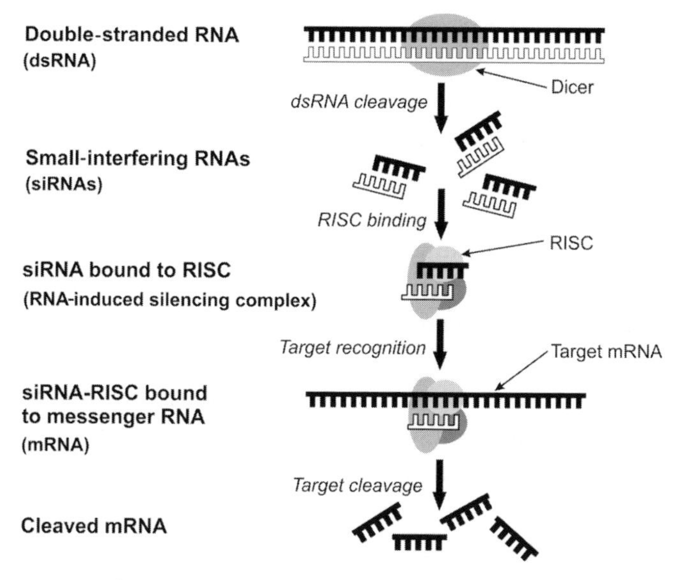

Figure 4.8 RNA interference. Double-stranded RNA in a cell (e.g. viral RNA) is bound by the enzyme Dicer, which cuts the RNA into fragments called small interfering RNAs (siRNAs). These siRNAs bind to the RNA-induced silencing complex (RISC), a group of enzymes that mediates recognition of mRNA complementary to the single-stranded siRNA. Once bound, RISC degrades the target mRNA, preventing gene expression. This is also known as gene silencing

genome-wide analysis of gene function. RNAi is also finding applications in the pharmaceutical industry, for example in the validation of drug targets.

However, there are many technical barriers to the use of RNAi as a therapeutic agent. A major problem is how to achieve effective and sustained delivery to a sufficient number of the target cells, given that RNAi molecules cannot readily cross cell membranes, are not replicated when cells divide, and break down rapidly in the bloodstream. One strategy to solve these problems involves using viral gene therapy vectors as expression systems to direct the production of precursor molecules, called short hairpin RNAs (shRNAs), that are processed to form siRNAs within the target cells. Alternatively, synthetic siRNAs can be conjugated with molecules such as lipids to aid their entry into cells.

Researchers reported recently that, using the viral vector approach, they had been able to effect some clinical improvement in mouse models of the genetic diseases spinocerebellar ataxia type 1 and Huntington's disease, both of which are caused by build-up of toxic mutant proteins in neurons. RNAi is also being investigated in animal models as a way of combating viral infections such as HIV and hepatitis, and of treating cancer, for example by use of RNAi molecules targeted against oncogenes. Early clinical trials in humans are underway to test the use of specific siRNAs in the treatment of age-related macular degeneration.

Because RNAi works by inhibiting gene expression there is a significant danger of unanticipated adverse effects, particularly where the aim is to reduce over-expression of a gene that has a normal physiological role, rather than to destroy expression of a mutant gene. It is also important to avoid perturbing the normal functions of the RNAi system in cellular metabolism. Questions such as when to begin treatment, how long treatment should last, and whether continuous, intermittent or transient treatment is needed must also be answered for each condition.

Despite its promise, clinical implementation of RNAi therapy seems likely to be some years away. RNAi faces many of the same problems encountered by gene therapy; in particular, how to combine high specificity and efficiency with low potential for adverse immune responses or tumorigenicity.

Stem cell therapy

Stem cells are cells that have the potential both for self-renewal and to differentiate into specialised cell types. Stem cells found in the early mammalian embryo, at around five to seven days after fertilisation, are able to give rise to virtually all the different cell types of the organism (Figure 4.9A). These embryonic stem (ES) cells are said to be 'pluripotent'. Stem cells are also found in the fetus, in umbilical cord blood, and in tissues of the adult organism, where they provide a pool of progenitor cells for the development and renewal of specific tissues such as the blood and the

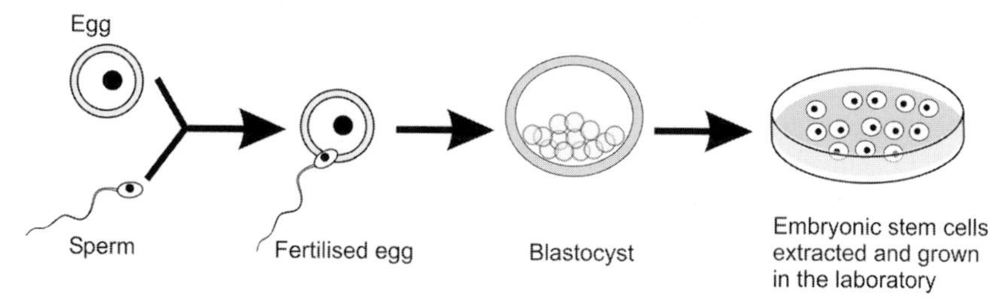

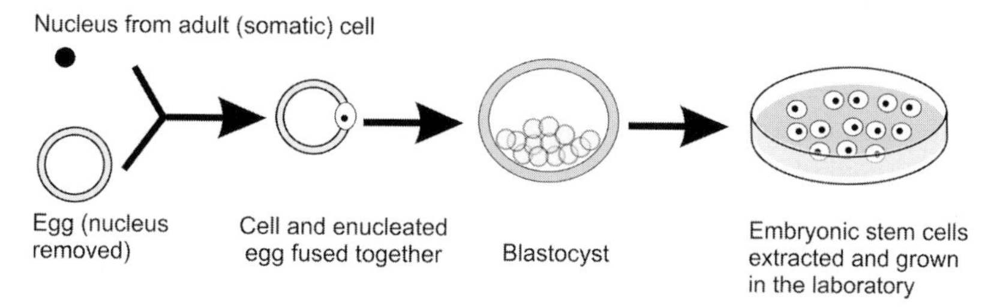

Figure 4.9 **A, B** Embryonic stem cells. The figure shows, in simplified form, the derivation of embryonic stem cells from an embryo produced by in vitro fertilisation (A), and from an embryo produced by cell nuclear transfer (B). In each case the embryo is allowed to develop to the blastocyst stage (about five to seven days after fertilisation). The blastocyst consists of an outer layer of cells (the trophoblast), which develops into the placenta, and the inner cell mass, which develops into the embryo. Embryonic stem cells are derived from the inner cell mass. Adapted from Department of Health (2000d). *Stem Cell Research: Medical Progress with Responsibility*, published 16/08/2000, product code 21925. Crown copyright (2000), reproduced with permission

nervous system. There is evidence that some non-embryonic stem cells are able, under appropriate conditions, to differentiate into cell types other than those of the tissue from which they are isolated, but the degree of their developmental plasticity is not yet clear.

Stem cell researchers hope that it might be possible to use stem cells, or specialised cell types differentiated from them, to repair organs and tissues damaged by injury or disease (Box 4.9). Stem-cell-derived transplants may be autologous (derived from the patient – only applicable in the case of adult and possibly cord blood stem cells) or allogeneic (derived from an unrelated but immunologically matched donor). Blood stem cells derived from umbilical cord blood are already used in children to treat several different types of leukaemia and some genetic diseases of the blood including Fanconi anaemia, thalassaemia and severe combined immunodeficiency disease.

Box 4.9 Possible uses of tissue derived from stem cells to treat disease

Cell type	Target disease
Neural (nerve) cells	Stroke, Parkinson's disease, Alzheimer's disease, spinal cord injury, multiple sclerosis
Heart muscle cells	Heart attacks, congestive heart failure
Insulin-producing cells	Diabetes mellitus
Cartilage cells	Osteoarthritis
Blood cells	Cancer, immunodeficiencies, inherited blood diseases, leukaemia
Liver cells	Hepatitis, cirrhosis
Skin cells	Burns, wound healing
Bone cells	Osteoporosis
Retinal (eye) cells	Macular degeneration
Skeletal muscle cells	Muscular dystrophy

From Department of Health (2000d). *Stem Cell Research: Medical Progress with Responsibility*, published 16/08/2000, product code 21925. Crown copyright (2000), reproduced with permission.

Current research is investigating the therapeutic potential of other stem cell types, both embryonic and adult. There is particular interest in the possibility of developing new treatments for degenerative or autoimmune diseases including Parkinson's disease, multiple sclerosis and type 1 diabetes. By yielding new insight into the molecular control of cell differentiation, stem cell research may also lead to the discovery of new drugs or biomolecular treatments to stimulate tissue repair or regeneration.

Other applications for stem cells are also being investigated, for example as sources of differentiated cell types for drug screening and toxicity testing, or as vehicles for drug delivery. These applications are of interest to the pharmaceutical industry.

Because of the developmental plasticity of ES cells, many researchers regard them as more promising than adult stem cells, and there has been some success in directing ES cells to differentiate into specified cell types. However, it is likely to be several years before cell transplants derived from ES cells are ready for mainstream clinical application. Difficulties that remain to be surmounted include the need to produce clinical-grade cell lines uncontaminated by infectious agents or by the animal products used in standard cell culture media, and to achieve stable and functional integration of transplants into target tissue, avoiding problems of immune rejection and tumorigenicity.

Cell nuclear transfer and 'therapeutic cloning'

Human embryonic stem cells are currently derived from surplus embryos donated by couples undergoing in vitro fertilisation treatment. Any stem cells, or cell types derived from them, that are transplanted into an unrelated recipient run the risk of causing a serious immune reaction and may be rejected. The process of cell nuclear replacement, or 'therapeutic cloning', has been suggested as a way of avoiding this problem by making it possible to derive ES cells that are genetically (and therefore immunologically) identical to the recipient. Cell nuclear replacement involves injecting the nucleus from a normal body cell into an oocyte (egg) from which the nucleus has been removed, thereby creating a construct that can be induced to behave as if it were a fertilised egg, dividing and developing into an embryo (Figure 4.9B). This is the same process that was used to create the first cloned mammal, Dolly the sheep, in 1996. The difference is that in 'therapeutic cloning' the aim is to use the cloned embryo to derive ES cells, not to implant it in a woman's uterus with the purpose of producing a cloned human being.

It seems unlikely that ES cell production by therapeutic cloning could be a feasible mainstream clinical strategy for producing immune-matched cell transplants. Human ES cell lines have not yet been produced by cell nuclear transfer, though some researchers have produced cloned embryos that have survived to the blastocyst stage. Claims by a South Korean scientist to have produced cloned human ES cells in 2005 were found to be fraudulent. Nuclear transfer (cloning) in animals is very inefficient, requiring use of large numbers of eggs to produce a single viable embryo; there are serious ethical problems in obtaining such large numbers of human oocytes, as oocyte donation entails significant health hazards for the donor. The cost involved in deriving patient-specific ES cells is also likely to be prohibitive.

However, ES cells derived from embryos produced by cell nuclear replacement may have uses in research. For example, cells derived from embryos produced using nuclei from patients suffering from various genetic or degenerative diseases may prove a useful model system for investigating the pathogenic processes in these diseases.

A more promising scenario for obtaining tissue-matched stem cells for transplant is to build up a bank of ES cell lines representing as many human tissue types as possible. It has been calculated that about 150 cell lines might be required to cover the majority of the population. The UK Stem Cell Bank has been set up as a repository for stem cell lines derived in the UK and for accredited lines derived elsewhere (see Chapter 7 for further information).

Genetics and infectious disease

Infectious diseases are a leading cause of death worldwide. They account for around 25% of deaths overall, and up to 45% of deaths in developing countries.

There are also growing indications that microbial infection may play a role in some common, chronic diseases. For example, it is now known that stomach ulcers are caused by infection with the bacterium *Helicobacter pylori*, while there are suggestions that chronic *Chlamydia pneumoniae* infections may contribute to cardiovascular disease.

Simple environmental and behavioural measures such as improved sanitation and 'safe sex' can make a major impact on infectious disease incidence. However, genetic research can also play an important role by elucidating the molecular basis of infection and the disease process, thereby identifying potential new targets for drug therapies or vaccine development. Many important pathogens have also developed resistance to standard drug treatments; molecular analysis can identify the mechanisms of drug resistance and may suggest ways of overcoming it.

Pathogen genetics

A major thrust of the worldwide genomics initiative has been towards the sequencing of pathogen genomes. More than 70 pathogen genomes have been sequenced, including those of the organisms implicated in such important diseases as tuberculosis, malaria, plague, leprosy, diphtheria, cholera and typhoid.

It will take several years for knowledge stemming from this research to be translated into validated medical applications, but genomic approaches are already flagging up potentially useful avenues for more detailed investigation. For example, research on the genome of the malaria parasite *Plasmodium falciparum* identified an unusual biochemical pathway for steroid synthesis and suggested that a drug known to inhibit a crucial step in a similar pathway operating in bacteria and plants might be useful in treating malaria. The drug, fosmidomycin, has shown promise in several clinical studies.

Common strains of the bacterium *Escherichia coli* are not normally very harmful to humans but strain O157:H7 is a highly virulent variant that can cause severe bloody diarrhoea and kidney failure. Comparison of the genomes of benign strains of *E. coli* with that of O157:H7 has identified a common set of about 4000 genes, and a set of 1387 genes found in virulent but not benign strains. Further analysis of these genes is underway, with the aim of identifying those encoding crucial virulence factors. This sort of comparative genomic analysis can also be used to identify genetic 'signatures', specific for different pathogens, that can be used as rapid diagnostic tests.

A striking recent illustration of the power of genomics in the service of communicable disease control has been the characterisation and sequencing of the coronavirus responsible for the severe acute respiratory syndrome (SARS) epidemic. Accurate diagnosis of SARS enables it to be distinguished from other diseases that have 'flu-like symptoms in their early stages, so that individuals suffering from SARS can receive intensive treatment and the disease can be more effectively contained. The avian 'flu virus is also under genetic surveillance in the hope that, if it mutates to a strain capable of human-to-human transmission, information about the genome sequence will aid diagnosis and perhaps also point to features that may be useful in developing an effective vaccine and/or therapy.

'Host' genetics

The process of infection involves not just the pathogen genome but also that of the host organism. The genomes of human populations have co-evolved with those of the pathogens that infect them, and resistance or susceptibility to infection has been a strong selective pressure in human evolution. A wide range of human genes, including the highly polymorphic genes of the immune system, are involved in human responses to pathogens. In some cases a single genetic variant appears to be significantly associated with susceptibility or resistance to a disease. A well-known example concerns the high prevalence of the haemoglobin S allele that causes sickle-cell disease in some African and Asian populations. The geographic distribution of this allele coincides remarkably closely with that of endemic falciparum malaria. It is thought that the sickle-cell allele is associated with resistance to malaria and that the high prevalence of the allele is due to the selective advantage it confers on heterozygotes.

In most cases, however, susceptibility or resistance to a specific disease is likely to be associated with variation in several genes, each of which has a relatively weak effect. So, just as with pharmacogenetics, the search for these genes has much in common with approaches used to identify the genes implicated in susceptibility to common disease, and shares the same difficulties and pitfalls. Nevertheless, association studies on some candidate genes have met with some success. For example, a specific polymorphism in the gene encoding the cell-surface receptor molecule CCR5 was shown to be associated with resistance to infection by human immunodeficiency virus (HIV). This gene was chosen for analysis because the receptor was known to be involved in entry of the virus into specific cells of the immune system. Resistant individuals are homozygous for a 32-base-pair deletion in the *CCR5* gene (Figure 4.10).

Similarly, the polymorphic proteins of the major histocompatibility complex are known to play an important role in immune responses to pathogens. Specific polymorphisms in some of these genes have been associated with resistance or susceptibility to diseases including pulmonary tuberculosis, HIV/AIDS, typhoid, leprosy and malaria.

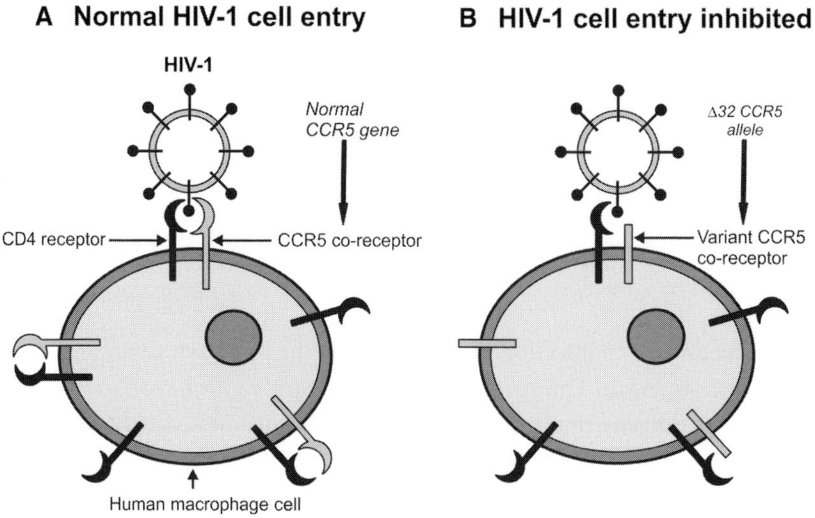

Figure 4.10 Genetic resistance to HIV-1 infection. Individuals homozygous for the Δ32 CCR5 allele show increased resistance to HIV-1 infection, due to structural changes in the CCR5 cell surface receptor that inhibit HIV-1 binding and entry

Genome-wide association studies to search for novel genes and gene families involved in responses to pathogens are underway but have not yet yielded robust, validated associations. Association studies face many difficulties, including the problem of ascertaining which individuals have been exposed to the disease-causing organism. Some success has been achieved by genome-wide linkage studies, which attempt to identify marker alleles that are shared more often by family members with a particular disease than would be expected by chance. This approach has identified genomic regions that may harbour genes affecting susceptibility to schistosomiasis and leprosy, for example.

As well as pointing the way to new drug targets and modes of treatment that will be applicable at the whole-population level, studies on genetic determinants of responses to infection may eventually enable the development of approaches targeted at individuals with specific genotypes. For example, vaccination might be targeted at people most susceptible to infection, or intensive treatment targeted at those whose genotype indicated that their infection was likely to lead to particularly severe disease. As with the other possibilities for new modes of disease management discussed in this chapter, these new approaches will require careful validation. Attention must also be paid to the need to protect the interests of those – perhaps minority ethnic groups – whose genotype may render them highly susceptible to infection but who constitute too small a market to be of interest to drug companies searching for new therapies.

Further reading and resources

Genetic testing and screening

Basic information is available on the Human Genome Project Information website of the US Department of Energy. More technical information about genetic testing may be found in Chapter 8 of Peter Sudbery's 2002 book *Human Molecular Genetics*.

Further information on clinical applications of genetic testing can be found in standard medical genetics textbooks such as *Emery's Elements of Medical Genetics* (Turnpenny and Ellard 2005), and *Principles of Medical Genetics* by Gelehrter and colleagues (1998). Grace, El Toukhy and Braude have published a recent review (2004) of the fast-moving field of preimplantation genetic diagnosis.

The section 'Assessing genetic tests for disease prevention' in *Human Genome Epidemiology* (edited by Khoury and colleagues, 2004b) has an excellent set of articles providing an overview of genetic test evaluation. For those interested in some of the underlying conceptual issues, papers by Kroese, Zimmern and Sanderson (2004), and by Sanderson *et al.* (2005b), deal with many of the important problems. Additional references on the evaluation of genetic tests, in the context of regulation of the availability of tests, are noted in the Further reading section of Chapter 7.

For a general review of genetic screening, see the review by McCabe and McCabe in the 2004 volume of *Annual Review of Genomics and Human Genetics*. 'Ethical issues concerning genetic testing and screening in public health', a 2004 paper by Hodge, is an interesting article weighing the balance between individual rights and public health benefits in the context of genetic testing and screening. Khoury and colleagues (2003), in the *New England Journal of Medicine*, have reviewed the range of current population screening programmes for genetic conditions in the US, and discuss the prospects for population screening for genetic susceptibility to common diseases. A review by Davey Smith *et al.* (2005) in the *Lancet* includes an assessment of the value of population screening programmes for genetic conditions. A briefing document, *Population Screening and Genetic Testing*, published by the British Medical Association in August 2005 contains some useful discussion but is muddled in its distinction between testing and screening.

Genetics and disease prevention

Juengst was the first to distinguish the concepts of phenotypic and genotypic prevention, setting out his discussion in a 1995 paper in the journal *Human Gene Therapy*.

For a recent review of the application of family tracing (cascade testing) to identify individuals affected by genetic disease, see 'Implementation of cascade testing for the detection of familial hypercholesterolaemia' by Hadfield and Humphries (2005), and 'Role of early case detection by screening relatives of patients with HFE-associated hereditary haemochromatosis' by Powell and colleagues (2005).

A recent review on hereditary non-polyposis colorectal cancer (a hereditary form of bowel cancer), including both genetics and clinical implications, has been published by Chung and Rustgi (2003). Burt and Neklason (2005) have reviewed clinical genetic testing approaches, and the difficult issue of deciding which individuals should be offered genetic testing, for several different types of inherited bowel cancer. Narod and Offit (2005) have reviewed hereditary breast cancer and the options for prevention and management. Suggestions for further reading on clinical guidelines and health services for families affected by hereditary cancers are given in Chapter 5.

There is considerable debate about the feasibility of the 'predict and prevent' scenario for using genetic information in disease prevention in the general population rather than a family-based setting. Some of the published literature arguing for and against the concept has been highlighted in the Further reading section of Chapter 1. Pharoah and colleagues' theoretical analysis of genetic risk profiling in breast cancer is published in *Nature Genetics* in the 2002 paper 'Polygenic susceptibility to breast cancer and implications for prevention'. Van Rijn, van Duijn and Slooter (2005) take a more sceptical view in a theoretical analysis of the potential application of genetic testing on risk assessment, secondary (pharmacogenetic) prevention and prognosis in common disease, using ischaemic stroke as an example. For a head-to-head argument on this issue, see the paper by Yang and colleagues (2003) in the *American Journal of Human Genetics*, arguing that testing for multiple disease-associated genetic variants could increase the clinical validity of genetic testing for common disease, a rebuttal by Janssens and colleagues (2005), and a further response by Yang *et al.* (2005).

Theresa Marteau and colleagues (1999) have carried out research on people's perception of genetic risk, their reactions to genetic risk information and the likelihood that they achieve an appropriate change in behaviour. For a brief commentary see 'Genetic risk and behavioural change' by Marteau and Lerman (2001). Lerman and Shields (2004) have reviewed the complex psychological reactions to genetic information, using the example of genetic testing for cancer susceptibility, and discuss how an understanding of these reactions might be used in order to maximise the benefits of genetic testing.

The CDC Office of Genomics and Disease Prevention (OGDP) in Atlanta is spearheading a research programme on the use of family history in disease prevention. Information on this research can be found on the OGDP website. Key papers explaining the rationale for the family history approach, and setting out the research that is needed to validate it, have been published by Yoon and colleagues (2002, 2003). Hunt, Gwinn and Adams (2003) have outlined the use of family history for prevention in the context of cardiovascular disease. Tyagi and Morris (2003) have developed a 'decision analytic framework' for assessment of family history as a tool for targeting preventive interventions.

'The emerging field of ecogenetics', by Costa, provides a useful introduction to ecogenetics, looking at some specific examples. Salanti, Higgins and White (2006) have published an analysis of evidence for a gene–gene–environment interaction involving the *NAT1* and *NAT2* genes and smoking in susceptibility to bladder cancer. A HuGE review of *GSTM1* polymorphisms, smoking and bladder cancer has been published by Engel and colleagues (2002). Maier (2002) has reviewed the evidence for genetic variants associated with susceptibility to beryllium sensitisation, and points out gaps in the current evidence base.

Details of the Environmental Genome Project (EGP), a National Institute of Environmental Health Sciences (US) initiative intended to improve understanding of human genetic susceptibility to environmental exposures, are available from the EGP website. The field of toxicogenomics – the use of genomics to investigate gene–environment interactions in toxicity and disease causation – is explored in 'Toxicogenomics and systems toxicology: aims and prospects' by Waters and Fostel (2004). Kelada *et al.* (2003) have reviewed the role of genetic polymorphisms in environmental health.

For comprehensive and balanced reviews on nutrigenomics, see 'Nutrigenomics, proteomics, metabolomics, and the practice of dietetics', by Trujillo *et al.* (2006) and 'Public health nutrition and genetics: implications for nutrition policy and promotion' by Darnton-Hill and colleagues (2004). Kaput *et al.* (2005) make a case for strategic collaborations among researchers and efforts to ensure that developing countries benefit from nutrigenomics research.

The website of the European Nutrigenomics Organisation, as well as displaying information on the work of this network, provides links to the websites of other related groups and institutes.

Genetics and disease management

For those interested in a thorough review of all aspects of pharmacogenetics, Weber's 1997 book, though now a bit dated, provides a comprehensive treatment. Briefer but more recent reviews include 'Pharmacogenetics – five decades of therapeutic lessons from genetic diversity', by Meyer (2004), and an editorial article from the *British Medical Journal* by Tucker (2004). Allen Roses presents an upbeat assessment, including analysis of the abacavir example, in a 2002 review in *Nature Reviews Drug Discovery*. A more sober assessment is provided by Sadee and Dai (2005), who discuss the obstacles to implementing pharmacogenetics in clinical practice. Little *et al.* (2005) review the epidemiological approach to pharmacogenetics. They outline the strengths and weaknesses of different study designs and stress the need to pool data across studies in order to achieve sufficient statistical power to test hypotheses. Walgren, Meucci and McLeod (2005) review current approaches to the discovery of genes implicated in drug responses, including candidate gene studies and whole-genome approaches. Brice and Sanderson have published a series of three brief reviews (2006a–c), at an introductory level, in the *Pharmaceutical Journal.*

Published papers and reviews on specific aspects of pharmacogenetics include a HuGE Review by Sanderson and colleagues (2005a) of the relationship between two *CYP2C9* alleles and warfarin response. Sconce *et al.* (2005) have presented an analysis of the potential for using a 'package' of genetic and phenotypic variants to predict a patient's optimum warfarin dosage. Recent papers containing information about the use of Herceptin® in breast cancer, and Glivec in chronic myeloid leukaemia, have been published by Emens (2005), and by Krause and Van Etten (2005), respectively.

PharmGKB is a web-based knowledge base of reported genotype–phenotype associations relevant to pharmacogenetics. Suggestions for further reading on policy aspects of pharmacogenetics are given in Chapter 7.

'Trends in microarray analysis', by Stears *et al.* (2003), reviews the technological basis of microarrays and their application in gene expression and proteomic analysis, as well as for genetic screening. 'Gene expression profiling: from microarrays to medicine', by Weeraratna and colleagues (2004), outlines the basis of the technique and clinical applications. 'Array of hope', an article by Philippa Brice in the *Health Service Journal,* reviews, for a general health-professional audience, the use of genetic profiling in cancer management and emerging issues surrounding transfer of the technique into clinical practice.

A range of general information on gene therapy is available from the Department of Energy (US) Human Genome Project website. 'The future of gene therapy' by Cavazzana-Calvo *et al.* (2004) provides a brief review of successes and failures in the gene therapy field and considers how to balance the risks and benefits. A 2006 paper by Ott *et al.* reports the recent successful gene therapy treatment of X-linked chronic granulomatous disease. The UK's Gene Therapy Advisory Committee has considered the issues surrounding gene therapy in utero. 'Gene therapy progress and prospects: bringing gene therapy into medical practice: the evolution of international ethics and the regulatory environment', by Spink and Geddes (2004), looks at the challenges posed by a constantly evolving science base and regulatory environment. The website of the *Journal of Gene Medicine* provides data on gene therapy clinical trials across the world. Information on gene therapy trials approved within the UK is available on the website of the Gene Therapy Advisory Committee.

For recent reviews on RNAi and its use as a therapeutic agent, see the papers by Downward (2004) in the *BMJ* and Stevenson (2004) in the *New England Journal of Medicine*.

There are many reviews and reports on the therapeutic potential of stem cells. Good starting points are a 2000 report from an expert group reporting to the Chief Medical Officer (Department of Health, 2000d) and pamphlets produced by the Medical Research Council and the Parliamentary Office of Science and Technology (2004b). The report of the House of Lords Stem Cells Committee (2002) also contains useful background information. Brivanlou and colleagues (2003) have recently set out the standards required from human embryonic stem cells. Taylor *et al.* (2005) have calculated the number of donor ES cell lines needed for tissue matching.

In an excellent recent review by O'Connor and Crystal (2006), gene therapy, RNA-based therapy and stem cell therapy are all considered as examples of 'genetic medicine', and their potential use to treat hereditary disorders is discussed.

'Genetics of susceptibility to human infectious disease' by Cooke and Hill (2001) is a broad-ranging review of the subject, whilst 'Genetic susceptibility to infectious disease' (Segal and Hill 2003) focuses more on how to study the genetic contribution of host factors to infectious disease pathogenesis. Kwiatkowski (2005) has reviewed genetic factors associated with resistance and susceptibility to malaria in different human populations, and discusses how this knowledge might be harnessed in the development of new vaccines. The Genome News Network website contains information about many of the pathogen genomes that have been sequenced. References cited in the Further reading section of Chapter 1 provide information about the potential of genomics and biotechnology to help combat infectious disease in the developing world.

5

Genetics in health services

In Chapter 4 we have discussed a variety of potential applications of genetic science in the treatment and prevention of disease. Many of these applications are still at the research stage; at present, the application of genetics in health services is largely confined to services for individuals and families affected by – or at risk of – relatively rare Mendelian diseases, chromosomal disorders, syndromes or congenital abnormalities. In this chapter we first review these services and then outline some of the challenges for service development that are likely to emerge in the coming decades as research on the genetic contribution to common disease begins to bear fruit.

It is important to keep in mind that, although individually rare, Mendelian diseases and chromosomal disorders collectively account for a significant burden of mortality and morbidity, especially in children. The genetic cause of around 1800 single-gene or chromosomal disorders is now known, and the number continues to grow rapidly. As knowledge has grown about single-gene causes of common disease such as breast cancer, increasing numbers of individuals have identified themselves as potentially at risk on the basis of their family history, and sought advice from genetics specialists. The workload of clinical geneticists, laboratory geneticists and genetic counsellors has grown at a rapid rate. It is vital, therefore, that funding for clinical genetics services is protected and that provision is made for the introduction of validated new tests and technologies as they become available, to improve services for patients.

Organisation of clinical genetics services in the UK

The organisation of clinical genetics services varies widely in different countries. In some, such as the UK, US, Canada and Australia, clinical genetics is recognised as a medical specialty whereas in others, including many of the countries of continental Europe, genetics services have tended to be provided by other specialists including gynaecologists and paediatricians.

In the UK the clinical genetics service receives referrals from primary care practitioners, other specialist services and occasionally also self referrals. Centres have developed as multidisciplinary regional centres of expertise based in teaching hospitals and serving a population of approximately 2–5 million. Most genetics centres consist of a clinical genetics service closely linked to molecular and cytogenetic laboratory testing services and an academic department of medical genetics.

Clinical genetics services in the UK are mainly outpatient based and usually delivered through a network of central, joint and district clinics allowing greater accessibility for patients and contact with other hospital staff throughout the geographic region. Organisationally strong links are usually made with other centres such as oncology, paediatrics, fetal medicine and haematology centres. Secondary and tertiary paediatric and neonatal services and tertiary adult services, such as those for neurology and ophthalmology, are often included in formal working relationships, sometimes through the provision of joint clinics. In addition, more recently working relationships are being established with primary care services and in some areas community genetics services have been developed.

The multidisciplinary clinical team

Clinical genetics departments are usually organised as a multidisciplinary team, with each referral being seen by appropriate members depending on the skills required. UK professionals working in the realm of medical genetics are represented by the British Society for Human Genetics, a federal organisation with four constituent groups (Box 5.1).

As well as consultant clinical geneticists and genetic counsellors, the multidisciplinary team also includes officers involved in data handling and genetic record facilities as well as sometimes support workers for people with genetic conditions. Some of these individuals are provided by voluntary organisations.

The clinical geneticist

Where referrals are for diagnostic purposes, they will require the skills of the consultant physician. Consultant geneticists are accredited medical specialists, having undertaken specialty training in clinical genetics after a period of general professional training in one of the basic disciplines, usually general medicine or paediatrics. Their specialist training covers basic theoretical genetics, counselling theory and practice, and a period of laboratory experience. Within genetics there is some degree of sub-specialisation into areas such as cancer genetics, dysmorphology and neurogenetics.

Box 5.1 Organisations representing medical genetics professionals in the UK

The British Society for Human Genetics (www.bshg.org.uk), founded in 1996, is a federation of four constituent groups:

- The Clinical Genetics Society (consultant clinical geneticists)
- The Association of Clinical Cytogeneticists
- The Clinical Molecular Genetics Society (laboratory molecular geneticists)
- The Association of Genetic Nurses and Counsellors.

The British Society for Human Genetics also includes three special interest groups: the Cancer Genetics Group, the Genethics Club and the Society for Genomics, Policy and Population Health. The organisation holds an annual conference, produces policy statements and is represented on the Joint Committee on Medical Genetics.

The Joint Committee on Medical Genetics was set up in 1998 to consider genetics services and their future, and to communicate with the Department of Health and the various Government advisory committees on issues concerning genetics. It represents the views of professional organisations and patient groups concerned with genetics: the British Society for Human Genetics, the Royal Colleges, the Faculty of Public Health Medicine, and the Genetic Interest Group. Reports on its work are published on the British Society for Human Genetics website: www.bshg.org.uk/JCMG/jcmg.htm.

The genetic counsellor

The clinical geneticist is now increasingly supported by genetic counsellors. In cases where the diagnosis is known, and medical history taking and examination will not be required, the patient may be seen by a genetic counsellor.

In the past most genetic counsellors came from a nurse specialist background, but practitioners are now entering the profession with an MSc in Genetic Counselling available at a number of higher education institutes within the UK. Genetic counsellors are now recognised as a distinct professional group with established requirements for training, accreditation and continuing professional development.

The clinical genetics consultation

Making a genetic diagnosis is central to the role of the clinical genetics service. Suspicion might be raised by a community paediatrician, for example, that a child's developmental delay or learning disability has an underlying genetic cause, possibility a chromosomal abnormality. This suspicion might be increased if the child has particular facial or other characteristics, or associated medical conditions such as a heart defect. The geneticist will see the child and parents, take a medical history and a family history and examine the child, to assess the likelihood that the condition has a primarily genetic cause. Where appropriate, they

Box 5.2 Medical databases for syndrome diagnosis

Several databases have been developed to provide comprehensive information for geneticists to assist in diagnosis and management of rare conditions. Examples include:

- Winter–Baraitser Dysmorphology Database – information on over 3400 dysmorphic, multiple congenital anomaly and mental retardation syndromes. For each, it includes details of the underlying genetic abnormalities, inheritance pattern, a comprehensive list of clinical features, links to Online Mendelian Inheritance in Man (OMIM), photographs and a full reference list from its database of over 35 000 references.
- Baraitser–Winter Neurogenetics Database – contains information on over 3250 syndromes involving the central and peripheral nervous system (not all genetic).
- GENEEYE – a comprehensive database of genetic ophthalmic conditions with information on all syndromes where there are eye features as well as many single congenital abnormalities such as macular dystrophies, rod-cone dystrophies and many others.
- DECIPHER (DatabasE of Chromosomal Imbalance and Phenotype in Humans Using Ensembl Resources) – collects clinical information about chromosomal microdeletions/duplications and inversions and displays this information on the human genome map. Submicroscopic chromosomal imbalances are a major genetic cause of developmental delay and learning disability, and may also cause multiple congenital abnormalities. The aim of the database is to capture the growing body of information on these chromosomal lesions and relate the position of the lesion to the clinical phenotype.

The dysmorphology, neurogenetics and GENEEYE databases are available from London Medical Databases (http://www.lmdatabases.com/index.html). DECIPHER (www.sanger.ac.uk/PostGenomics/decipher/) is maintained at the Wellcome Trust Sanger Institute.

will discuss with the family what tests might be done in order to make a diagnosis. Various resources are available to aid the geneticist in making a diagnosis (Box 5.2). Diagnostic tests such as DNA-based and cytogenetic tests may raise complex issues of interpretation, both technically and in terms of the clinical implications of test results. For example, if a chromosomal abnormality is found in a child with learning disability, the clinician will try to determine whether it is likely to be causal. If the abnormality is not one that is known to be associated with learning disability, this assessment will involve examination and testing of the parents to determine whether the abnormality is inherited or has arisen de novo and, if inherited, whether the parent displays similar phenotypic features. The consultant will explain the interpretation of the test result to the parents and discuss its implications with them. Once a diagnosis is made, the consultant may refer the child to appropriate services for care and management of the condition.

Unlike other clinical services, genetics takes the family, rather than the individual, as the unit of care. Often, an important component of the clinical genetics consultation is the calculation and communication of risk: usually, the risk that a genetic disease diagnosed in one family member will also affect another member such as an unborn child. Sometimes calculation of risk is relatively straightforward and requires little more than a knowledge of Mendelian inheritance. But factors such as delayed age of onset, incomplete penetrance, variable expressivity and the use of linked DNA markers rather than a direct gene test (see Chapter 4) can result in the calculation becoming much more complex and here special knowledge and skills are required.

For communication to parents, risks need to be quantified, qualified and placed in context. Professionals need to be skilled in knowing how to communicate the size of the risk, avoiding common misconceptions and comparing the risk with other risks of similar magnitude that patients are likely to experience. They also need to be able to describe the other facet of risk, namely the nature of the long-term burden associated with the disease. This will include likely clinical manifestations, whether a condition can be treated, and whether it is associated with pain and suffering. It may be difficult to give precise information if the disease is characterised by variable expressivity. Finally they also need to be able to discuss whether prenatal diagnosis or other preventive action is available. Many genetic conditions, however, are very rare: being able to give such advice might well involve the geneticist in searching the internet for the necessary information – a skill which is very much part of the clinical role – and then explaining it in detail and in writing to parents and other members of the clinical team involved in care.

The genetic consultation aims to be non-directive; that is, to provide parents and patients with the necessary information and to support them in the process of decision-making in as neutral a way as possible. Clinical geneticists and genetic counsellors also accept an important responsibility to offer advice and services to extended family members who might also be at risk. Contact with family members is usually made only with the consent and cooperation of the index (proband) patient or family. It may involve dealing with individuals over a wide geographic area and certainly across boundaries of healthcare systems within the UK. In Chapter 6 we discuss some of the ethical and legal issues that may be faced by the clinical genetics team.

Following initial work with families there may often be a need for re-referral, for example at times of further distress, or when new cases arise in the family, or where other family members are concerned about their own children. Some genetics services maintain contact through a register (discussed further later in this chapter in 'Genetic registers'), but others make it clear to patients and their family doctors that a referral back to the service will sometimes be necessary, and under what circumstances.

The extent to which genetics services provide ongoing support to people with genetic disorders varies. Some services do become involved in the follow-up, support and coordination of surveillance for specific genetic conditions, such as some inherited cancers. In other clinical areas, such as haemophilia or haemoglobinopathy services where the genetics counselling element is provided within the specialist haematology service, genetics services might not remain closely involved. Elsewhere genetics support should be available as a resource to those caring for patients with long-term genetic conditions. This can be achieved through joint clinics or by the attachment of genetic counsellors to the clinical service (for example, genetic counsellors attached to cystic fibrosis services).

Cancer genetics

The close association of genetics services with cancer research and clinical oncology practice began with the development of disease registers and preventive programmes for rare single-gene-determined cancers such as familial adenomatous polyposis (FAP, a form of inherited colon cancer) and syndromes such as multiple endocrine neoplasia, an autosomal dominant disorder with typically high frequency of peptic ulcer disease and primary endocrine abnormalities involving the pituitary, parathyroid and pancreas. These specialised services originally arose because of the need to provide systematic surveillance and treatment for family members of people with the condition. The genetic aspects of the work were then greatly accelerated by the identification of the genes involved in these diseases and mutations that were associated with the cancers. This meant that relatives could be tested so that only those who carried the harmful mutations needed to undergo the onerous surveillance programmes.

Subsequently, single gene subsets of common cancers such as breast cancer and colorectal cancer have been described (see Chapters 2 and 4 for further information). These cancers cannot always be distinguished pathologically from the group as a whole and, though possession of the mutation will not invariably lead to disease, the risk is such that surveillance or prophylactic measures are justified in family members who carry the harmful mutations. Although these cancers represent a small proportion of the total burden of cancer, the high overall incidence of cancer in the population means that the number of people potentially identifying themselves as at risk, on the basis of their family history, is considerable.

Growing numbers of referrals of such individuals by general practitioners have led to a steadily increasing workload for specialist genetics services over recent years and to the setting up of various triage systems (discussed later in this chapter) to ensure that only those patients who were likely to benefit from specialist genetics advice – those at the highest genetic risk – were referred to the genetics service. The clinical genetics team advises these individuals and their families on their risk and, where appropriate, arranges genetic testing for mutations known to be associated with familial cancers. In most cases, as discussed in Chapters 2 and 4, a mutation must first be identified in an affected family member before testing can be offered to other members of the family who are at risk.

Cardiac genetics

Genetic conditions that affect the cardiovascular system include single-gene defects that lead to conditions such as long QT syndromes, Marfan syndrome, hypertrophic cardiomyopathy and familial hyperlipidaemias, and chromosomal anomalies such as Down syndrome, other trisomies, and 22q11 deletion (diGeorge) syndrome. Structural heart malformations causing congenital heart disease occur in 7/1000 live births. In addition, multiple genes and gene–environment interactions are implicated in the development of essential hypertension, stroke and ischaemic heart disease.

Increasingly the geneticist and cardiologist work closely together, sometimes in joint clinics, to reach a detailed diagnosis, make recommendations on management and provide genetic counselling to the patient and family members. For example, when congenital heart disease consists of a complex heart defect or occurs in the presence of another anomaly or a positive family history, there is a need to involve the geneticist to look for an underlying genetic abnormality and provide advice about prognosis, management and risk of recurrence.

Cardiomyopathies (both hypertrophic and dilated) are another group of structural cardiac abnormalities for which the input of a geneticist is commonly sought. The clinical approach to these patients requires a full cardiological examination, ECG and echocardiograms with exercise testing. As well as assisting with the primary diagnosis through genetic testing, geneticists also have an important role to provide information and sometimes predictive testing to family members and to advise on the possibilities of antenatal testing.

Sudden cardiac deaths occurring in previously healthy infants, children, adolescents and young adults may be caused by inherited arrhythmia syndromes due to mutations in potassium channel and sodium channel genes. Diagnosis relies on close working of the cardiologist and geneticist and, specifically, an evaluation of the personal medical history, family history and genetic tests (mutations in potassium channel genes or sodium channel genes are found in about 70% of cases). Where a mutation is identified, cascade testing of families can be offered to see if they also possess the abnormality. At risk family members can then be reviewed by a cardiologist and advice given on natural history and measures to avoid risk.

Neurogenetics

Certain neurological disorders that affect children and adults are genetically determined, and include single-gene disorders such as Huntington's disease or tuberous sclerosis where there is a high risk to family members. Known as neurogenetics, this special area forms a significant part of the workload of adult and paediatric neurologists as well as that of the geneticists who receive referrals for diagnosis and genetic counselling of family members. Increasingly, molecular tests are used in primary neurological diagnosis. Many services hold joint clinics between neurologists and geneticists, some of which are purely diagnostic while others have a management orientation as well. Good access to laboratory services specialising in these conditions is also an important element of the service.

Although all neurologists and clinical geneticists will encounter neurogenetic disorders, the wide range and large number of conditions, many of which are very rare, and the need for specialised confirmatory diagnoses have increased the importance of specialist neurogenetics clinics, usually based in tertiary centres. These may be generic in nature or specific, most commonly for neuromuscular disorders or for Huntington's disease, but across the country there are also management clinics for disorders such as neurofibromatosis, tuberous sclerosis and ataxias.

Clinical geneticists are also often closely linked and extensively involved in the management and therapeutic aspects of people with these neurogenetic conditions. In these centres it is usual to find multidisciplinary teams involving appropriate therapies such as occupational therapy and physiotherapy in the case of neuromuscular disorders or psychiatry in Huntington's disease. Because the diseases are so complex, and involve many different systems, the professionals in these highly specialised clinics are able to provide support highly tailored to individuals. This will include recognition of specific genetics issues, provision of specialist assessments for other agencies involved in care, monitoring of systemic complications and specialist care during concomitant medical treatments, and provision of information and support to patients and their families.

Genetic registers

Some clinical genetics departments within the UK maintain genetic registers. Registers may be disease specific, such as those for Huntington's disease, familial cancers, muscular dystrophies or fragile X syndrome, or they may be general with disease-specific tags.

The clinical role of genetic registers is to maintain contact with families and facilitate follow-up. For example, a register might be used to contact young patients when they reach adolescence and need to discuss the implications of a genetic diagnosis for themselves and for any children they might want. Where there is a need for long-term surveillance, such as in the case of some familial cancers, the register may be used to initiate and facilitate the appropriate surveillance protocol. For example, in families with familial adenomatous polyposis, the register might be used to contact family members at an appropriate age to initiate regular colonoscopy, which detects early bowel polyps that are the precursors of bowel cancer. A register might also be used to provide a call-recall system to ensure mammography for patients with *BRCA1* and *BRCA2* mutations who have an increased risk of breast cancer.

Although these examples show that there are many possible advantages to patients of being on a register, such registers are not in widespread use in the UK at present. Barriers to their use include issues of data protection and informed consent, lack of sustainable funding, and the possibility that they might impose or imply an obligation to follow-up family members that cannot be fulfilled because of resource constraints.

Laboratory genetics services

Laboratories are an integral component of the clinical genetics service and also serve other specialties and the screening programmes. They generally include molecular genetic and cytogenetic laboratories and they can also include biochemical genetics laboratories. Testing at present is mostly for chromosomal abnormalities and single-gene mutations that can be highly predictive of disease and have implications for family members as well as the individual being tested. There needs to be a close relationship between the laboratory staff and clinicians in order to ensure that any test that is offered is appropriate for the individual patient and that adequate and appropriate pre-test and post-test counselling is undertaken. For this reason laboratories have normally developed within or in close proximity to the clinical genetics services. However, this may change in future, as there is incorporation of new technology and a wider range of tests. In particular as more monogenic subsets of common diseases are being identified the laboratory diagnostic service will have to interface with a widening range of other medical specialties.

Molecular genetics

Clinical molecular genetics as a specialty has developed over the past 10 years and there is at least one laboratory in each NHS Region. Clinical molecular geneticists are scientists who, supported by technicians, provide diagnostic services in collaboration with the local clinical genetics service. Typically laboratories provide a service for the most frequently requested tests, such as tests for cystic fibrosis and fragile X syndrome, plus a number of specialised services for rare disorders on a

Box 5.3 The UK Genetic Testing Network

The UKGTN aims to provide high-quality and equitable services for patients and their families in the UK who require genetic advice and diagnosis. It offers access to a range of expert advice and appropriate tests via local genetics centres as the clinical interface and gateway to the network.

The UKGTN is overseen by a steering group whose role includes:

- Confirming criteria for participation in the Network and identifying providers that meet these criteria
- Developing criteria for the choice, evaluation and prioritisation of tests
- Reviewing the provision and distribution of NHS testing services
- Encouraging work to increase the appropriateness of requests for tests
- Horizon scanning to inform policy and commissioning
- Maintaining an interest in the quality of service delivery
- Encouraging cooperation with other networks that offer testing services, such as the biochemical testing and haemophilia testing services.

subnational or national basis. Such is the pace of change in molecular genetics that clinical scientists working in this area are constantly involved in developing, evaluating and introducing new services and in research arising from this work. Some of the testing technology currently in use in clinical molecular genetics laboratories is described in Chapter 4.

In 2000, a report on *Laboratory Services for Genetics* (Department of Health 2000c) highlighted variable provision of molecular genetic testing across the UK and recommended some rationalisation of services, particularly in the provision of tests for very rare conditions. The UK Genetic Testing Network (UKGTN) was set up in 2002 to take a strategic role in the provision of molecular genetic testing within the NHS (Box 5.3). The UKGTN approves specific genetic tests for provision within the NHS, using evaluation criteria along the lines of those discussed in Chapter 4. Two National Genetics Reference Laboratories have also been designated, with a remit to develop and evaluate new testing technologies, develop new systems for quality assurance, and provide advice to government and other bodies.

Testing for several haematological disorders including haemoglobinopathies (sickle-cell disease and thalassaemias), haemophilias, haemochromatosis and factor V Leiden (which is associated with a tendency to venous thrombosis) are carried out predominantly or partly in pathology laboratories. These tests tend to be ordered by specialist haematologists rather than by clinical geneticists. One aim of the UKGTN is to encourage better coordination and cooperation between the UKGTN and other laboratories and networks offering molecular genetic testing within the NHS.

Cytogenetics

Cytogenetic laboratories undertake a wide range of investigations on peripheral blood, bone marrow, amniotic fluid and chorionic villus samples, and other tissues including tumour and haematological malignancy samples. The main patient groups are pregnant women known to be at risk through antenatal screening programmes, babies and children with birth defects or learning disability, and patients with leukaemia. Other groups include males and females with reproductive problems, such as recurrent miscarriage. As outlined in Chapter 4, cytogenetic testing involves the analysis of chromosomes using an increasing range of techniques. Traditional karyotype analysis (see, for example, Figure 2.10) has in recent years been augmented by special techniques such as fluorescence in situ hybridisation (FISH; see Figure 2.16), which uses fluorescently labelled DNA probes to detect or confirm gene or chromosome abnormalities that are beyond the resolution of routine cytogenetic examination. Array-based comparative genomic hybridisation (array CGH) is a comparatively new cytogenetic technique enabling much higher resolution than routine microscopy. Other high-resolution techniques included in most laboratory repertoires include testing for microdeletions, looking for microscopic changes near the ends of chromosomes (known as the subtelomeric regions), and the use of chromosome 'paints' (labelled probes specific for different chromosomes) to detect chromosomal rearrangements.

Biochemical genetics

In the UK at present there are 17 specialist biochemical genetic laboratories undertaking testing on blood, urine and tissue to diagnose inherited metabolic disease. The tests are largely chemically based and include assays of metabolites and enzymes. Some specialised techniques are used including high-pressure liquid chromatography and tandem mass spectrometry. Some laboratories also provide selected molecular-genetic testing for inherited metabolic disease to complement the biochemical tests.

The role of the biochemical genetics laboratory includes advice on testing, provision of specialist assays for diagnosis, interpretation of results and further testing, extended family testing, antenatal diagnosis, and testing to monitor disease progression and assess the effectiveness of disease management. The service includes confirmation of presumptive positives from screening programmes (for example, neonatal phenylketonuria screening). In many centres, the biochemical genetics laboratory is intimately linked with the newborn screening service, with shared accommodation, staff and equipment.

Staff members include both medical and scientific consultants, who direct and manage the service and are supported by specialised clinical and biomedical scientists. Clinical scientists are responsible for method selection and development, the quality and reporting of results and clinical liaison, participating in outpatient clinics and ward rounds as part of a multidisciplinary team. Biomedical scientists undertake a large part of the specialist technical work.

Some services closely associated with genetics centres

Inherited metabolic disease

Inherited metabolic diseases are a group of over 500 genetic conditions caused by defects in genes encoding functional enzymes or other proteins involved in metabolism. These defects can cause severe disruption of metabolic processes in the body, such as those concerned with energy conversion, manufacture or breakdown of proteins, or management and storage of fats and fatty acids. The result is that patients have either a deficiency of metabolites essential for health, or sometimes have an accumulation of unwanted or toxic products. The diseases can manifest in damage to many organ systems, and many of these conditions lead to severe learning or physical disability and death at an early age. Phenylketonuria (PKU), a condition for which testing is possible at birth, is a typical example of an inherited metabolic disorder.

The diagnosis and management of these diseases requires specialised biochemical laboratory testing and highly complex and skilled clinical care. Often babies present as a metabolic emergency and will die without treatment with a specially produced diet which excludes the harmful components. Dietary and sometimes drug management needs to be followed throughout the patient's life with constant surveillance and management of the disease, as it severely affects other organs such as the heart, kidneys, joints and nervous system. Because of the familial component of the condition, it is also necessary to check whether other family members are at risk.

The conditions are individually rare, but collectively are thought to amount to about 1 in 1000 live births, according to a recent needs assessment and review of services for people with inherited metabolic disease in the UK (Burton 2005). Increasing numbers of patients are surviving into adolescence and adulthood as a result of earlier detection, for example through expanded neonatal screening programmes, and improved treatment (including specific replacement therapies, such as imiglucerase or Cerezyme® for Gaucher disease).

It is important that children and adults have access to specialist care for diagnosis, acute and long-term management of their condition and support through the many crises that can occur. This requires close integration of clinical and laboratory services. The specialist laboratory services are included within the genetic services definition and include also neonatal screening diagnostics and genetic testing. There are two main centres in the UK providing a holistic clinical service, which includes neonatal and paediatric intensive care, cardiology, neurology, nutritional teams and genetic services. These centres are Great Ormond Street Hospital for Sick Children and the Manchester Willink Biochemical Genetics Unit, which cares for children and adults. The centres provide some regional outreach and have developed shared care arrangements.

A number of other smaller regional centres are emerging but overall across the UK there are many small-scale providers and large inequities in services. Services for adults with inherited metabolic disease are particularly lacking. This means that, as children reach adolescence and young adulthood, adult services to which they can transfer are rare; inappropriately, many either stay with the paediatric service or are lost to follow-up.

Haemoglobinopathies

Haemoglobinopathies are a range of genetic conditions in which the haemoglobin molecule is defective as a result of an abnormality in one of the genes involved in manufacture of haemoglobin. The most notable haemoglobinopathies are sickle-cell disease and thalassaemias. These diseases are inherited in a Mendelian recessive fashion (see Chapter 2). Sickle-cell disease most commonly affects people whose ancestors originate from Africa, Asia, Middle and Far East and the Mediterranean. However, cases have been found in White English since the advent of neonatal screening in some regions of the UK. Thalassaemia is particularly prevalent in communities of Mediterranean, Asian and Far Eastern origin.

Sickle-cell disease has an unpredictable clinical course with a differing level of complications affecting many organs of the body. These complications can be very severe and require considerable expertise on the part of healthcare providers in assessing and managing routine care. Individuals and their families often become expert in managing the disease and are able to limit the occurrence of crises through, for example, maintenance of hydration and antibiotic prophylaxis. Families need long-term contact with services to assist them in management of the condition and to provide advice on genetic aspects.

Patients with thalassaemia require lifelong regular blood transfusion, and drug treatment to eliminate the excess iron that is acquired by repeated transfusions. Bone marrow transplantation from a matched donor can sometimes cure the condition but the success rate is unpredictable.

There are approximately 50 specialist Sickle Cell and Thalassaemia Centres/ Services nationwide. The majority are managed and staffed by specialist nurses and a few have a multidisciplinary team of professionals that may include nurses, doctors, social workers and psychologists. They offer a range of resources that includes information literature, visual aids, advice, counselling, client support and antenatal diagnostic services.

Inherited bleeding disorders

The management of patients and their families with inherited bleeding disorders in the UK provides a good example of a specialist service where laboratory and clinical genetic elements are integral and essential components. Recent advances in molecular laboratory techniques now mean that it is possible to provide most patients and family members with reliable genetic information. Such information can help to ensure optimal management for the patient and also provide the best possible basis for informed decision-making for family members who are carriers.

Inherited bleeding disorders, including haemophilia A (factor VIII deficiency), haemophilia B (factor IX deficiency) and von Willebrand's disease (a defect in blood platelet function) are rare lifelong conditions resulting from specific genetic defects in the blood clotting proteins, or in the blood platelets. These disorders are complex to diagnose and to manage and require long-term and close follow-up and often costly treatments.

The management of people with inherited bleeding disorders is undertaken in the UK in specialist centres. There is a two-tier structure with Comprehensive Care Centres (CCC) providing the highest level of care and networking with more local centres. The CCCs provide lifelong care for people with these disorders and their families with a comprehensive programme that includes administration of prophylactic therapy, provision of coagulation concentrates and specialist support and therapy including rheumatological and orthopaedic care and support at critical times such as during pregnancy.

The haemophilia service must be underpinned by a high-quality laboratory service and in the UK a laboratory network, the UK Haemophilia Genetic Laboratory Network, has recently formed as a consortium of laboratories, mostly associated with haemophilia CCCs to ensure uniform high standards of testing and turnaround time. This network is represented on the UK Genetic Testing Network – a relationship that, in its turn, ensures close collaboration between haemophilia genetic testing and clinical genetics.

The way in which genetic counselling services are offered through a haemophilia service varies between different centres, often depending on the knowledge, skills, experience and qualifications held by individual members of the multidisciplinary team. A recent report of the United Kingdom Haemophilia Doctors Association (Ludlam *et al.* 2005) suggested that, with more options now available for diagnostic and carrier testing, families need access to specialist counselling expertise outside the main care centre, in order to avoid problems of privacy and conflict of interest that may arise when medical staff know several family members well as a result of frequent contact through the centre.

The role of voluntary organisations

Genetic diseases are frequently lifelong chronic diseases affecting many systems of the body. As many of these diseases are very rare, patients and their families can often feel isolated and lacking in support from people who understand the realities of living with the disease. In the UK there are over 100 voluntary organisations which aim to provide support for families affected by genetic disease. These vary from small organisations focusing on specific conditions such as Gaucher disease, to larger organisations such as The British Heart Foundation or Cancer Research UK, where genetics is a small proportion of the organisation's work. Some organisations support a range of related but individually rare conditions. For example, CLIMB (Children Living with Inherited Metabolic Diseases) provides services for all inherited metabolic diseases, while Unique supports those with any rare chromosome disorder.

A key activity of many of these organisations is the provision of information, aimed at patients and their families but useful also for the non-specialist professional. The information is usually written or endorsed by clinical experts with a particular research interest in the field. It is presented so as to be as reassuring as possible and not to confront people with medicalised or shocking images of the condition. Most voluntary organisations also provide a facility for people to gain personal support by telephone, or even by putting people in contact with somebody nearby with experience of the condition. As well as this, some provide an internet facility for people to exchange experiences about the condition, and also tips on how they have coped with problems. Such websites enable people to be in contact on a worldwide basis.

Some organisations are able to provide specialist support workers who work alongside other health professionals in the clinical setting. They may provide practical and emotional support around the time of diagnosis and also liaison with other agencies such as education or social services, sometimes operating as key workers for their patients. They may also be able to promote social interaction in meetings or social gatherings or even holidays.

On a wider basis, all voluntary organisations aim to promote awareness of the genetic condition, and many also fund research. They also provide an important function in ensuring that their members are kept up to date with research findings, often through a regular newsletter.

Two larger, overarching organisations also exist to support and represent the interests of families affected by genetic diseases. The Genetic Interest Group was founded in 1989 as a national (UK) alliance of voluntary organisations with an interest in genetics. It now has a membership of over 130 organisations. Its purpose is to coordinate action on issues of common concern, primarily to improve support and services for people affected by genetic disorders and to advance knowledge and understanding about genetic disease.

Contact a Family provides support for parents with a child affected by a serious disability or rare syndrome; many of these conditions are genetic in origin. The charity puts affected families in contact with one another, campaigns for improved services and social provision for families with severely disabled children, and provides information and advice on a wide range of issues. Contact a Family's online medical directory contains medical information covering more than 900 different rare disorders.

Commissioning of genetics services

The UK NHS consists of bodies that provide health services, and bodies responsible for the commissioning of these services; that is, for assessing the health service needs of a specific population and allocating resources to meet those needs. In other countries the term 'commissioning' may not be used but other arrangements exist to fulfil a similar function, for example reimbursement mechanisms or the requirements imposed by health maintenance organisations.

The organisational arrangements for commissioning of health services in the UK have tended to be subject to frequent change, usually driven by political imperatives. The policy introduced by the 2002 reorganisation known as *Shifting the Balance of Power* devolved responsibility for commissioning to a very local level, the Primary Care Trusts (PCTs), which serve populations of around 100 000 people.

These arrangements created considerable difficulty for medical genetics services, which are classified as specialised services. The Department of Health defines specialised services as those with low patient numbers but which need a critical mass of patients to make treatment centres cost-effective. Currently, 36 specialised services are designated within the Specialised Services National Definitions Set (Medical Genetics is definition number 20).

A national advisory group, the Genetics Commissioning Advisory Group (GenCAG), has a remit to consider strategic issues for medical genetics and coordinate national activity and service development. It works closely with the Health Technology Assessment programme and the National Institute for Health and Clinical Excellence in the evaluation of new technologies and services and with the UK Genetic Testing Network in the evaluation of genetic tests and the coordination of test provision.

GenCAG performs a useful function in providing a strategic overview for the commissioning of genetics services but ultimate responsibility and authority for commissioning remains at a local level. Because, by definition, patients needing access to specialised services are rare, there tend to be few within any one local commissioning area and it has proved difficult to engage commissioners to recognise the importance of these services or to allocate sufficient resources to them. Attempts to address this problem by establishing collaborative commissioning arrangements involving groups of 10–15 PCTs have not been universally successful, leading to lack of coherence, and difficulties in implementing national programmes such as that of the UK Genetic Testing Network. Plans for the merging of PCTs into larger bodies may alleviate some of these problems. In May 2006 the Department of Health published an independent report of a review on specialised commissioning, in which it was recommended that there should be a National Specialised Services Commissioning Group to provide oversight and coordination of the commissioning arrangements, and a comprehensive review of the Specialised Services National Definitions Set.

Whatever mechanisms are in place for the commissioning of genetics services, those responsible for commissioning need a transparent system within which to operate, and a sound evidence base for their decisions. Although considerable progress has been made in developing the evidence base, for example in establishing an evaluation system for genetic tests, further progress needs to be made.

Population screening programmes for genetic conditions

As discussed in Chapter 4, screening programmes are systematic programmes aimed at reducing the risk of a disease or reducing its harmful effects. They differ from other health services in being proactive and aimed at healthy people who have not sought medical advice over symptoms or other concerns. They can be aimed at whole populations, or, more commonly, sub-populations identified on the basis of such factors as age, reproductive status (for example, pregnant women) or ethnic minority group.

Screening programmes for genetic disease may be carried out in the neonatal period, antenatally or, in the case of carrier screening, at any stage of life, for example in adolescents or in young adults considering having children (see Chapter 4, Box 4.1).

Box 5.4 outlines the screening programmes that are currently available (or in the process of being established) in the UK at a national level. The UK policy position on screening is kept under review by the National Screening Committee. All current national population screening programmes for genetic disease fall into the antenatal or neonatal category.

Box 5.4 Genetic screening programmes in the National Health Service (England and Wales)

- **Down syndrome screening** is offered to all pregnant women before 20 weeks of gestation. From April 2007, all pregnant women should be offered a screening test with a detection rate above 75% and a false-positive rate of less than 3%.
- **Newborn bloodspot programme** including phenylketonuria, congenital hypothyroidism, cystic fibrosis and sickle-cell conditions. This programme is supported by the UK Newborn Screening Programme Centre, which is also considering the possibility of screening for other inherited disorders such as medium chain acyl CoA dehydrogenase deficiency (MCADD) within the UK.
- **Sickle-cell and thalassaemia programme.** The antenatal screening programme offers carrier screening to all women as part of early antenatal care, ideally with results available before the end of the first trimester. The form of screening offered for sickle-cell disease varies locally depending on the local population prevalence of haemoglobin variants. Neonatal screening for sickle-cell disease is offered as part of the newborn bloodspot screening programme.

Antenatal Down syndrome screening

The screening test used in screening programmes for genetic diseases may or may not involve DNA analysis. For example in antenatal Down syndrome screening, measures of the levels of two to five specific biochemical markers in maternal serum in the first and/or second trimester are combined with the woman's age to give a risk estimate for Down syndrome in the fetus. An additional screening marker used in some centres is nuchal translucency in the first trimester: ultrasound is used to measure the collection of fluid in the space between the skin and the cervical spine of the fetus; fetuses with Down syndrome tend to have higher nuchal translucency measurements.

Women in higher risk categories after the screening test, usually those with a risk calculated as greater than 1 in 250 (around 5% of those screened), are then offered a diagnostic test, which is usually a full karyotype on cells obtained at amniocentesis or chorionic villus sampling.

Some controversy surrounds the choice of method for the diagnostic test for Down syndrome. Full karyotyping may detect chromosomal anomalies other than trisomy 21; some of these (such as other trisomies or major structural abnormalities) will be clearly pathological but others may be of uncertain clinical significance, creating serious counselling difficulties. More specific diagnostic tests have been developed that detect only the three major trisomies (trisomies 13, 18 and 21). These tests, which are also much more rapid than karyotyping, are based on the use of highly sensitive molecular techniques such as quantitative fluorescent

PCR (see Chapter 4). Some clinicians suggest that these tests should be adopted as the standard form of diagnostic testing, while others think that it is necessary to carry out full karyotyping in addition.

Haemoglobinopathy screening

Antenatal carrier screening for sickle-cell disease and thalassaemia is offered to all pregnant women during the first trimester of pregnancy, as part of their routine antenatal care. The initial screening test is a full blood count, which includes mean corpuscular haemoglobin (MCH). A low MCH indicates an increased probability that the mother is a carrier of thalassaemia, and further analysis of the type and quantity of haemoglobin is carried out. If these tests indicate that the woman is a carrier, her partner is also offered testing. If both parents prove to be carriers, they are offered antenatal diagnostic testing to determine whether the fetus is affected.

The antenatal carrier screening programme for sickle-cell disease varies in different areas of the country, depending on the population prevalence of the condition. Universal laboratory screening to detect haemoglobin variants is offered in high prevalence areas. In areas where the population prevalence of haemoglobinopathies is low, laboratory screening for sickle-cell disease may only be offered to women who are identified, on the basis of a questionnaire, as belonging to an ethnic group at high risk of this condition.

Neonatal screening for sickle-cell disease is carried out by biochemical tests for haemoglobin variants in neonatal blood spot samples. An initial positive result is confirmed by a follow-up test using a different method. All babies are screened. The screening test detects carriers as well as affected babies; a health technology assessment study is currently underway to determine the best way of informing parents about their child's carrier status.

Neonatal cystic fibrosis screening

Newborn screening for cystic fibrosis (CF) has been available for several years in Northern Ireland, Wales and Scotland, and in some regions of England. A variety of different protocols have been used in the various laboratories.

In 2004 the decision was taken to extend neonatal screening to all babies born in the UK. The current protocol specifies the tests to be carried out on bloodspots taken as part of the newborn bloodspot programme. An initial biochemical test [the immunoreactive trypsin (IRT) test] is followed, if the test is positive (above the 99.5th centile), by DNA testing for four of the most common CF mutations. Infants with two CF mutations are referred with a presumptive diagnosis of the condition. If one CF mutation is found, further DNA testing for a panel of around

30 mutations, combined with IRT testing of a second bloodspot, is used to identify those babies with a high likelihood of having the disease.

If no mutation is found, only those babies with very high IRT results (above the 99.9th centile) are tested further: an IRT test on a second bloodspot is used to distinguish those with a likely diagnosis of CF from those in which the disease is not suspected.

Neonatal screening for inborn errors of metabolism

The UK newborn bloodspot screening programme includes screening for phenylketonuria, a rare recessive disorder caused by deficiency of the enzyme phenylalanine hydroxylase. Early identification of affected babies allows initiation of a low-phenylalanine diet and avoids the permanent brain damage that would otherwise occur. Screening for phenylketonuria is generally carried out at present using the biochemical Guthrie test.

The technique of tandem mass spectrometry can also be used to detect phenylketonuria and, in addition, a range of other rare inborn errors of metabolism including medium chain acyl CoA dehydrogenase deficiency (MCADD). For these diseases, too, early treatment is beneficial to prevent permanent disability and there has been strong pressure for the introduction of neonatal screening. For most of these conditions there is currently insufficient clinical evidence on the natural history of the disease, the effectiveness of treatments or the sensitivity and specificity of the tandem-mass-spectrometry-based test to warrant introduction of a universal screening programme. A recent health technology assessment review has, however, recommended introduction of neonatal MCADD screening in the UK and a pilot screening programme is underway.

Population carrier screening in specific communities

As a result of founder effects, some ethnic groups have an elevated prevalence of certain recessive genetic diseases. An example is the neurodegenerative disorder Tay Sachs disease (TSD) in the Ashkenazi Jewish community, where 1 in 25 individuals is a carrier (compared with around 1 in 250 in the general population). Such communities may benefit from the availability of population screening to detect carriers of the condition.

Caused by deficiency of the enzyme hexaminidase A, TSD is characterised by loss of motor skills and progressive neurodegeneration resulting in death usually by the age of four years. Community-based carrier screening for TSD has been available in the Ashkenazi Jewish community in the UK for over 30 years. Screening was initially based on biochemical measurement of the hexaminidase A enzyme. In the last decade, the cloning of the *HEXA* gene and the identification of more than 80 associated TSD-causing mutations has permitted molecular diagnosis in many instances.

Carrier screening programmes for TSD have been encouraged and promoted by Jewish community organisations by, for example, visits to schools and youth groups to raise awareness and holding screening sessions in schools, youth groups and universities. In some communities individuals are screened as teenagers. Where communities have systems of arranged marriages, information on individuals' carrier status is held on a computer database, and when matchmakers are looking for a potential spouse the database is consulted to avoid matches between carriers. Information on individuals is not released, in order to avoid stigmatisation. This approach enables the community to reduce the risk of affected babies without the need for prenatal testing and termination of pregnancy.

It was the first genetic condition for which community-based screening for carrier detection was implemented in the UK. The TSD experience can be viewed as a prototypic effort for public education, carrier testing and reproductive counselling to avoid fatal childhood disease. Such programmes can only be successful if they have the approval and support of the community involved.

Genetics in mainstream medicine

As the options for diagnosis and management of genetic diseases improve and expand, and in particular as highly penetrant single-gene subsets of common disease are more widely recognised, genetics is moving outwards from the specialist genetics centre to become a feature of mainstream medical services. Genetics advice and expertise in this setting may increasingly be provided by specialists from other disciplines who have received additional training in genetics, backed up by the experience and resources of the specialist clinical genetics and laboratory services. Genetics is, in effect, becoming a component of a multidisciplinary approach to disease diagnosis and management.

Genetics in other specialist services: the multidisciplinary approach

The multidisciplinary model, with genetics as a component part, is already well established in some services within the NHS. Examples of multidisciplinary clinics in neurogenetics and cardiac genetics have been described earlier in this chapter. Multidisciplinary ophthalmology genetics clinics are also in operation in some regions, and other services are being developed.

Some projects to extend this model are underway as part of a programme of service development work supported by funding made available as a result of commitments in the Government's 2003 Genetics White Paper *Our Inheritance our Future* (see Chapter 7 for further details about the White Paper policy initiatives). For example, a multidisciplinary approach to services for renal genetics is being trialled. As around 12% of patients attending nephrology outpatient clinics have a primary renal genetic disorder (the most common being autosomal dominant polycystic kidney disease), such disorders constitute a significant part of the service's workload.

The multidisciplinary clinic, taking referrals from GPs, hospital clinicians or nurse specialists, brings together a specialist nephrologist, urologist, clinical biochemist and geneticist, together with a renal nurse specialist, genetic counsellor and renal dietician, to provide an integrated service to patients. Genetic tests and/or other biochemical and radiological investigations are offered as appropriate, and arrangements for effective management and follow-up are put in place.

Genetics is also being introduced in other clinical settings. For example, cascade testing (also known as family tracing; see Chapter 4) to identify affected relatives of people with familial hypercholesterolaemia is currently being piloted by selected lipid clinics in the UK. To date, this condition has been significantly underdiagnosed, as cardiologists have tended to concentrate on treatment of the index patient and have not in general considered the implications for other family members. If audit of the pilot centres shows that the approach has been successful, it will be rolled out as a service throughout the country.

Development of service models for cancer genetics

As discussed earlier in this chapter, the demand for service provision for people whose family history indicates an increased risk of cancer has grown significantly in recent years. Ways of addressing this need have grown up in an ad hoc manner across the country but during the last few years attention has turned to the need to establish a rational service model at a national level.

A general framework for the development of cancer genetics services was suggested as long ago as 1996, in the report *Genetics and Cancer Services* (known as the 'Harper report'). This report recommended a three-tier model for cancer genetics services:

- Initial risk assessment by the primary care team, with provision of information and support to those whose family history does not indicate an increased risk.
- Incorporation of genetics expertise into multidisciplinary hospital-based cancer units, providing management and services for those identified as at 'moderate' risk but also able to identify and refer high-risk genetic forms of cancer.
- Specialist cancer genetics services which should primarily see those at high genetic risk but also act as a source of expert advice to other parts of the service and carry out research.

This general framework for cancer genetics services was endorsed in the 2000 NHS Cancer Plan.

In 2004 this approach became formal policy for familial breast cancer in the NHS in England and Wales, with the publication of guidelines by the National Institute for Health and Clinical Excellence. The guidance makes recommendations on the assessment of risk (including genetic testing), surveillance for women at increased risk, management plans including prophylactic options and psychological support, referral, and information and support for families.

A similar graded approach, with management dependent on risk calculated from family history information, has been adopted in some regions of the UK for familial colorectal cancer. National guidance may be issued at some point.

A programme of new services for people with a family history of cancer is being trialled as one of the Genetics White Paper projects. This approach, a partnership programme between the Department of Health and the charity Macmillan Cancer Relief, focuses on community outreach, particularly in areas with high proportions of ethnic minorities and high levels of social exclusion, with the aim of improving access to familial cancer services for those at high risk.

National Service Frameworks

As new evidence-based applications of genetic knowledge and technologies emerge, their incorporation into clinical policy through mechanisms such as the National Service Frameworks (NSFs) will be a key indication of their recognition as a component of mainstream healthcare. The NSFs were established to improve services through setting national standards to drive up quality and tackle variations in care.

Few of the early NSFs include any specific mention of genetics although some make passing reference to the role of family history as a risk factor, particularly in the case of early-onset disease. In several of these disease areas, however, there is now a growing body of evidence concerning the best way of identifying and managing people with single-gene forms of the disease. As this evidence based strengthens, it is important that standards of care for such patients (and, where relevant, their families) should be included in revisions of the relevant NSFs.

As an example, recognition of the importance of genetic conditions has led to the incorporation of standards for patients and families affected by sudden cardiac death within a 2005 revision of the 2000 NSF for Coronary Heart Disease. The new chapter recognises that sudden cardiac death in young people may be indicative of an inherited heart arrhythmia or cardiomyopathy. It specifies that an expert post-mortem should be carried out to ensure accurate diagnosis, with retention of tissue for possible genetic testing (dependent on legal consent). It also requires that NHS services should have systems in place to identify family members who may be at risk and provide them with personally tailored diagnosis, treatment, information and support.

Other candidate conditions for formal recognition within existing NSFs include services for patients with familial hypercholesterolaemia in the NSF for coronary heart disease, and recognition and management of people with maturity-onset diabetes of the young in the NSF for diabetes.

Some of the more recently published NSFs recognise genetic conditions in their first editions. The NSF for children, young people and maternity services (2004), for example, acknowledges in Standard 5 (for children and young people who are ill) that genetic diseases are responsible for a high proportion of childhood disease and disability. It sets out several requirements for services, including strengthening of access to clinical genetics services and other services such as haematology and pre-conception services; provision of support and information to siblings of children with genetic disorders; and ensuring that health and social care staff are trained to recognise families who might benefit from genetics services and information. Standard 8, for disabled children and those with complex health needs, does not mention genetics specifically. However, many of its recommendations – for example on access to effective procedures for prompt assessment and diagnosis, integrated care by a multidisciplinary team, support for families and carers, access to the Expert Patient programme, and smooth transition from paediatric to adult services – are highly relevant to children with genetic disorders.

Similarly, the NSF for long-term neurological conditions (2005) sets out standards that are applicable to all such conditions, whether primarily genetic or multifactorial. The important contribution made by genetic conditions (including Huntington's disease, muscular dystrophy, the ataxias and Charcot–Marie–Tooth syndrome) to the total burden of long-term neurological disease is acknowledged by their inclusion in a table, accompanying the service standards, of the prevalence of various neurological disorders in the UK.

Genetics in primary care

The primary care team already has an important role in the provision of services for genetic conditions (Box 5.5). Perhaps the main area in which genetics currently arises in primary care is in the context of reproduction. Primary care practitioners must be aware of the range of antenatal screening programmes available, and be able to advise couples about their options. This is particularly important where the primary care practice serves a racial or ethnic group with a high prevalence of a particular genetic disease, such as sickle-cell disease.

In some situations it may be appropriate to advise couples about options for pre-conception carrier testing. Examples include testing for carrier status for Tay Sachs disease in Jewish populations, or for beta-thalassaemia carrier testing in Cypriot communities.

Box 5.5 The role of the primary care team

Areas in which the primary care team can contribute to current genetics services include:

- Antenatal and neonatal population screening programmes for genetic conditions: support and assistance in provision of information
- Carrier screening programmes in some communities: support and assistance in provision of information
- Supporting patients affected by genetic conditions, and their families
- Recognising conditions or clusters of symptoms that could have a genetic cause, and referring to specialist services
- Assessing patients concerned about a family history of common disease: taking a family history, estimating risk and providing reassurance or referral as appropriate.

Primary care services may also play a role in care for families with children who have genetic disease, helping parents manage the more routine aspects of childhood health care such as immunisations and treatment of common illnesses, and working in partnership with the relevant genetic and other specialist services.

Better recognition and management of single-gene disease in adults is also an important task for primary care. Examples include hereditary haemochromatosis, genetic heart arrhythmias and familial hypercholesterolaemia.

The primary care practitioner also has a role in identifying those who may be at risk of disease with a major genetic component, providing advice and reassurance where appropriate and referring those who can benefit from specialist advice and consideration of testing.

For example, primary care services are usually the first port of call for people worried about a family history of cancer. The general practitioner (GP) needs to be able to take and interpret an accurate family history and decide whether referral to the cancer genetics service is appropriate. Many surveys have found that GPs feel ill-equipped to take on this role. Various proposed solutions to this problem include the development of computer-based decision support tools to estimate risk based on family history data, and new service models involving nurse-led outreach from genetics centres.

As mentioned in Chapter 4, it has been suggested that family history could potentially be used much more proactively to identify those most susceptible to common disease. The primary care clinic is the obvious setting for this approach. However, as discussed in Chapter 4, further research is needed to demonstrate clinical benefits from the use of family history to target prevention. If such research does indicate benefits, primary care practitioners will need appropriate training and the necessary financial resources will need to be allocated.

As one of the Genetics White Paper initiatives, funding has been allocated for new initiatives in primary care genetics, including a programme of funding for 10 GPs with a Special Interest in Genetics. The role of these GPs is to provide a source of expertise on genetics for local service-commissioning groups, to act as a route for liaison with the specialist genetics service, to promote awareness of genetics within the primary care team, and to offer training to primary care colleagues.

The future of genetics in clinical services

As we move towards a greater understanding of the multiple genetic and environmental factors that predispose to common chronic diseases such as diabetes, rheumatoid arthritis, Alzheimer's disease and coronary heart disease, health professionals will increasingly need to incorporate genetics into their everyday clinical practice. New applications will arise from the ability to carry out rapid and inexpensive large-scale genetic analyses and relate genetic determinants to disease risk in population subgroups. As discussed in Chapter 4, this may allow targeting of screening, surveillance, preventive advice or prophylactic treatment, as well as better prediction of clinical course, identification of subgroups of clinical disease and optimal treatment choices.

General practitioners and others in mainstream medicine will be at the forefront of using and interpreting genetic test results in relation to common chronic diseases. Only the more complicated questions are likely to be referred to genetics specialists. Practitioners will need to have a thorough understanding of the evidence base in order to be able to guard patients against misleading or unhelpful tests or interventions.

Perhaps the earliest impact will come from pharmacogenetics. As discussed in Chapter 4, there are still many hurdles to be overcome before pharmacogenetic testing becomes a reality in mainstream medicine, but already service implications are being considered. Many questions will need to be resolved, including who will be responsible for selecting, administering and interpreting pharmacogenetic tests, how and where test results will be stored and who will have access to them. As some genetic tests are likely to be relevant to more than one drug, robust information systems may help to avoid wasteful repeat testing. The nature of pharmacogenetic (and other genetic) information should also be considered in the design of new electronic health record systems to ensure that these systems have the required technical capability.

The advent of pharmacogenetics may signal new roles and responsibilities for the pharmacist. Other health professions will also be affected by advances in genetics. Dieticians, for example, may make use of genetic analysis in formulating dietary guidelines tailored to individual patients. Specialist nurses may take on new roles such as the recording and interpretation of family history information within the primary care team, and perhaps some aspects of risk communication and counselling.

The emergence of new clinical roles will have implications for manpower and capacity planning within health services and, crucially, for the education of health professionals. These aspects of policy development for genetics will be discussed further in Chapter 7.

It seems likely that the evidence base for new genetics-based technologies and interventions will largely be established by existing mechanisms such as health technology assessment and bodies such as the National Institute for Health and Clinical Excellence. Programmes of translational research will also be needed to trial new service models; the active involvement of patients in such service development research will be essential.

In addition, however, as we stress repeatedly throughout this book, the holistic approach of public health genetics, integrating scientific and clinical knowledge with insights from the humanities and social sciences, will be needed to ensure that scientific advance proceeds in tandem with service capability, appropriate regulation and social acceptability.

Further reading and resources

Organisation and development of genetic services

Two brief reviews by Donnai (2002), and Donnai and Elles (2001), provide an excellent overview of clinical genetics services in the NHS, and the roles of clinical genetics professionals. Policy considerations in the development of genetics services can be traced through several publications of the Royal College of Physicians throughout the 1990s.

An early analysis of genetics services, written for health service managers and commissioners, may be found in *Population Needs and Genetic Services*, published in 1993 by the Department of Health. This document contains an often-quoted table listing estimated numbers of patients with various genetic diseases, and their relatives, who may require advice and testing through the clinical genetics service in a hypothetical district with a population of 250 000. McCandless and colleagues (2004) have documented the major role of genetics in paediatric illness.

Landmark reports that have affected the development of genetics services include *Laboratory Services for Genetics* (Department of Health 2000c; the 'Bobrow report').

The activities of the UK Genetic Testing Network – including the development of 'gene dossiers' for the evaluation of genetic tests, a list of tests approved for NHS use and a list of UKGTN laboratories – are detailed on the UKGTN website. The two National Genetics Reference Laboratories have a joint website portal. Much useful information on DNA testing in the NHS, including reports on the numbers of tests performed by laboratories associated with the Regional Genetics Centres and the conditions tested for, is provided on the website of the Clinical Molecular Genetics Society. For further reference material on genetic test evaluation, see the Further reading section at the end of Chapter 4.

Voluntary organisations

The website of the Genetic Interest Group (GIG) contains patient-oriented information about genetics services in the UK, and an online archive of GIG policy documents. The Contact a Family website includes its database of medical conditions and information about accessing the services the charity provides.

Commissioning of genetics services

Current Department of Health guidance on commissioning arrangements for specialised services is available from the Department of Health (2003c). The Specialised Services Definitions Set Number 20 (Medical Genetics) sets out the range of services that are currently classified as 'core genetic activity' and are largely carried out by the Regional Genetics Laboratories.

Population screening

The website of the UK National Screening Committee documents policy development for population screening programmes in the UK. Detailed information about the evidence supporting screening programmes is collected by the Screening Specialist Library, which is part of the National Library for Health. A health technology assessment review of the use of tandem mass spectrometry in neonatal screening for inborn errors of metabolism has recently been published by Pandor *et al.* (2004).

Recommendations of the European Society of Human Genetics with respect to genetics services and screening programmes and other issues are available, along with reviews, in a 2003 special issue of the *European Journal of Human Genetics*.

Information about current NHS antenatal and neonatal screening programmes is available from several different sources. Current recommendations on antenatal Down syndrome screening have been published by the National Collaborating Centre for Women's and Children's Health (2003), as part of guidelines covering all antenatal care for pregnant women, and are available on the website of the Royal College of Obstetricians and Gynaecologists. Ogilvie *et al.* (2005) have compared rapid testing methods and full karyotyping in the diagnosis of Down syndrome.

Information about the NHS Sickle Cell and Thalassaemia Screening Programme is published on the website of the lead organisation developing the programme, the Department of Public Health Sciences at King's College London. The website of the UK Newborn Screening Programme Centre covers screening programmes using the neonatal bloodspot, and the Centre's activities in developing a quality assurance and performance management framework for these programmes.

Information about the community programme for Tay Sachs disease carrier screening is available on the website of the Guy's and St Thomas' NHS Trust, which runs this programme for the National Health Service.

A Health Technology Assessment Programme review by Green *et al.* (2004) provides an informative analysis of the psychosocial aspects of antenatal and neonatal screening programmes and identifies areas in which such programmes are weak.

Genetics in mainstream medicine

The implications of advances in genetics for the future development of health services have been considered in *Genetics and Health*, Zimmern and Cook's 2000 report of the Nuffield Trust Genetics Scenario Project. The Genetics White Paper *Our Inheritance, our Future: Realising the Potential of Genetics in the NHS* (Department of Health 2003a) sets out current Government policy initiatives for genetics, including commitments for service-related initiatives. Information about current service development projects can be found on the website of the NHS National Genetics Education and Development Centre and on the Department of Health's Health Services Research Programme in Genetics website.

A 2004 paper by Scheuner and colleagues makes the case for better recognition and management of single-gene subtypes of common diseases. Information about the UK pilot programme for cascade testing for familial hypercholesterolaemia is available on the project's website (London IDEAS Department of Health Familial Hypercholesterolaemia Cascade Testing).

Current UK guidelines for the management of women with a family history of breast cancer are available on the website of the National Institute for Health and Clinical Excellence. Similar guidance was published in 2005 by the US Preventive Services Task Force. No national guidance has so far been agreed in the UK for the management of individuals with a family history of bowel cancer.

Rose and Lucassen's 1999 book *Practical Genetics for Primary Care* provides an excellent guide for general practitioners wishing to increase their knowledge and improve their professional practice. The NHS National Genetics Education and Development Centre website features useful information for health professionals who are applying genetics in their practice, including a list of regional genetics centres, information on genetic tests, and instructions on how to construct a pedigree. GenePool, the genetics section of the National Library for Health, also provides information for non-specialist clinicians. Firth and Hurst's 2005 book *Oxford Desk Reference – Clinical Genetics*, although written primarily for clinical geneticists, contains a wealth of information of value to clinicians from other specialties.

The report of a recent workshop on the future of genetics in primary care is available on the website of the London IDEAS Genetics Knowledge Park (2004). Qureshi and colleagues (2004) have also discussed the current, medium and long-term prospects for genetics in primary care, suggesting ambitiously that primary care practitioners will eventually carry out routine personalised genetic risk assessments for their patients. Burke (2004) has reviewed future challenges for primary care practitioners surrounding genetic testing and related issues, while a recent review by Grice and colleagues (2006) has assessed the potential scope for the application of pharmacogenetics in primary care.

A September 2004 special issue of the journal *Primary Care* (Acheson and Wiesner 2004b) contains several articles devoted to the theme of genetics in the (US) primary care setting. Acheson and Wiesner (2004a) present an overview, while other reviews tackle subjects including cancer genetics, taking a family history, pharmacogenetics, and the role of the primary care practitioner in the care of patients with genetic conditions. An article by Whelan *et al.* (2004) encourages primary care practitioners to 'think genetically', describing a variety of 'red flags' that should alert them to the possibility of an underlying genetic diagnosis.

Hilary Burton's 2003 report *Addressing Genetics, Delivering Health* discusses future genetics-related roles of health professional groups. For other documents discussing service policy for the future, and references on genetics education for health professionals, see the Further reading section at the end of Chapter 7.

6

Ethical, legal and social implications of genetics

No book about the role of genetics in health care would be complete without a discussion of the ethical, legal and social implications (often shortened to the acronym 'ELSI') of genetic science. Hardly a week goes by without debate about the possible moral and social consequences of our greater understanding of – and perhaps also temptation to meddle with – our genetic make-up.

In this chapter, we discuss those aspects of genetics that have led to its current position in the spotlight of such intense ethical scrutiny. In general, we concentrate on the conceptual issues and arguments, while the options for the development of public policy on these issues may be found in Chapter 7. However, there is inevitably some overlap and readers interested in a particular issue should consult the relevant sections of both chapters for a full picture.

While not underestimating the importance of ethical, legal and social concerns raised by genetics, we try to approach them within the framework of an understanding of genes as an important, but by no means the only, factor affecting health and other human characteristics. Many of the current concerns that have been raised about genetics can, we believe, be at least to some extent allayed if we avoid the twin pitfalls of genetic determinism and genetic reductionism.

Genetic determinism and reductionism

Genetic determinism is the belief that it is our genes, and only our genes, that 'make us who we are'. Such beliefs may be reinforced by some of the language used by genetic scientists to describe (or perhaps hype) their work. The human genome project has attracted a particularly large dose of hyperbole: 'the book of life', 'the blueprint for life', 'decoding humanity', to pick just a few of the many metaphors that have been used.

There is no doubt that genetic factors make an important contribution to 'who we are'. It is entirely due to our genome that we are human beings, and not mice or bananas. The striking similarity of monzygotic twins, whose genomes are identical at the time when twinning occurs, shows that the genome plays an important role. We have also all noticed family resemblances in appearance and personality.

As we have discussed in Chapter 2, however, the relationship between the genome and the organism is not a straightforward one of input and output: at every stage of the unfolding of the genomic 'programme' during development, there is interaction with, and feedback from, the environment that surrounds cells, tissues, organs and, ultimately, the developing organism. Although the genomes of monozygotic twins are identical at the outset, they will not remain so throughout life: each twin will almost certainly acquire a different set of mutational and epigenetic changes that will influence a range of characteristics including how their body functions and what diseases they develop. The twins will also experience different environmental influences, beginning with their position in the mother's uterus, their experience at birth, the infectious illnesses they suffer during childhood, and continuing into and throughout adult life as they take on different occupations, live in different places, marry different people and perhaps move in different social circles.

Virtually every human characteristic, as we have stressed repeatedly throughout this book, is the result of interaction between genomic endowment and environmental influences. It is vital to keep this in mind when thinking about the ethical implications of knowledge about genetics, as an approach based on genetic determinism runs the risk of overstating the ethical dangers of this knowledge.

A related pitfall is genetic reductionism: the tendency to oversimplify the relationship between a genetic factor and a phenotypic trait. Again, as we have seen in Chapter 2, no gene works in isolation but as part of a complex network with an equally complex system of controls. In recent years, molecular biology has begun to move on from a reductionist emphasis on gene sequences towards a systems approach and a renewed emphasis on the importance of epigenetic mechanisms in development, normal physiology and disease. Although the phrase 'gene for X' is still often used as a convenient shorthand by scientists, it is almost always an over-simplification and, like the language of genetic determinism, can distort the debate about ethics.

The reasons for the persistence of genetic determinism and reductionism are largely related to the history of genetics. The earliest research studies in genetics concentrated on simple traits inherited in a Mendelian fashion. The first human genetic diseases to be studied were highly penetrant conditions caused entirely, or almost entirely, by mutations in single genes. The genes implicated in these conditions were among the first to be mapped and sequenced, and indeed

Mendelian diseases and chromosomal disorders remain the primary focus of current clinical genetics services, as we have seen in Chapter 5.

Perhaps inevitably, the idea has taken root that the lessons learned from such diseases can be applied wholesale when thinking about the role of genetics in all human characteristics, including common disease. In fact highly penetrant single-gene diseases are a poor model in this respect. To take one example: Huntington's disease is often used as a paradigm in discussions about genetic testing for late-onset disease. Ethical issues including the right to know and not to know, the effects of genetic knowledge on other family members, the testing of children, and the psychological effects of a 'genetic death sentence' have been extensively debated in connection with this disease. In the case of Huntington's disease, a single genetic lesion *is* highly deterministic and *does* have a direct relationship with an untreatable late-onset disease (though even in this case, there can be phenotypic variation in the condition, depending on the length of the tract of repeated sequence that causes the condition). Genetic testing can change a prior risk of 25% or 50% based on family history to (virtually) 100% or zero. There is no doubt that for those families affected by Huntington's disease issues around genetic testing cause particularly agonising problems and decisions.

By contrast, however, no genetic factors associated with common disease are as predictive as the Huntington's disease mutation, apart from those associated with the rare single-gene subsets of these diseases. It should follow, then, that for most people, worries about potential ethical and social problems arising from genetics – although they do not disappear entirely – should be similarly tempered.

Geneticisation

Related both to genetic determinism and genetic reductionism is the concept of geneticisation, a term coined by social scientists to describe what they see as the negative consequences of an increasing tendency to frame disease in genetic and molecular terms, to invoke genetic causes for disease, and to incorporate genetics into medical practice.

Geneticisation may be thought of as a subset of the broader phenomenon of medicalisation: a trend towards medical models for a range of human attributes and conditions, some of which were not previously considered as 'diseases'. Pregnancy and childbirth, for example, have become increasingly medicalised, with the availability of a wide range of tests and scans to detect abnormalities (many of them genetic) in the fetus or newborn baby. The area of mental health has also provided fertile ground for medicalisation: many types of behaviour that were once seen as part of the normal spectrum have become regarded as pathological and acquired medical 'labels'. Genetics increasingly forms part of the explanation for the causes of such conditions.

In its most extreme form, geneticisation may equate a predisposing genotype with the disease itself. An example can be found in the often quoted statement that haemochromatosis is the most common genetic disease in Anglo-Celtic populations. The predisposing genotype is indeed common but the prevalence of clinical haemochromatosis is very low. The danger of equating genotype with disease is that many people may be unnecessarily labelled as ill and in need of treatment.

The geneticisation of a condition may also have consequences for how the condition is perceived by those affected by it: how serious they feel it is, their attitude to treatment and their relationships with other family members. An example is congenital absence of the vas deferens, a form of male infertility that is now known to be linked to specific mutations in the gene associated with cystic fibrosis: men who would once just have thought they were infertile are now faced with a genetic explanation for their condition that appears to bring it within the realm of a completely different and much more serious disease.

It is important to be aware of the pitfalls of geneticisation, and to be sensitive to the social and psychological impact of introducing genetics into people's concepts of health and illness, but it is also important not to go to the other extreme by denying that genetic factors are relevant to the description of diseases and their causes.

The legacy of eugenics

Many concerns about the application of genetics in health care, particularly in the area of reproductive choice, can be traced back to worries about the notorious practice of eugenics. In the late nineteenth and early twentieth centuries, Darwin's theory of evolution by natural selection and survival of the fittest, combined with strong beliefs in a hereditary basis for physical, psychological and moral qualities, led to the idea that humans could take evolution into their own hands and 'improve' the human gene pool by encouraging those people judged to be the 'fittest' to breed, while discouraging or even forbidding procreation by the genetically 'unfit'. The name 'eugenics', meaning 'good breeding', was coined by British scientist Francis Galton (a cousin of Darwin) to encapsulate this idea.

In the early part of the twentieth century, eugenics movements (Figure 6.1) were established in many countries throughout the industrialised world, including the US, Sweden and Britain. In Britain, the emphasis was primarily on encouraging the upper and middle classes, who supposedly possessed desirable genetic characteristics, to have many children. In the US, however, 'negative eugenics' gained ground with the enactment, on eugenic grounds, of legislation to limit the immigration of racial and ethnic groups deemed to be genetically inferior. Even

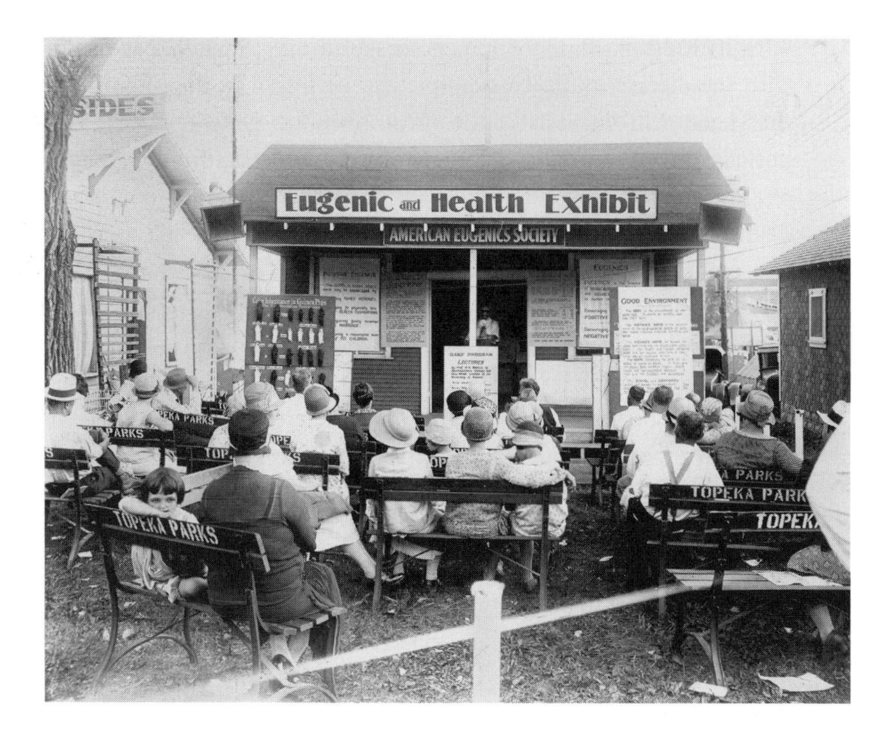

Figure 6.1 American Eugenics Society exhibit, 1929. Eugenic and Health Exhibit at the Kansas State Free Fair, Topeka Park, US. American Philosophical Society, Fitter Families Collection (2000), 1286. Reproduced with permission

more perniciously, in the belief that characteristics such as homelessness, alcoholism, sexual promiscuity or 'feeble-mindedness' were genetically based, many States passed laws allowing the forced sterilisation of individuals accused of having these characteristics. The result, over a period of about 50 years, was the involuntary sterilisation of around 60 000 people.

In Europe, Sweden had a eugenic sterilisation programme that ended as late as the 1960s. Under the Nazi regime in Germany, eugenic policy plumbed even greater depths in the 1930s as it was used to justify the murder of thousands of people, including children, with conditions such as learning disability, epilepsy or mental illness. The mass slaughter of entire racial and ethnic groups such as Jews and gypsies was also based on belief in the genetically based racial purity of the (imaginary) 'Aryan' race.

The practice of eugenics by selective breeding, forced sterilisation and even murder has rightly been widely condemned as cruel and immoral, and the idea that preventing socially disadvantaged groups from having children would somehow produce a genetically 'fitter' population has been discredited. Most western countries now espouse values of individual freedom and autonomy that are at odds with state-enforced reproductive decisions. Some countries, including China and Taiwan, have current laws that seem to run counter to these principles; for example, part of China's Maternal and Infant Health Care Act appears to require couples at risk of passing on a genetic disease to undergo antenatal diagnosis though it is unclear to what extent these laws are enforced. It should be borne in mind that social attitudes in China are different from those in the west: social responsibility is considered a stronger moral value than individual rights so parents may feel they have an obligation to avoid having a child that is likely to be a burden to the rest of society.

In the remaining sections of this chapter we will attempt a rational debate of some of the ethical and social issues that are commonly raised in connection with genetics. Many of these issues fall into one of three main areas: the role of genetics in reproductive choice, the uses of genetic information, and the use of human embryos in research and therapy. We will also outline the major ethical, legal and social issues affecting the practice of clinical genetics and discuss current evidence concerning public attitudes to genetics and genetic science.

Genetics and reproductive choice

Traditionally, much of the debate about genetics has centred on its applications in human reproduction: to what extent can we, or should we, control the genetic characteristics of the children that are born? Debate on this issue tends to be highly emotional, partly because it touches on a fundamental human attribute – the desire to bear children and to give them every possible advantage in life – and partly because it is closely associated in many people's minds with eugenics.

Antenatal genetic testing and screening

Does the current availability of antenatal testing for genetic disease, accompanied by the option of abortion if the fetus proves to be affected, constitute eugenics? Some argue that it does. As evidence for their conclusion they point, for example, to assessments of the effectiveness of antenatal screening for Down syndrome in reducing the birth prevalence of this condition. It is hard to escape the conclusion that there is indeed at least an element of eugenic thinking at work here (though note that reducing the birth prevalence of a largely sporadic condition such as Down syndrome will not affect the gene pool or the rate at which the mutation causing the condition arises).

It may be useful to make a distinction between ends and means. It is difficult to argue that it would be a bad thing if devastating diseases such as Huntington's disease were no longer present in the population. A eugenic approach would forbid individuals who are at risk to have children, or insist that they undergo antenatal diagnosis and abort affected fetuses. This is very different from making available testing, antenatal diagnosis and selective termination to those who request it. The argument is that the availability of genetic testing and selective abortion is morally acceptable as long as the reason is to allow individuals to exercise reproductive choice, and state coercion is not involved.

In practice, most of those at risk of transmitting serious autosomal dominant conditions such as *BRCA*-related breast cancer or Huntington's disease do not seek antenatal diagnosis and abortion to avoid transmitting the disease to the next generation, so the population frequency of these mutations is unlikely to have decreased. In the case of recessive diseases, the availability of antenatal diagnosis has virtually no impact on the frequency of the alleles in the population because it does not select against carriers, and most affected individuals do not have children. It would be hard, then, to argue that eugenics is at work here.

It seems that informed reproductive choice is generally the reality in the case of rare genetic diseases affecting families who consult clinical genetics services. The situation may be different where there is a population screening programme for a genetic condition. The quality of information and counselling can be considerably poorer in this situation. Many couples experience antenatal screening programmes as something more akin to a medical conveyor belt than an opportunity to exercise free choice based on individual needs and values, and some have suggested that there is a presumption on the part of medical professionals that affected babies will be aborted.

Limits to reproductive choice?

As genetic factors associated with a wider range of conditions are discovered, what limits should there be on the use of this knowledge for reproductive choice? Should individuals and couples be entitled to make their own decisions, or should society decide where the limits should lie?

Most surveys of public opinion indicate that the majority of people think governments should restrict the use of antenatal testing to the detection of serious diseases. There is less consensus, however, on how to define 'serious'. Life-limiting and untreatable congenital diseases come within most people's definition, but conditions such as achondroplasia or congenital deafness – which are untreatable but in a supportive society are compatible with a normal or near-normal life – are controversial in this context. In societies where abortion on essentially 'social' grounds is legal it may be difficult to argue that couples should not be allowed to decide when they think a disability is serious enough to warrant abortion.

In contrast, some people who have such disabilities feel that this attitude encourages discrimination against the disabled by implying that they do not have a right to exist. Some go further, arguing that disability is not an objective condition but a socially constructed concept. They may regard their condition as a social and cultural identity – perhaps even one that they would like to choose for their own children by the use of antenatal genetic testing. The question of whether such a choice should be allowed by society is a difficult one. Regulatory agencies have tended to take the position that the interests of the child are paramount, and that it is not in a child's interest to be born with a disability. There is a clear logical flaw in this argument, however, in that the alternative option for that particular child is not to be born without the disability, but not to be born at all.

So far, genetic testing can only be used to find out whether a baby has a specific genetic disease: either a disease for which that particular couple is at risk, or one (such as Down syndrome) that has a sufficiently high birth prevalence to warrant population screening. In the future, as testing technology becomes cheaper, the range of conditions for which routine antenatal screening can be offered may increase. Society will then have to decide what limits to impose.

Genetic enhancement

If antenatal genetic testing can be used to select against specific genetic conditions, could it also be used to select in favour of others? The development of pre-implantation genetic testing means that, at least in principle, the answer to this question is 'yes'. Pre-implantation genetic testing (see Chapter 4, Figure 4.1) has already been used to select babies whose tissue type matches that of an older sibling needing matched cord blood or bone marrow to treat a life-threatening disease.

If a desired trait is associated with a specific and readily identifiable genetic variant(s), then pre-implantation genetic testing to select for such a trait is technically feasible, provided the variant(s) is (are) actually present in one or both parents and thus has a chance of being present in the offspring. In reality, the situation will rarely be straightforward. First, very few traits that people are likely to want to select for will be strongly associated with a single or even a few specific genetic variants. If more variants are involved, simple probability works against effective selection. To take a speculative future scenario: if, say, ten genetic variants had been identified that together were known to be associated with above-average intelligence, the combined chances that all ten variants (or even most of them) were present in one or other parent *and* that all ten (or even most of them) had been inherited by any single embryo out of the relatively small number available to the couple would be vanishingly small. In vitro fertilisation itself also has a low success rate. Couples attempting to use pre-implantation genetic diagnosis to achieve genetic enhancement would almost certainly be disappointed.

If the trait is a simpler one – say, red hair – genetic selection will be much simpler, but even in this case it will only be possible if the parents actually carry the genetic variant(s) responsible.

If pre-implantation genetic testing and selection for desired characteristics is unlikely to be successful in all but a handful of situations, what about genetic manipulation to introduce such characteristics into an embryo? At present, this lies within the realms of science fiction, and is illegal in many countries. Genetic manipulation of animals has been achieved, but only for relatively simple and genetically well-defined traits. Manipulation of many genes simultaneously would be technically extremely difficult. Most genetically manipulated embryos would probably not develop to term, and those that did so might well have unexpected abnormalities that would become apparent after birth or in later life.

In addition to such technical problems, the same theoretical considerations that argue against eugenics by selective breeding also apply to enhancement by genetic manipulation: because the genetic contribution to characteristics such as intelligence, abilities and behaviour is so complex and is modulated by environmental influences, genetic manipulation on any feasible scale would be a very blunt tool with which to try to influence such characteristics.

When it comes to scientific developments, it is sensible never to say 'never': it is possible that there will be at least some situations in which genetic enhancement will become a realistic possibility. It seems likely, however, that interventions of this sort would be expensive and thus likely to be available only to those able to pay for them. In debating its ethical stance on this issue, society will need to confront the question of whether there is any ethical difference between seeking to enhance a child's attributes or chances in life by manipulating its environment (paying for private education, perhaps) and attempting to achieve the same result by manipulating its genes. The ethical arguments here revolve around questions of social justice, and whether particular options should be prohibited if they cannot be made available to all.

Genetics and assisted reproduction

Assisted reproduction technology, in particular the use of donated gametes (sperm and eggs) or embryos, raises some issues relevant to genetics. One concern is whether children born as a result of the use of donated gametes or embryos have a right to know who their genetic parents are. There are potentially competing interests here. On the one hand, it can be argued that knowledge of one's genetic parentage may be important both in the context of personal identity and also because an individual may have medical reasons for needing family history information or perhaps even DNA samples from their genetic parents. On the other hand, if donors are compelled to allow their identity to be disclosed, they may feel they have lost their right to privacy and they may be deterred from donation, thus decreasing the availability of treatment for infertile couples.

Other questions concern the use of genetic testing in conjunction with assisted reproduction. For example, should gamete donors be tested for carrier status for genetic diseases? If so, what should be the extent of testing? Current UK policy on this issue is discussed in Chapter 7.

Reproductive cloning

In 1996 the first cloned mammal was produced: Dolly the sheep was created by inserting the nucleus of a somatic cell into an unfertilised egg from which the nucleus had been removed, and stimulating the resulting cell to divide and produce an embryo as if it had been fertilised by a sperm (see Figure 4.9). Dolly had the same genetic make-up as the sheep from which the somatic cell nucleus was taken. Over the last decade, several different mammals have been cloned including agricultural animals and domestic pet species.

Some people have called for reproductive cloning to be permitted in humans. It could, for example, be the only way for some infertile couples to have a biologically related child. Opponents fear that a child who was genetically identical to an existing (or even a dead) person could face potentially severe psychological problems with personal identity and relationships, and might face unreasonable expectations. Strong religious objections have also been expressed. Cloning technology is also far from perfect: it is a very inefficient process requiring the use of hundreds of eggs to create one successful embryo, and many cloned animals are born with congenital medical problems. The long-term health of cloned animals can also not be guaranteed.

For these reasons reproductive cloning is generally considered ethically unacceptable and is banned in many countries. However, public opinion on the issue may change over time, particularly if the technical and safety problems can be overcome and if some benefits are perceived. Some commentators question the assumption that individuals produced by cloning would suffer severe harm. It has also been pointed out that, although genetically identical to another person, an individual produced by cloning would be likely to experience a completely different environment from that person; the assumption that they would be an 'identical person' relies on a very deterministic understanding of genetics.

Embryo research and embryonic stem cells

Research on human embryos first arose in the context of artificial reproduction technology, where it enabled development and improvement of in vitro fertilisation procedures. Later, manipulation of human embryos also became essential for developing the technique of pre-implantation genetic diagnosis and for the derivation of embryonic stem cells.

The use of human embryos has always been controversial. At one end of the spectrum is the belief that the embryo, from the moment of conception, is a person in its own right with the same moral status as an adult human. At the other is the view that an embryo is simply a collection of cells with no moral status at all.

A compromise view is that the embryo acquires full personhood, and the moral rights that go with this status, by gradual stages during the process of development from conception to birth. It follows that it might be ethically acceptable, under certain circumstances, to use embryos for research. In the debate about embryo research, the formation of the primitive streak has been suggested as a key cut-off point. This event, the appearance of a surface thickening that marks the first visible organisation of the embryo, occurs at around 14 days after fertilisation.

A commonly held view is that embryos do have moral value but it might be permissible to use embryos that are surplus to in vitro fertilisation treatments and would otherwise be destroyed. It has been argued that it would be immoral *not* to use such embryos if their use might lead to the development of treatments that could improve the lives of existing human beings.

A further ethical debate surrounds the use of cell nuclear replacement ('therapeutic cloning', see Figure 4.9) to create embryos for the derivation of stem cells. Some people feel an instinctive distaste for what they regard as an 'unnatural' process. Another frequently heard argument is that perfecting techniques for cell nuclear replacement will inevitably lead to human reproductive cloning; the counter argument is that society does have the ability to impose limits on the uses of technology and that there would be no beneficial progress at all if the 'slippery slope' argument were allowed to prevail.

An even more contentious issue is that of human/animal hybrid embryos produced by transfer of a human nucleus into an oocyte from another mammal. It has been suggested that such embryos would be useful for various types of research and for deriving human embryonic stem cells without the need to use scarce and precious human oocytes. The creation of human/animal hybrids is currently illegal in the UK (see Chapter 7) and, again, is regarded as anathema by many people, raising questions of how we define both an 'embryo' and what is considered 'human'. Although initial reactions to the concept of human/animal hybrid constructs tend to be very negative, it is possible that public opinion could change if benefits are perceived and effective safeguards are proposed.

If human embryos and gametes (eggs or sperm) are used for research or in the development of therapies, an important ethical principle is that they should be ethically sourced: donors should not be coerced either directly or indirectly, and should give valid consent after provision of appropriate information and counselling. The appropriate level of financial compensation for donors is controversial. Some people think, for example, that a woman should not be expected to donate eggs (an unpleasant and potentially harmful procedure) without financial reward, while others feel that payment in this situation would be an unacceptable inducement.

Current UK policy on the use of embryos and cell nuclear replacement is discussed in Chapter 7.

Genetic information

There has been much debate about genetic information: how it may be used, and the degree of protection that should be afforded to it. But what do we mean by 'genetic information'? The Human Genetics Commission (2002) has defined personal genetic information as 'information about the genetic make-up of an identifiable person, whether derived directly from DNA (or other biochemical) testing methods or indirectly from any other source'. Defined in this broad way, genetic information about a person may be obtained from features of their genotype, or phenotype (for example, sex or ABO blood group) or family history.

Such a broad definition may make it difficult to distinguish between genetic information and any other type of personal biological information. Observing that a person is female or has red hair, for example, would allow an inference about an aspect of their genetic make-up but it would be difficult to argue that this 'genetic information' is particularly sensitive unless, perhaps, it were to be used in a forensic context. On the other hand, if the definition of genetic information is restricted to information derived from direct analysis of the genetic material (DNA, RNA or chromosomes), a different set of difficulties arises. Such a definition would exclude family history, which is often used to make predictions about genetic conditions. It would also exclude phenotypic features used to diagnose genetic diseases. For example, adult polycystic kidney disease is a condition that may be diagnosed either by a DNA test or by renal ultrasound. The importance and consequences of the genetic information for the patient are the same, regardless of how it was derived.

These examples suggest that, although the term 'genetic information' cannot logically be restricted to information derived from DNA or chromosomal analysis, it is not sensible to propose that all genetic information is equally sensitive. Its sensitivity will depend on its diagnostic or predictive power and on the seriousness of the condition to which it relates. In the case of highly penetrant single-gene disorders such as Huntington's disease, the genetic information provided by a DNA test is highly predictive and the condition devastating. The information provided by a family history of this disease, although less accurate than a DNA test result, is also serious and highly sensitive for the individual. By contrast, the genetic information provided by a test for weakly penetrant polymorphisms implicated in, say, susceptibility to coronary heart disease will in most cases be no more predictive or serious in its consequences than risk predictions derived from factors such as age, sex, body mass index, blood lipid profile and smoking status.

The idea that genetic information is in some way special – different from other types of personal and/or medical information – is sometimes known as 'genetic exceptionalism'. We will examine the arguments for and against genetic exceptionalism in more detail; we will then consider some of the situations in which genetic information is likely to be used, and the issues raised by these uses. These issues generally revolve around concerns about privacy, confidentiality and consent, together with the potential for unfair discrimination. In Chapter 7 we will consider in more detail the policy responses to these issues.

Genetic exceptionalism

Several features of genetic information have been invoked in support of genetic exceptionalism:

- The familial nature of genetic information. We share 50% of our genes with each of our first-degree relatives, and smaller but still significant percentages with more distantly related family members. For this reason, genetic information about one person can give at least an indication of the likely genetic make-up of a close relative.
- DNA-based genetic information is remarkable for the specificity with which it can be used for the purpose of identification. This is the basis for the technique of DNA fingerprinting, widely used in forensics and paternity testing. Moreover, the use of the polymerase chain reaction means that DNA analysis is exquisitely sensitive: only a tiny biological sample such as a smear of saliva or a single hair root is sufficient to derive DNA-based information about the person from whom the sample came.
- Genetic information has the potential to predict ill health. In some situations, genetic information may be used to predict future disease in a currently asymptomatic person, whilst other types of medical information are based on existing phenotypic features.
- A person whose genetic endowment has increased their risk of a particular disease has no control over their genotype and indeed may have no notion that they are at increased risk.

The list of arguments in favour of genetic exceptionalism is powerful but, on closer inspection, caveats emerge.

- Several of the arguments apply only to genetic information related to highly penetrant single-gene diseases (including the single-gene subsets of some common diseases). This, as we have pointed out earlier in this chapter, is at present the only type of genetic information that has predictive value beyond that of phenotypic and lifestyle information. It is also the only type of genetic information that has clear significance for other family members.
- Few of the characteristics of genetic information are unique to this type of information. Other non-genetic sources of medical information may have considerable predictive value. For example, families often share many attributes other than genes that may affect their health: socioeconomic status, geographic location and infectious disease experience, to name just a few.
- Individuals have no control over their genes, but they may also have little effective control over other health-related exposures such as growing up in a smoke-filled environment or with a poor childhood diet. Environmental factors such as these may actually have a less reversible effect than that of some genetic 'exposures'. Individuals with familial hypercholesterolaemia, for example, can reduce their risk of heart disease to near-normal levels with appropriate treatment, but the effects of passive smoking or poor diet in childhood may be lifelong.

For all of these reasons, attempts to devise a blanket protection for genetic information while at the same time being fair, logical and consistent are doomed to fail. Nevertheless, the general perception in society, fuelled at least in part by the rhetoric of some scientists, is that genetic information is special and powerful, and therefore potentially dangerous. Acknowledging the social reality of this situation is not an argument for making genetic exceptionalism the basis of public policy but it is an argument for ensuring that policy development is approached in such a way as to maintain public confidence.

Establishing a rational basis for using and protecting genetic information will also have a 'future-proofing' function. As we learn more about the genetic variants that predispose to common disease, how these factors interact with each other and how genetic risk is modulated by lifestyle, the predictive value of genetic information may increase. It is important, therefore, that we give thought to how genetic information may be used to improve human health without compromising such important values as psychological well-being and social justice.

Genetic databases

There are two main types of database containing genetic information about individuals: disease-based databases and population databases. Disease-based databases hold information about individuals suffering from a particular disease; increasingly, genotype information is being added to these databases, for use in association studies comparing the genotypes of individuals with and without the disease.

Population genetic databases include forensic DNA databases (which raise many ethical issues but lie outside the scope of this book), and databases used in research studies on the relationships between genetic factors, lifestyle variables and disease. (The approaches used in such studies are discussed in detail in Chapter 3.) Recently, interest has grown in establishing very large population genetic databases of this type. In the UK, for example, the Biobank project (see Box 3.3) aims to collect genotypic, medical and lifestyle information about 500 000 healthy volunteers between the ages of 40 and 69. The health of these individuals will be monitored over the next 15–20 years, and various research studies using the database and DNA samples will attempt to relate outcomes such as disease incidence and death to genotypic and lifestyle features. Within this large, prospective study, nested case–control studies may also be carried out, comparing groups of individuals who have developed a specific disease with matched controls who have not.

Biobanking initiatives are also under way in several other countries including Iceland, Estonia, Finland, Japan, Canada and the US. Table 6.1 compares the characteristics of some of these projects.

There are concerns about the ethical governance of projects involving the use of personal information, particularly medical information. These concerns relate mainly to issues of consent, feedback of findings to participants, the role of the commercial sector, and security and confidentiality of personal (including genetic) information.

As a general principle, it has been recommended that the ethics and governance of all such projects should be subject to oversight by a group independent of both the funders and the research groups involved in use of the database. Arrangements of this nature have been put in place for UK Biobank and most similar projects (Table 6.1).

Consent

By their very nature, prospective initiatives such as Biobank, birth cohort studies or the banking of samples for future pharmacogenetic research cannot specify precisely all the possible future research studies that may be undertaken using samples and genetic and other data. It is therefore extremely difficult to satisfy, at the outset, the requirements for informed consent, namely that the individual knows and understands the nature of the study and has freely agreed to participate.

Two possible solutions have been suggested to this problem. One is that, at the stage of enrolment in the project, participants give their general consent to a fairly broadly worded description of the types of studies envisaged, and agree that their

Table 6.1. Examples of large population-based DNA collections

	Iceland DeCode Biobank	Estonian Genome Project	UK Biobank	GenomEUtwin	CARTaGENE	Generation Scotland
Size (no. individuals)	270 000	1 065 000	500 000 aged 40–69	Total resource 800 000 twin pairs. Studies are on subsets of this resource (e.g. MORGAM cohort of 80 000 individuals)	60 000–65 000 aged 24–75	50 000
Aims	Identify gene variants related to common disease	Genetic research; public health surveillance related to genetic variants to be developed	To study gene–environment interactions in common disease	Influence of genetic and non-genetic factors on 5 complex traits: obesity, stature, coronary heart disease, stroke and longevity	Map Quebec population genetic variation of medical relevance; genomic research towards clinical applications	Identify gene variants associated with 10 major common diseases prevalent in Scotland
Further description	Three linked databases: genealogical, health and DNA	Genotype and phenotype (health status) database of Estonian population	DNA and medical records. Resource for nested case–control studies	International collaboration; mostly uses existing cohorts and samples	Will not access medical records or other phenotypic information	Family-based linkage studies and case–control studies. DNA samples and medical records
Follow-up	Through health database	Through health database	Partial follow-up through medical records; more detailed follow-up for sub-groups	Yes	Semi-longitudinal study	As required

Table 6.1. (cont.)

	Iceland DeCode Biobank	Estonian Genome Project	UK Biobank	GenomEUtwin	CARTaGENE	Generation Scotland
Ethical governance	Supervision by national ethics committee	Ad hoc specific ethics committee	Specific Ethics and Governance Council	Governance protocol under development	Specific ethics committee. Governance details developed through open workshops	Separate oversight committee
Informed consent	Opt out for health and genealogical data; informed specific consent for biological samples	Volunteer (opt in) participation, with a restricted opt out option	Initial written consent for overall participation; re-consent for specific nested projects; option to withdraw	New consent required in case of existing samples	Informed consent and multi-layer options	Volunteer (opt in) participation with initial informed consent. Details of any subsequent consent for specific studies not yet specified
Confidentiality	Complex structure for protection of data	Coded and encrypted data	Key-coded data; different kinds of data in different unconnected machines	Coded information; no link with any identifying information in the database	Double-coded information	Will use existing systems for confidential linking of medical records
Commercial aspects	12 years exclusive rights to DeCode	Plans are to market products and access to information through Egeen (public foundation) to private companies	Yes, but no exclusive rights. Conditions for commercial access not yet fully defined	None	No private ownership – possible access for private sector under specific agreements	Partnership with biotech and pharmaceutical industries on drug development

with permission from Macmillan Magazines Ltd, copyright 2004.

samples and data may be used for all future research studies approved under the ethical and governance arrangements for the overall project. In this model, those charged with ethical oversight of the project take responsibility for protecting the interests of participants and the general public.

A second solution requires separate consent from participants for each use of their information or sample. Such a procedure, however, is cumbersome and expensive. As long as participants are free to opt out of the project at any stage, a compromise solution may be to inform people about new projects that have been approved and leave it to them to opt out should they wish to do so. It would be relatively straightforward to exclude a specific individual's sample or data from a future study or studies; however, it would be virtually impossible to destroy data used in past studies, and participants should be made aware of this fact.

Views about the nature and adequacy of different forms of consent hinge on the reason for seeking consent in the first place. If the goal is to prevent harm, then broad or generalised consent combined with the freedom to opt out at any stage would appear to be adequate. However if, as some believe, the purpose of consent is to achieve absolute personal autonomy, it follows that specific consent would be needed for every use of the sample or of genetic or other information derived from it.

Confidentiality

Projects involving large computer databases raise inevitable questions about the security and confidentiality of information. It is generally accepted that questions of confidentiality do not arise if information is irreversibly stripped of all attributes that would enable it to be linked to a specific individual. In the case of genotypic information, however, this may be impossible to achieve: as more and more information is accumulated about each sample, the possibility of matching a record to a specific person will increase. There seems no ready solution to this problem other than rigorous attention to computer security, though it is doubtful whether complete security is achievable.

Even if it were, irreversible anonymisation would negate the whole rationale of a prospective project such as Biobank, where future information about health outcomes for an individual will need to be added to existing data about that person. In such a situation, the usual solution is to encode the personal identifiers in some way; researchers given access to the data have only the coded identifier, while a trusted third party (such as an ethics oversight committee) is the custodian of the key to the code. This system has been given various names including pseudo-anonymisation and reversible anonymisation. Its effectiveness depends, of course, on the security of the code and the probity of all those responsible for the steps involved in adding incoming information to the database.

Concerns have also been voiced about who should be allowed to have access to information and samples held by research facilities such as Biobank. The Human Genetics Commission (2002) recommended that law enforcement agencies should not be allowed to use biomedical research databases for forensic purposes. The Commission was concerned that allowing police access to this information would lead to difficulties in recruiting participants for research. In its response, the UK Government (2003) did not accept this recommendation, stating that it believed the current legal arrangements for access to research databases under the Police and Criminal Evidence Act contained sufficient safeguards to prevent improper access.

In the future, databases containing genetic information are likely to spread beyond the realms of research. Pharmacogenetic testing, for example, will generate genetic information that will need to be stored in some way and accessed by appropriate clinicians and patients themselves. Many healthcare organisations in developed countries are working towards implementing electronic health records that will detail key features of an individual's medical history and treatment. It is important to ensure that these systems are capable of including genetic data where appropriate and that effective safeguards are in place to protect the security of all the sensitive personal information they contain.

Role of the commercial sector

The commercial sector, in particular the pharmaceutical industry, has shown increasing interest in the use of human sample collections and genetic databases for research and development purposes. For example, collections of DNA and genetic information are being established by some pharmaceutical companies for possible use in pharmacogenetics and pharmacogenomics research. The people invited to contribute to these collections are usually those enrolled in clinical trials of new drugs.

The role of the commercial sector in biobank projects is controversial. The secretive nature of pharmaceutical research and development prompts fears about commercially owned biobanks. An individual in a clinical drug trial who consents to a sample being retained for future pharmacogenetic research will probably have very little knowledge (and no control) over the uses to which their sample and data will be put, especially if the original company goes out of business or is bought out by a different company. The right to opt out in the future may have little practical value if samples cannot be traced or have crossed national boundaries. The only practical solution to this difficulty seems to be to place an obligation on the company requesting the sample to make it clear that the donor will have no control over its future use; any individual unhappy with this situation would be free to deny consent. People's fears about misuse might be alleviated to some extent, however, if companies adopted a policy of greater transparency about their activities, as they have recently been forced to do with regard to clinical trials.

There is also disquiet about the prospect of allowing commercial organisations to have access to publicly owned and funded biobank resources. Surveys of public opinion routinely find that most people are opposed to the use of public assets for private profit. Nevertheless, it is clear that the commercial sector has an important role to play in realising the benefits of genomic medicine (only pharmaceutical companies, for example, produce new drugs). Bioscience industry is also an important sector of the economy in many western countries, including the UK, contributing to national wealth and thereby to the nation's ability to fund healthcare development.

The plans for UK Biobank allow commercial access to the resource. No company will be granted exclusive rights to samples or data, and commercial users will have to adhere to Biobank's ethical framework, but other aspects of the arrangements with commercial users have yet to be specified in detail. One problematic area may be that of intellectual property and ownership of discoveries arising from use of the resource; it may be difficult to decide at what point a sample or a set of data has been transformed by a user into a patentable 'invention' that can be 'owned' by that user. This difficulty is likely to apply to academic users as well as commercial ones.

A related question concerns possible benefit sharing: should a company that has derived profit from products developed as a result of access to a biobank resource return part of that profit to the resource, or even to the set of individuals whose samples and data were used? The idea of benefit sharing seems superficially attractive but only in a very small number of clearly defined cases is it likely to be possible to trace the development of a drug or other healthcare intervention directly back to samples or data relating to specific individuals, or to decide what proportion of the profit was due to access to the biobank resource. A more feasible approach may be to levy an up-front fee for commercial access to the biobank. At a more general level, it will be important to foster partnerships between government and industry, in which access by industry to public resources, and a favourable climate for research and development are conditional on industry's agreement to make new drugs and interventions available to the health service at affordable prices. The role of the commercial sector in healthcare policy for genetics is discussed further in Chapter 7.

Feedback to participants

Projects such as Biobank have been established in the hope that they will yield information about relationships between genetic and lifestyle factors that have a significant impact on health. If this promise is fulfilled, should participants be informed of any findings that may be relevant for their health or medical treatment? Some take the view that it would be unethical not to do so. Others have argued that feedback to individual participants would not only be far too expensive and onerous, but could be misleading and even do harm. The reasoning behind this stance is that the findings from population-level projects such as Biobank will be probabilistic in nature and further tiers of analysis and validation will be needed to assess their usefulness at the level of the individual. Issues of quality control are also important: while it is in the interests of research laboratories to make every effort to generate accurate results, they are not subject to the same stringent assessment as clinical testing laboratories and the possibility of mistakes is higher.

All commentators agree on the importance of continued communication with participants at a general level, however. It has been suggested that general bulletins about the progress of research studies using resources such as Biobank would be effective in informing participants about significant new developments; any who were concerned about implications for their personal health would be encouraged to consult their own doctor.

Genetic discrimination

Many concerns about genetic information relate to the potential for use of this information to justify unfair discrimination against individuals or groups on the basis of their genetic features. Two potential arenas for discrimination are often discussed: insurance and employment. In addition, there is disquiet about the possible use of genetics to stigmatise particular racial or ethnic groups.

Genetic information and insurance

There are two types of insurance system: solidarity-based insurance and mutual insurance. In a solidarity system (of which the UK's National Health Service might be considered an example), insurance premiums are not based on risk. Rather, all those covered by the system may pay equal premiums, or premiums may be based on some other factor, such as income, that is not directly related to risk. In mutual insurance, by contrast, individuals applying for insurance cover are assessed on the basis of their risk for the outcome they are seeking to insure against, and the premium they pay is set accordingly. If the insurer judges that the risk is unacceptably high, cover may be refused.

Mutual insurance, which is the model in operation for life insurance and products such as income protection and critical illness cover in many countries, depends on the principle of 'utmost good faith'. That is, the person seeking insurance must disclose any information known to him or her that has a bearing on their risk. If this principle is breached there is the potential for 'adverse selection', which occurs if people who know they are at increased risk (but do not disclose this knowledge) are more likely to take out insurance, or to seek higher-value policies. This has the effect of increasing the number and/or value of claims above the expected level calculated by actuaries when the insurance product was developed. Insurers argue that adverse selection is unfair to other policy holders and that a significant level of adverse selection could make some types of insurance product unviable.

The principle of utmost good faith in mutual insurance, and concerns over the potential for adverse selection, have led many in the insurance industry to argue that, if genetic information is a significant predictor of risk, and if this information is known to an applicant for insurance, it should be disclosed. In effect this already happens in many countries, including the UK and the US, where insurers routinely seek family history information from applicants. Actuarial tables are used to relate this information to risk and a premium is set accordingly or cover refused. (It should be noted that, in practice, insurers do not attempt a fine level of accuracy in assessing risk but rather assign applicants to one of a few fairly broad risk bands. In the UK around 95% of applicants for life insurance in connection with a mortgage loan obtain insurance at standard rates.)

Much of the opposition to the use of genetic information by insurers is based on the concern that people will be deterred from seeking genetic information that may be relevant to their health because of fears that they will be denied access to affordable insurance. In the US these fears are particularly acute because health care is largely funded by private insurance and, in addition, health insurance for many people is linked to their employment contract.

It may turn out that fears about the use of genetic information in insurance underwriting can largely be allayed. There is no doubt that those at risk of serious single-gene diseases such as Huntington's disease face great difficulty in obtaining various types of risk-rated insurance. This will continue to be the case as long as insurers are allowed to use family history information. The use of genetic test results should actually improve the situation for at least some members of these families in that those who test negative can be offered insurance at standard rates.

For most people, genetic information will have only a modest impact on risk. If the predictive value of genetic information turns out to be low in all but a small minority of people, insurers may feel that they can afford to ignore it. If they are allowed to use it, its impact on premiums would be correspondingly small in most cases. Insurers have not so far argued that they should be allowed to *require* applicants to undergo any genetic test; as long as neither applicant nor insurance company possesses any genetic test information, the principle of utmost good faith is not breached and adverse selection will not occur.

In the future there may be people whose family history and current health give no cause for concern but for whom genetic testing reveals a substantially increased risk of disease. These people would be likely to encounter problems with obtaining affordable insurance if insurers were allowed to use predictive genetic test results, and societies will have to decide whether they are prepared to allow this. If insurance is regarded as a social good, many think it is not acceptable to discriminate against people on the basis of characteristics over which they have limited control. Various solutions are possible, including subsidies or other special measures to assist those at elevated risk because of genetic factors. It seems reasonable to point out, though, that people have little or no control over many other factors that affect insurable risks, such as their age or the type of area in which they live, and yet society accepts differential premiums for various types of insurance, based on such factors. The 'genetic exceptionalist' argument in the case of insurance therefore needs careful justification.

Alarm about genetic testing and insurance also needs to be tempered by consideration of the reasons that would lead an individual to undertake a genetic test in the first place. Experience with genetic testing for Huntington's disease has shown that, unless effective treatment or prevention is available, most people opt not to be tested. It follows that the main rationale for genetic testing (apart from in the context of reproductive choice, discussed earlier) is to assess risk of a treatable or preventable condition. Provided such treatment or prevention is actually undertaken, it will be likely to modify risk and so be a factor that insurers should take into account. There is some evidence that this has indeed proved to be so in the case of familial hypercholesterolaemia, a highly penetrant genetic condition that is very effectively treated by the statin drugs. Several companies are now prepared to insure people with this condition at standard rates, or only modestly elevated premiums, if there is evidence that they are complying with risk-lowering treatment (Figure 6.2).

Insurance companies have a responsibility to keep up-to-date with scientific and medical advances, to continually assess the evidence base for their practices, and to modify these practices appropriately. In practice, it may turn out that the predictive value of new phenotypic biomarkers is substantially higher than that of DNA sequences. It remains to be seen how the insurance market will evolve if it becomes possible to predict future disease risk accurately – by whatever means – in healthy asymptomatic people.

Genetic information and employment

Three main purposes have been suggested for the possible use of genetic information in decisions related to employment:

- Health and safety (for example, to gauge susceptibility to hazards in the work place)

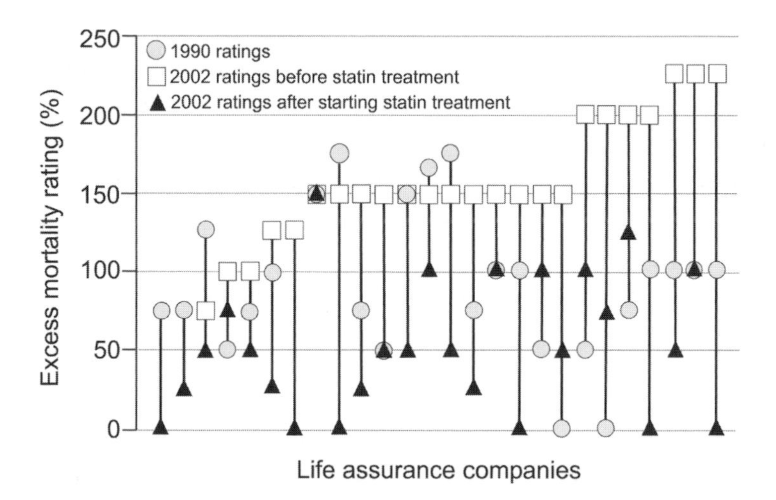

Figure 6.2 Effect of statin treatment for familial hypercholesterolaemia on life assurance. Percentage excess mortality ratings applied by 24 life assurance companies in 1990 and 2002, before and after starting statin treatment. From Neil, H. A. *et al.* (2004). *BMJ* 328, 500–1. Reproduced with permission from the BMJ Publishing Group

- To assess capacity to carry out a key component of the job
- To help judge whether prospective employees were likely to have long periods of illness and absence from work.

The current state of knowledge is such that there are very few examples of scientifically justifiable uses of genetic information in the context of employment. Virtually all of them relate to existing medical or other conditions that have a direct genetic cause; for example, people who are colour blind (a genetically determined condition) are not eligible to train as aircraft pilots. Except in the case of rare, adult-onset Mendelian diseases, genetic information is not at present sufficiently predictive to judge the likelihood of future illness. Even when the predictive value of genetic information is high, it does not necessarily provide grounds for refusing employment in a specific job: a person in his early twenties who carries the Huntington's disease mutation would be likely to have at least two decades of disease-free working life.

It is known that susceptibility to some environmental hazards, including occupational hazards specific to certain industries, has a genetic contribution. In Chapter 4 we gave the example of susceptibility to lung disease resulting from contact with beryllium-containing materials in the nuclear industry. Is there a case for screening people likely to come into contact with these compounds and advising those who are particularly susceptible to avoid their use or seek other employment?

The ethical issue under consideration here is whether it is right to determine a level of exposure that is 'safe' for all, including those who are most susceptible, or to allow different levels of exposure depending on an assessment of individual genetic risk. If genetic testing gave a perfect measure of risk then perhaps the latter course of action would be justifiable. In practice, however, individual risk is likely to be affected by factors other than genetic ones and an employer who sought to justify higher exposure for some workers on the basis of a genetic test would be likely to find themselves on shaky ground. In general, substances that are highly toxic to some individuals are also far from harmless to others, and the first line of action of employers, wherever possible, should be to remove the hazard rather than the worker.

Justice and the 'genetic underclass'

Some commentators have suggested that a growing understanding of the contribution of genetic factors to ill health could lead to the identification of a group of people who suffer severe social disadvantage as a result of their genetic constitution. Such a 'genetic underclass', it is suggested, might be denied access to insurance and employment opportunities, and experience discrimination and stigmatisation in many areas of life.

Although society must be aware of the potential for this scenario, and be alert to any indication that it is coming to pass, such doom-laden predictions are probably unduly pessimistic. As we have stressed repeatedly, the predictive value of genetic information for most people is likely to be limited. There may be some who discover that genetics has 'dealt them a bad hand of cards' but it is to be hoped that this discovery will generally be made only when effective treatment or prevention is available. Where this is not the case, social measures might be justified to protect those who discover that they are at a genetic disadvantage. Legislation to protect the rights of disabled people shows that this can be achieved where there is the social will to do so. It will be important to outlaw any coercive genetic testing, particularly for conditions that are not treatable.

Turning the argument the other way round, there may also be fears that the *advantages* of new genetic interventions and technologies may be available only to a privileged few who have both the knowledge that they exist and the means to afford them. These people might be able to use genetic or phenotypic biomarker testing, together with assessment of environmental and lifestyle factors, to gain a better measure of their disease risk and an indication of the most effective preventive measures. They might also have access to pharmacogenetic testing to indicate the best drug and dosage for any medical conditions from which they suffer. Perhaps, eventually, they might even be able to make use of genetic technology to choose specific genetic characteristics in their offspring. In this scenario, the 'genetic underclass' would be those who are denied the benefits of genetic technologies.

The ethical arguments here are essentially the same as for any other expensive new medical technology. Society must decide which interventions it is prepared to make available to all, which should be rationed, and which should be prohibited. Such judgements will not be 'once and for all' but will change in the light of many factors including accumulating evidence for the effectiveness or otherwise of interventions, changing costs (the costs of genetic tests, for example, are likely to fall) and shifting societal values.

Genetics and racial discrimination

In the context of research on human genetic variation, there have been attempts to find out whether specific genetic factors can be identified that can be correlated with racial or ethnic groups defined by physical appearance, geographic origin or social and cultural features.

There is clear evidence that some genetic variants show different prevalence in different human populations. The birth prevalence of the genetic disease Tay Sachs disease, for example, is higher in Ashkenazi Jews than in other populations, while sickle-cell disease is particularly prevalent in Afro-Caribbeans and some other groups. Such findings are not restricted to disease-related genetic variants. As mentioned in Chapter 4, for example, variants associated with pharmacogenetic characteristics may also be present at different frequencies in different populations.

Given such examples, and the extreme sensitivity that surrounds the concept of race, some fear that attempts may be made to justify racial discrimination, or reinforce damaging racial stereotypes, on genetic grounds. Such discrimination is explicitly condemned in statements from many different international bodies concerned with human rights and health. It is invariably pointed out that, with only about 0.1% difference between the genomes of any two human individuals, regardless of race, there is far more that unites than divides us. Nevertheless, it is important to address the issue of genetic variation between populations in order to ensure that the potential benefits of genetics for medical care are not denied to minority or disadvantaged groups.

Another concern is the provision of appropriate genetic testing and population screening services. Such services have already been developed for some populations. The examples of neonatal and antenatal screening for sickle-cell disease, and carrier screening for Tay Sachs disease in Ashkenazi Jewish communities, have been discussed in Chapter 5. It is generally accepted that programmes such as these are not discriminatory if they are offered in a non-coercive way and are acceptable to the group concerned.

Many argue that it is inequitable not to make provision, in the development of genetic services, for population subgroups with specific needs. An important issue for public health is the question of how to target population-level programmes appropriately. As discussed in Chapter 5, universal neonatal screening for cystic fibrosis and sickle-cell disease has been introduced in the UK, even though the risk for these conditions varies widely between different populations. The decision has been made – and it is an ethical one insofar as it concerns both the allocation of public money and the provision of health care appropriate to each individual – that it is better to offer the tests to all than to take the chance of missing some cases by targeting specific self-defined racial or ethnic groups.

In healthcare services in general, the goals and standards that are adopted tend to be those of the majority population and these may not always be accepted by minority groups. Some extremely sensitive issues can arise, for example in attitudes to consanguineous marriage and the potentially increased risk of autosomal recessive diseases. It may be difficult to strike a balance between ensuring that services are available to all and that people know about them, and appearing to impose interventions on minority groups.

In the US, epidemiological research studies funded by the National Institutes of Health must include representation of minority groups, for example African Americans and Hispanics. This policy has been criticised, however, as potentially encouraging stereotyping and stigmatisation if it leads to assumptions about health status and appropriate treatment being made on the basis of racial grouping (see Box 6.1 for a controversial example). Genetic studies have also shown that racial categories based on self-reporting and observable physical characteristics are very much over-simplified, particularly in countries such as the US, where more than two centuries of immigration and inter-marriage have led to significant levels of racial admixture. Some genetic variants of likely medical importance show a rough correlation with such simple categories but many others do not, so it will generally be unsafe to make assumptions based on racial appearance alone.

Box 6.1 Genetics and race: the BiDil example

The drug BiDil was approved in June 2005 by the US Food and Drug Administration (FDA) for the treatment of heart failure in patients who identify themselves as African Americans. Approval was based on review of the results of the African American Heart Failure Trial, which presented evidence that the drug was effective in this group of patients. Corresponding evidence for its effectiveness in other self-identified racial groups in the US (such as 'Whites' or 'Hispanics') is not at present available.

The BiDil decision is controversial. Critics argue that it may deny the drug to many people who would benefit from it, because it uses self-identified race as a (very imperfect) surrogate for whatever genomic or other variants are implicated in response to the drug. Those who agree with the FDA's decision point out that the alternative would have been to refuse to licence the drug altogether, thus depriving African Americans of a potentially useful therapy.

Ethical and legal aspects of clinical genetics

In the remainder of this chapter we will discuss some ethical and legal issues that arise in clinical genetics; that is, in the context of the clinical genetics services for patients and their families that we have described in Chapter 5. It is important to emphasise that as a general rule these ethical and legal dilemmas are specific to this context and will not be relevant in the eventual application of genetics in the context of common disease.

The general principles of medical practice – the physician's duty of care, the autonomy of the patient, and the patient's right to privacy and to have their medical information kept confidential, for example – apply equally to clinical genetics. Difficulties can arise, however, as a result of the familial nature of genetic information in the context of highly penetrant Mendelian disease or certain chromosomal disorders; for example, respect for one person's autonomy may undermine the autonomy of a close relative.

Several professional organisations, including the UK's Joint Committee on Medical Genetics (which includes representatives of the British Society for Human Genetics and of several Royal Colleges including the Royal College of Physicians and the Royal College of Pathologists; see Box 5.1 in Chapter 5) and the American College of Medical Genetics, have developed guidelines to help clinical professionals faced with ethical problems. In some cases, court judgements have established legal precedents but contradictory rulings may confuse rather than clarify the clinician's understanding of his or her legal responsibilities.

In many situations, no hard and fast rules can be put forward. Clinicians must attempt to judge each case on its merits and to weigh up the likely harms and benefits of different courses of action.

Confidentiality versus the duty to warn

Clinicians have a professional duty, and a legal obligation under the common law, to keep information about their patients confidential. In most countries, however, this duty is not absolute: a clinician may breach confidentiality if disclosure is necessary to prevent harm to the patient or to others, or if it can be shown to be in the public interest.

In the context of clinical genetics, difficulties may arise if genetic information about a patient has implications for other family members but the patient refuses to allow the information to be divulged to them. In many countries including the UK, US and Australia (France is an exception), a physician who decided to inform at-risk relatives would be protected legally providing three conditions were met: that all reasonable steps had been taken to persuade the patient, that the information related to a disorder with serious and imminent consequences, and that the disorder was treatable or preventable.

The difficulty for clinicians is to decide on the definitions of 'serious' and 'imminent'. If a woman has had a genetic test that reveals a pathogenic mutation in one of the *BRCA* genes but does not wish her close relatives to be informed of this, does the clinician have a duty to over-rule her wishes, given that at-risk female relatives may wish themselves to be tested and perhaps to take preventive measures such as prophylactic mastectomy and/or oophorectomy if they test positive?

In situations such as this, the clinical geneticist would generally try to persuade the patient to allow their information to be disclosed. In the face of persistent refusal the clinician might decide that breach of confidentiality was justified. However, such decisions have very rarely been tested in the courts so there is little case law to guide geneticists. In practice, research suggests that clinicians very rarely attempt to inform relatives without their patient's consent, even if there may be very good reasons for doing so.

The right not to know

Some people do not wish to be informed of their genetic risk of disease. It is imperative therefore, and a cardinal principle of clinical genetics, that no pressure is placed on an individual to undergo genetic consultation or diagnosis.

Circumstances can arise in which genetic information about one family member inevitably reveals information about another person who has declared a wish not to know this information. For example, a person who has a grandparent with Huntington's disease and who wants to have a predictive genetic test may have an at-risk parent who does not wish to know his or her genetic status. If the person has a test and tests positive, it is likely to be very difficult for the parent to avoid knowing that he or she is also destined to develop the disease. There is no solution to this problem that protects the autonomy of all concerned; all clinicians can do is to try to help the family to come to some agreed resolution.

There is also no satisfactory way of protecting the right of a person not to know about their genetic risk if a close relative is affected by a condition with a strong genetic basis. The very act of asking someone if they wish to have this information removes their 'right not to know'. Again, the problem can be approached by trying to balance potential benefit and potential harm: if the condition in question is a serious but treatable one and the risk to close relatives is high, it might be assumed that relatives will wish to know about their risk. If, on the other hand, the risk is uncertain and the condition untreatable (as, for example, in the case of the *APOE4* allele and risk of Alzheimer's disease – a test that is not in current clinical use), the balance of benefit would be against informing relatives.

These general guidelines are in accordance with a growing body of evidence on the uptake of genetic tests by at-risk individuals. Uptake of predictive testing for Huntington's disease, where no prevention is available, has been low; most people prefer to cling to the hope that they will be unaffected rather than risk losing all hope with a positive test. By contrast, there has been much higher uptake of testing for *BRCA1* and *BRCA2* gene mutations in families at high genetic risk of breast cancer, because action can be taken to reduce the risk.

Consent to genetic testing

The legal requirements for securing consent for genetic testing depend on whether the test is carried out for the purpose of medical diagnosis or treatment, or for research.

The common law governs the former, provided the test is carried out on a tissue sample from the patient themself and the purpose is the clinical benefit of that patient. Clinical geneticists try hard to ensure that patients who are offered a genetic test are properly informed about the nature of the test and its implications for themselves and their family.

If, however, a test result is needed from an affected relative – as is usually the case with DNA testing for the *BRCA1* or *BRCA2* mutations associated with breast cancer risk – the provisions of the Human Tissue Act 2004 (UK Government 2004c) apply: 'qualifying consent' is required for holding material that consists of or includes human cells ('human bodily material') with the intention of analysing any human DNA in the material. So if a relative refuses to give a sample of blood or other tissue for DNA analysis, or to allow DNA to be extracted from an existing sample for the purpose of testing, that refusal is absolute and must be respected, even if another person's health or well-being depends on that consent being given. The relevant sections of the Human Tissue Act, which came into force in 2006 and is discussed in a more general context in Chapter 7, apply throughout the UK.

If a tissue sample from the relative has already been obtained but the donor is untraceable or it has not been possible, after reasonable attempts, to discover whether he or she is willing to consent or not, then the person in whose interests the DNA test would be carried out can apply to the Human Tissue Authority, a statutory body set up under the provisions of the Human Tissue Act, which may 'deem consent' in this situation if it fulfils certain criteria.

Where DNA is needed from a relative who has died, the taking and analysis of samples is regulated by the wishes of that relative immediately before they died. If no decision was made, consent may be granted by a 'qualifying relative' (see Box 6.2).

The Human Tissue Act will initially have limited effect because it is not retrospective and does not apply to DNA itself (because DNA does not fall under the definition of 'bodily material') or to information derived from DNA analysis. This means that, if a sample of extracted DNA (with no cellular material), or sequence

Box 6.2 Qualifying relatives who may give consent for DNA testing of a sample from a person who has died

- Spouse or relative
- Parent or child
- Brother or sister
- Grandparent or grandchild
- Child of a brother or sister
- Step-father or step-mother
- Half-brother or half-sister
- Friend of long standing

For the purposes of genetic analysis alone, the consent of any qualifying relative is sufficient. However, the Human Tissue Act also regulates the removal, use and storage of tissue. For these purposes, the relationships are ranked such that consent should be obtained from the person who is at the top of the list. Where two or more people have equal ranking it is sufficient to obtain the consent of any of them.

information that can be used to derive a test result, is available from a relative, then use of that sample and/or information derived from it is governed by the common law and law relating to data protection, confidentiality and human rights, not by the Human Tissue Act. As discussed earlier in this chapter, the legality of using DNA or disclosing information obtained from it in this situation is not clear but clinical genetics practice supports its use in certain exceptional circumstances where it is likely to prevent the serious injury or death of another, if there is no alternative way to secure their welfare.

The Human Tissue Act also requires qualifying consent if DNA in bodily material is held for analysis for research. Most, if not all, clinical DNA tests are developed through research projects involving patients. In such projects, and particularly in the case of tests that are in transition between research and service, the distinction between medical diagnosis and research may not be a clear one in practice. It is advisable for clinicians offering DNA tests in a mixed clinical/research context to ensure that their consent procedures comply with the requirements of the Human Tissue Act.

Testing of children

The guiding clinical principle for considering genetic testing of a child is that child's best interests. In 1994, the UK Clinical Genetics Society (one of the constituent societies of the British Society for Human Genetics or BSHG) issued guidelines for genetic testing in children. Similar principles have also been set out in guidance by various groups such as the UK Government's Advisory Committee on Genetic Testing (1998) and the Human Genetics Commission (2002). Genetic testing of children is likely to be justified, for example, in the case of treatable, early-onset diseases such as familial adenomatous polyposis, where guidelines recommend testing at the age of 12. Genetic testing may also be undertaken to provide a definitive diagnosis of congenital genetic disease (such as cystic fibrosis or Duchenne muscular dystrophy) so that effective management of the disease may be undertaken as quickly as possible. In the case of diseases such as these, there may be an additional benefit to parents in the form of information needed to make informed choices about future pregnancies.

Testing for late-onset disorders for which no effective preventive treatment is available, or where treatment or preventive measures can safely be delayed until adult life, should not in general be considered until the child is old enough to make an autonomous decision. The BSHG guidelines state that it is also unlikely to be justifiable to test children for carrier status for recessive disorders or for balanced familial chromosomal rearrangements if the only reason is to enable them to make reproductive choices in the future. It should be noted that the current neonatal haemoglobinopathy screening programme in the UK is not in line with the BSHG guidelines, as for technical reasons both affected infants and carriers are identified. The Human Genetics Commission has recommended that efforts should be made to develop tests that do not reveal carrier status where this is not the purpose of the screening programme.

Generally, the common law supplemented by the Human Tissue Act governs the requirements for seeking consent for genetic testing of children. If the child is considered competent to decide for him/herself, then his or her consent is required. Existing case law in Britain allows the maturity of the child, and his or her level of understanding of the specific situation, to be taken into account; 16 is the age at which a person may give valid consent to a medical procedure but some children are considered capable of making an independent decision at an earlier age.

If the genetic testing is carried out for a range of purposes set out in the Human Tissue Act, such as providing information for the benefit of another family member, the Human Tissue Act follows the common law in stating that the consent of a competent child will prevail. If the child is unwilling or unable to make a decision, the Act states that those with parental responsibility can give consent on his/her behalf. If the child has died, another qualifying relative can give consent on the child's behalf, provided there is no reason to believe that the competent child has refused consent.

Testing of adults lacking capacity to consent

Adults who are unable to make autonomous decisions because of permanent or temporary mental incapacity require additional protection.

Until recently in England and Wales this protection was enshrined in the common law, which provided that medical treatment (including genetic testing) of someone who is unable to give valid consent is lawful provided it is deemed to be in the best interests of the person concerned, taking into account any views expressed by the person before becoming incapacitated. These principles have been incorporated into statutory law in England and Wales by the Mental Capacity Act (2005) and to a lesser extent, in Scotland, in the Adults with Incapacity (Scotland) Act (2000). The latter is currently under review. An important principle in the Mental Capacity Act is that a person is assumed to have capacity (that is, to be capable of making decisions him/herself) unless proved otherwise. In addition, a person who lacks capacity is not treated as unable to make a decision about a particular matter unless all practicable steps to help him or her have been taken without success.

A clinician treating a person lacking capacity must, when considering the person's best interests, take into account all relevant circumstances, including the person's past and present wishes and feelings, and any beliefs and values likely to influence the person's decision if they had capacity. The Mental Capacity Act also sets out a duty to consult a range of individuals including a specific named person, a carer or other person interested in the patient's welfare, a person who has been appointed Lasting Power of Attorney, or a court-appointed deputy. A new Court of Protection is to be established that will safeguard the interests of adults lacking capacity.

Difficulties may sometimes arise in the interpretation of a person's 'best interests'. Testing as part of medical diagnosis or treatment will usually be justified if it is likely to entail no significant harm and as long as the person has not expressed a wish not to be tested or not to have a sample taken.

Where genetic testing in the context of familial analysis is likely to yield scientific or medical information relevant to others, the taking of a sample for testing will have to satisfy the requirements of the Human Tissue Act 2004, as discussed earlier in this chapter. The final form of regulations and codes of practice to be made under the Mental Capacity and Human Tissue Acts are yet to be determined. Draft regulations deem consent in circumstances in which the lawful storage and use of material from incapacitated persons for the benefit of others is in the best interests of the person lacking capacity. Existing common law cases suggest that it may be in the patient's own best interests for information derived by DNA testing to be used for other family members where there is or is believed to be a genetic disorder in the patient's family. Similarly, it may be in the patient's own best interests to donate tissue for the benefit of a sibling if the patient is the only suitable donor.

Public perceptions of genetics

Advances in genetic science are not taking place in a vacuum but within a social and political context. *Genetics and Health*, the report of the Nuffield Trust Genetics Scenario Project, published in 2000 by Zimmern and Cook, identified two main drivers affecting the development of genetic medicine: the capacity of science to deliver the promised benefits, and public acceptability.

Opinion polls suggest that applications of genetic science to human health and medical care generally command high levels of public approval. For example, a poll commissioned by the Human Genetics Commission and conducted in 2000 by the polling organisation MORI found that, in a sample of about 1000 adults representative of the social profile of the UK, nearly 90% agreed with the statement that developments in genetic science will bring cures for many diseases. People did not give blanket approval to all uses of genetics, however. There was considerable disquiet about aspects of genetics that were thought to be 'tinkering with nature', particularly in the context of reproduction and the possibility of modifying the genetic characteristics of unborn babies. Approval was also limited for many non-medical uses of genetic information, for example by employers or insurance companies, but was very high for the use of genetic information in a forensic context. Except in the case of forensic use, explicit informed consent for each use of a person's genetic information was considered vital.

Continuing public approval, or at least acceptance, will be essential if the potential of genetic science to contribute to improved human health and welfare is to be achieved. As experience with genetically modified crops has shown, lack of public acceptance can effectively bring specific applications of science to a halt. It is cause for concern that, although the MORI poll showed high levels of approval for the use of genetics in medicine, it also revealed that around 70% of those polled had little or no confidence that regulation was keeping pace with developments and research.

This level of disquiet may indicate, as some other surveys have shown, a widespread perception that genetics has advanced further than is actually the case. For example, many people think that genetic information can already be used to predict the likelihood of common disease, and that the use of genetic testing to select unborn babies with characteristics such as high intelligence is imminent. Those who have a role in keeping the public informed about developments in genetic science, including scientists themselves as well as journalists and others, have a responsibility to ensure that they give a measured and accurate account of the significance of new research findings. 'Hype' about genetics could lead to unrealistic expectations of benefits on the one hand, and unrealistic fears on the other. Both will undermine public confidence and could have the effect of withdrawing social and political support for further research.

Further reading and resources

Several books concerned with general ethical issues raised by genetics are discussed in Chapter 1 and listed in the Further reading section at the end of that chapter. For current information and commentary on ethical, legal and social implications of genetics, the Bioethics Today, BioNews and Public Health Genetics Unit websites are good sources. All these organisations also produce online newsletters.

A database of bioethics literature is maintained online by the Kennedy Institute of Ethics at Georgetown University in the US. The Wellcome Library has developed BioethicsWeb, a portal to internet resources in biomedical ethics.

For examples of current ELSI research in the UK, see the web portal to the ESRC Genomics Network, and the website of the Ethox Centre in Oxford.

Genetic reductionism, geneticisation and eugenics

Sakar (1998) has published a comprehensive critique of genetic reductionism. For discussions of geneticisation by two social scientists with somewhat different views about the phenomenon and how it can be studied, see the review by ten Have (2001) and response by Hedgecoe (2001). Melzer and Zimmern (2002) have discussed genetics and medicalisation.

Daniel Kevles, in his 1995 book *In the Name of Eugenics: Genetics and the Uses of Human Heredity*, traces the history of eugenics and the uses of human genetics, from the founding of the eugenics movement by Francis Galton to modern day genetic engineering. Buchanan *et al.* (2000), in *Chance to Choice: Genetics and Justice*, also address the ethical issues underlying eugenics, as well as the application of genetic technologies to humans, asking how these technologies should affect our understanding of distributive justice, rights and obligations of parents and the meaning of disability. Kerr and Shakespeare (1999) argue that eugenic thinking is still at work in current attitudes to testing and screening for genetic diseases.

Genetics and reproductive choice

Contributors to *The Future of Human Reproduction: Ethics, Choice and Regulation*, edited by Harris and Holm (1998), explore different areas of reproductive choice, contrasting private choice and public regulation. A recent review by Knoppers and colleagues (2006) explores socio-ethical and legal issues raised by pre-implantation genetic diagnosis. In *Human Fertilisation and Embryology: Regulating the Reproductive Revolution*, authors Robert Lee and Deryck Morgan (2001) review the regulation of assisted conception, including embryo research and cloning.

The *Journal of Medical Ethics* has on several occasions hosted debate on the nature of disability and the question of whether genetic intervention (such as selective abortion or gene therapy) on a fetus affected by a severely disabling genetic condition is morally justified. Examples are the papers by Harris and by Reindal in 2000.

A 2004 consultation paper and 2006 report from the Human Genetics Commission set out many of the questions surrounding attitudes to genetics and reproductive decision-making, exploring the moral and ethical issues in their own right but also in the context of the provision of health services. The effect of likely future developments, such as non-invasive prenatal testing technology, is also discussed.

Genetics and assisted reproduction

Emily Jackson has published an excellent discussion on matters related to assisted reproduction technology and embryo research in her 2001 book *Regulating Reproduction: Law, Technology and Autonomy*. Papers by McGee *et al.* (2001) and Patrizio *et al.* (2001) in the journal *Human Reproduction* set out the ethical and other arguments for and against mandatory disclosure to children conceived with donated gametes.

Arguments for and against the ethical acceptability of human reproductive cloning have been explained succinctly in a 2002 commentary by Brock in *Science* magazine. References for legal and policy responses to the cloning issue are outlined in Chapter 7.

Embryo research and embryonic stem cells

Several bioethics groups have commented on the ethical issues surrounding embryo research, cloning technology and embryonic stem cells, including the Nuffield Council on Bioethics and the European Group on Ethics in Science and New Technologies. Mulkay's 1997 book presents a comprehensive discussion of the debate about the moral status of the human embryo; for a shorter account, see the Lockwood's 2001 paper in the journal *Human Fertility*. Steinbrook (2006) has recently summarised some of the ethical questions surrounding egg donation, from a US perspective.

Genetic information

Murray's book chapter "Genetic exceptionalism and 'future diaries': is genetic information different from other medical information?" coins the term 'genetic exceptionalism' and details the arguments surrounding the belief that genetic information is special. A 2003 paper by Green and Botkin in *Annals of Internal Medicine* concludes that genetic tests are not different from other types of medical test but that all tests that may result in distress or stigmatisation should be carried out with great caution. Zimmern's (2001b) paper in *Genetics Law Monitor* explores the concept of 'genetic information' and the different meanings the term can have. Richards provides a sociological perspective in his 2001 paper 'How distinctive is genetic information?'.

Chapter 7 of the latest edition of *Mason and McCall Smith's Law and Medical Ethics* (Mason and Laurie 2006) is a detailed discussion of the current legal position regarding genetic information in the UK, covering issues including antenatal testing, individual and family interests in genetic information, the right to know and not to know, other parties' interest in genetic information (such as insurers and employers), and research involving genetic material.

In *Genetic Databases: Socio-Ethical Issues in the Collection and Use of DNA*, editors Richard Tutton and Oonagh Corrigan (2004) have brought together articles on subjects such as the attitudes of donors to biobanks and ethical questions surrounding informed consent procedures. In her article, 'Regulating genetic databases: some legal and ethical issues', Jean McHale (2004) outlines some of the legal and regulatory issues involved in genetic databases. Knoppers and Fecteau (2003) have outlined the case for regarding human genomic databases as a 'global public good'. For specific information on the governance of selected European and non-European biobanks, see Ann Cambon-Thomsen's 2004 review in *Nature Reviews Genetics*. A wealth of information about current population biobank projects can be found on the P3G Observatory web pages of the Public Population Project in Genomics, an international consortium that aims to promote collaboration, knowledge sharing and best practice among biobank projects. The current ethical and governance framework for the UK Biobank can be accessed on the project's website. Bronwyn Parry's book *Trading the Genome: Investigating the Commodification of Bio-Information* explores the issue of commercial access to population biobanks.

Genetic discrimination

The Human Genetics Commission's 2002 report *Inside Information* sets out the debate about many uses of genetic information, including the potential for genetic discrimination in the context of insurance, employment, medical research and forensic investigation.

For opposing views on the use of genetic information in insurance underwriting, see, for example, the papers in *Science* by Nowlan (2002), and by Hudson and colleagues (1995). The issues are discussed in detail in a 2001 report by McGlennan, albeit from an industry point of view. Two papers by Humphries and colleagues (Neil *et al.*, 2004; Hunter and Humphries 2005) report on the insurance industry's willingness to take risk-reducing behaviour into account in underwriting policies for people affected by genetic diseases.

The European Group on Ethics in Science and New Technologies has issued a well-considered opinion on genetic testing in relation to employment. A 2004 review in the *Annual Review of Public Health*, by Brandt-Rauf and Brandt-Rauf, gives a comprehensive discussion of the ethical, legal and social issues from a public health perspective.

The literature on genetics and race is complex and confusing. Risch and colleagues (2002) have argued that racial categorisation in biomedical and genetics research is useful and scientifically justified. Readers should consult the reference list of their paper, which is available free online from PubMed Central, for counter arguments. A useful web page on the website of the University of Nottingham's Institute for the Study of Genetics, Biorisks and Society collects together articles on the debate about the drug BiDiL.

Ethical and legal aspects of clinical genetics

Guidance and policy statements on many aspects of clinical genetics may be found on the websites of professional genetics groups including the British Society for Human Genetics, the American Society of Human Genetics, the American College of Medical Genetics and the European Society of Human Genetics. Chapter 7 of *Mason and McCall Smith's Law and Medical Ethics* (Mason and Laurie 2006) is an authoritative account of current UK law on many topics relevant to genetics in clinical practice.

Guidelines on consent and confidentiality in clinical genetics practice are set out in a 2006 paper by the Joint Committee on Medical Genetics.

Chadwick, Levitt and Shickle (1997) have explored the right to know, and the right not to know, genetic information about oneself. For issues related to genetic privacy, such as the tension between confidentiality and the duty to inform relatives, see Graeme Laurie's 2002 book, *Genetic Privacy: A Challenge to Medico-Legal Norms*. The issue of genetic privacy is also explored in a 2003 review by Sankar.

A commentary on regulation of the use of human tissue, in the context of the Human Tissue Act, may be found in a 2005 paper by Kathleen Liddell and Alison Hall 'Beyond Bristol and Alder Hey: the future regulation of human tissue'. Information about development of the Codes of Practice for the Human Tissue Act can be found on the website of the Human Tissue Authority.

In *The Genetic Testing of Children*, editor Angus Clarke (1998) has brought together a number of articles that explore genetic testing in the context of whether such actions promote the welfare of the child. Contributions include articles on predictive genetic testing for children, and adult attitudes towards and children's understanding of genetic testing and its implications.

The Troubled Helix: Social and Psychological Implications of the New Human Genetics, edited by Marteau and Richards (1999), explores, often from the patient's or family's perspective, many of the difficult ethical and social issues encountered in clinical genetics services.

Public perceptions of genetics

Several papers by Richards and colleagues (1996, 1997) have explored lay perceptions and understanding of genetics and genetic concepts. The results of a MORI poll on public attitudes to genetics, undertaken on behalf of the Human Genetics Commission (HGC), are available on the HGC website.

Reports arising from a European citizens' and stakeholders' conference on the *Ethical, Legal and Social Aspects of Genetic Testing: Research, Development and Clinical Applications* (European Commission, 2004a) suggests an emerging consensus on these issues in Europe, at least among those (clinical professionals and patient representatives) with direct involvement in clinical genetics.

7

Policy implications

'Policy' is defined by the *Collins English Dictionary* as 'a plan of action adopted by a person, group or government'. In the context of this book, the scope of 'policy' is very broad: it encompasses the course of action adopted by society in all those areas that affect the impact of advances in genetics on health services and health care. In most cases policy on a particular issue is not static but is constantly being reassessed and adjusted in the light of new developments or social attitudes. Some areas are so new that no current policy exists and a number of options are under consideration. Policy for the application of genetics in health services does not develop in isolation but within a much broader national and international context. Nor, in the modern world, can policy be determined in a top-down, directive way, by government departments insulated from external influences.

In this chapter, we first outline how government policy for genetics is developed and implemented in the UK and describe the current advisory and regulatory framework. We then discuss the international 'climate' for policy on genetics.

The middle sections of the chapter deal with the development of the policy framework in the UK in some key areas: reproductive decision-making, consent to genetic testing and analysis, privacy and confidentiality of genetic information, protection against unfair discrimination, regulation of the availability of genetic tests, pharmacogenetics, regulation of gene-based and cellular therapies, clinical trials and intellectual property rights in the bioscience sector.

The final section of the chapter moves away from legislation and other modes of regulation as we consider other important 'drivers' for genetics policy. These include the state of the research base, public health policy, the attitudes of citizens to the role of science and technology, the 'genetic literacy' of health professionals and of the wider society, the role of the commercial sector and national economic priorities.

Our discussion of policy issues covers developments up to June 2006 and is based primarily on the UK but on some issues we draw comparisons with developments and attitudes in other countries. This chapter should be read in conjunction with the preceding chapter (Chapter 6), in which we have outlined the conceptual basis of some of the ethical issues that must be addressed by policy makers.

How government policy for genetics is developed in the UK

The development of genetics policy at a strategic level in the UK is the responsibility of the national (Westminster) government. Within the civil service, it falls mostly within the remit of the Department of Health. Other departments also have a role to play, for example the Department of Trade and Industry, the Department for Education and Skills and, of course, the Treasury. The Policy Unit within the Prime Minister's Office, and the Cabinet Office also have an interest in developments in biotechnology and genetics.

In Scotland, Wales and (eventually) Northern Ireland, the devolved administrations have responsibility for some aspects of health policy for their populations. In genetics, for example, policy for the development and delivery of genetics services is a devolved responsibility, as are aspects of funding for research and development. In Scotland, legislation on some broader issues that affect the application of genetic science in health care, for example confidentiality, informed consent and use of human tissue, differs in some respects from the legislation in force in England and Wales.

The Department of Health's Genetics, Embryology and Assisted Conception Branch supports policy development in five main areas: stem cells and cloning; science, safety and regulation in genetics; ethics; NHS services for genetics (in England); and services, policy and regulation in assisted conception. It also provides the secretariat for three major non-statutory national advisory bodies in the area of genetics (see below), and is the main point of contact, within the Civil Service, for the statutory Human Fertilisation and Embryology Authority and Human Tissue Authority. These bodies have a UK-wide remit. Civil servants in the Department of Health also make representations on behalf of the UK Government to international bodies such as the European Commission and the United Nations.

Other areas of the Department of Health's activity that impinge on genetics include the Research and Development Programme, Connecting for Health (the agency responsible for delivering the National Programme for Information Technology), the Information Policy Unit, NHS organisation policy (affecting NHS structure and policy for commissioning services in England), and policy for patient and public involvement.

In the Department of Trade and Industry, the Bioscience Unit (part of the Business Group) and the Office of Science and Innovation (OSI) take the lead on aspects of policy related to genetic science; much of their remit is UK-wide. The Bioscience Unit focuses on research and development policy and technology

Box 7.1 The 2003 Genetics White Paper: *Our Inheritance, our Future. Realising the Potential of Genetics in the NHS*

The 2003 White Paper announced a raft of measures, supported by £50 million of investment over three years, to strengthen existing genetic services and plan for a time when genetics and genetic technology will increasingly be integrated into a broad range of health services. Funding commitments included allocations for:

- Basic research (particularly on gene therapy and pharmacogenetics)
- Increasing capacity in genetics services
- Improving services for single-gene subsets of common disease (for example, familial hypercholesterolaemia and familial cancer)
- Education and training of health professionals
- The development of information technology systems to support the use of genetic data in health care.

These commitments apply specifically to England; the devolved administrations in Wales and Scotland are responsible for deciding whether to fund similar initiatives for their populations.

transfer; regulation and intellectual property rights; and fostering the development and competitiveness of small firms in the biotechnology sector.

The OSI is headed by the Chief Scientific Adviser, who advises Government on matters concerned with science, engineering and technology; the OSI is also the Civil Service 'home' of the Director General of the Research Councils. The work of the OSI includes allocation of science funding via the Research Councils, stimulating knowledge transfer from academia to industry, improving the quality and use of science advice across Government, managing the UK's involvement in EU science and technology initiatives, and encouraging public interest and engagement in science. The OSI supports the work of the Council for Science and Technology, the UK's top-level advisory body to the Prime Minister and the First Ministers of the devolved administrations in Scotland and Wales, on strategic and cross-cutting science and technology issues.

The Government's most important specific policy initiative for genetics has been the Genetics White Paper *Our Inheritance, our Future. Realising the Potential of Genetics in the NHS*, published in June 2003 by Department of Health (2003a) (see Box 7.1).

The advisory and regulatory system for genetics

In formulating policy for genetics, Government receives advice and input from a variety of groups and organisations (Box 7.2). Some of these are statutory agencies

Box 7.2 The advisory and regulatory framework for human genetics in the UK

A large number of statutory, advisory and professional groups contribute to the advisory and regulatory framework for genetics. The following list of examples is not exhaustive.

Parliamentary bodies
House of Commons Committee on Science and Technology; House of Lords Committee on Science and Technology

Statutory bodies
Human Fertilisation and Embryology Authority; Human Tissue Authority; Medicines and Healthcare Products Regulatory Agency

Government advisory bodies
Human Genetics Commission; Gene Therapy Advisory Committee; Genetics and Insurance Committee

Non-government advisory bodies
Nuffield Council on Bioethics

Health service bodies
National Screening Committee; Genetics Commissioning Advisory Group; UK Genetic Testing Network; National Institute for Health and Clinical Excellence

Professional groups
Joint Committee on Medical Genetics; Royal Colleges; British Society for Human Genetics; Royal Society; Academy of Medical Sciences; British Medical Association

Policy research and analysis groups
Institute for Public Policy Research; Centre for Policy Studies; Public Health Genetics Unit; ESRC Genomics Policy Forum; Science and Technology Policy Research Unit

Funding organisations and charities
Research Councils; Wellcome Trust; Cancer Research UK

Organisations representing industry
Association of British Insurers; Association of the British Pharmaceutical Industry

Patient and consumer groups
Genetic Interest Group; Disability Alliance; Consumers' Association

Lobby and 'watchdog' groups
GeneWatch; Genetics Alert; Comment on Reproductive Ethics

with executive functions (for example, the Human Fertilisation and Embryology Authority and the Medicines and Healthcare Products Regulatory Agency) while others act in an advisory capacity (for example, the Human Genetics Commission). Parliament is engaged in the process both through debates in the

Houses of Parliament and through the work of Standing Committees of parliamentarians (for example, the House of Commons Science and Technology Committee). In addition, ad hoc groups are from time to time established to consider specific issues and report to Government. The Government is obliged to respond to all reports and recommendations issued by the official advisory and parliamentary committees.

The three major advisory bodies to the Government specifically in the area of genetics are the Human Genetics Commission, the Genetics and Insurance Committee and the Gene Therapy Advisory Committee. The statutory Human Fertilisation and Embryology Authority (HFEA) is responsible for regulating embryo research and assisted reproduction in the UK. Some aspects of this role are closely relevant to genetics; for example, the HFEA licenses pre-implantation genetic diagnosis treatments and clinics, and the derivation of embryonic stem cells. The Human Tissue Authority has responsibility for overseeing compliance with the Human Tissue Act. In 2008 the HFEA and the HTA will merge to form a new regulatory authority, the Regulatory Authority for Tissue and Embryos.

As discussed in Chapter 5, a variety of specialist advisory groups also support genetics-related work in the NHS at a directly operational level. These include the National Screening Committee, the Genetics Commissioning Advisory Group and the UK Genetic Testing Network Steering Group. The National Institute for Health and Clinical Excellence, an independent body that makes recommendations to the NHS on treatments and health care that merit NHS funding, has also done some work in the area of genetics, for example on guidelines for the identification and management of genetic risk in breast cancer.

In addition to these sources of official advice and regulation, the Government takes note of reports and representations from a plethora of non-governmental groups including professional organisations, patient and consumer groups, industry representatives, 'watchdog' and lobby groups, policy research institutes, academics, research funding and many others.

The international context for genetics policy

Most regulation and legislation affecting genetics originates either in the UK or the European Union (the UK is obliged to incorporate EU Directives into national law) but there also is a wider international context for policy development. For example, there have been several attempts to achieve international consensus on ethical standards for applications of genetics in human health and medical care. International bodies such as the United Nations agencies, the Council of Europe, the World Medical Association and others have all formulated guidelines and protocols (Box 7.3).

For example, in 1997 the United Nations Educational, Scientific and Cultural Organisation (UNESCO) drew up the *Universal Declaration on the Human Genome and Human Rights*, which was adopted by UNESCO's General Conference later that year and endorsed by the United Nations General Assembly in 1998. The Declaration affirms the dignity of each individual human being, regardless of his or her genetic endowment, and sets out ethical principles for the conduct of research, treatment or diagnosis related to characteristics of a person's genome. It calls upon states to outlaw discrimination based on genetic characteristics if such discrimination would have the effect of 'infringing human rights, fundamental freedoms and human dignity'.

These principles are reiterated in UNESCO's 2005 *Universal Declaration on Bioethics and Human Rights*, which sets out principles relating to human dignity, autonomy and individual responsibility, consent (including protection for those lacking capacity to consent), privacy and confidentiality, respect for cultural diversity, non-discrimination, and sharing benefits within society and the international community. The Declaration encourages states to establish national ethics committees, foster bioethics education and promote international cooperation to encourage the sharing of scientific and technological knowledge.

The World Health Organization has also published several documents related to ethical issues in human genetics, including *Review of Ethical Issues in Medical Genetics* (2003b). The Review builds on an earlier consensus document published in 1998, and discusses ethical principles that should govern the practice of medical genetics, including genetic counselling, presymptomatic and susceptibility testing, antenatal and pre-implantation testing, and population genetic screening.

An international institution that has been particularly active in genetics and related areas is the Council of Europe. This organisation, not to be confused with the European Union, was founded in 1949 with a remit to defend human rights, parliamentary democracy and the rule of law, and develop Europe-wide agreements to standardise members' social and legal practices. Its 45 members include all 25 members of the European Union. Council of Europe Conventions are not legally binding upon member states unless actively incorporated into national legislation.

In 1998 the UK Government adopted the 1953 Council of Europe's Convention for the Protection of Human Rights and Fundamental Freedoms, incorporated into national law as the Human Rights Act (UK Government 1998). Several provisions of this law could have a significant impact on health policy. Article 2

Box 7.3 Examples of international reports and policy declarations in genetics, biomedicine and bioethics

United Nations Educational Scientific and Cultural Organisation (UNESCO)

- *Universal Declaration on the Human Genome and Human Rights* (1997)
- UNESCO Report of the International Bioethics Committee on confidentiality and genetic data (2000)
- Report of the International Bioethics Committee on *The Use of Embryonic Stem Cells in Therapeutic Research* (2001)
- Report of the International Bioethics Committee on *Preimplantation Genetic Diagnosis and Germ-Line Intervention* (2003)
- *International Declaration on Human Genetic Data* (2003)
- *International Declaration on Bioethics and Human Rights* (2005)

World Health Organization

- Statement of expert advisory group on ethical issues in medical genetics: *Proposed International Guidelines on Ethical Issues in Medical Genetics and Genetic Services* (1998)
- *Statement of the WHO Expert Consultation on New Developments in Human Genetics* (2000)
- *Human Genetic Technologies. Implications for Preventive Health Care* (2002)
- *Genetic Databases: Assessing the Benefits and the Impact on Human and Patient Rights* (2003a)
- *Review of Ethical Issues in Medical Genetics* (2003b)
- *Genetics, Genomics and Patenting DNA. Review of Potential Implications for Health in Developing Countries* (2005)

Council of Europe

- *Convention for the Protection of Human Rights and Fundamental Freedoms* (1953)
- *Convention on Human Rights and Biomedicine* [1997; includes additional protocols on cloning (1998), transplantation (2001) and biomedical research (2005)]

Organisation for Economic Cooperation and Development (OECD)

- *Guidelines for the Protection of Privacy and Transborder Flows of Personal Data* (1980)
- *Genetic Testing. Policy Issues for the New Millennium* (2001)
- *Quality Assurance and Proficiency Testing for Molecular Genetic Testing. A Survey of 18 OECD Member Countries* (2005)
- *Guidelines for the Licensing of Genetic Inventions* (2006)

World Medical Association

- *Ethical Principles for Medical Research Involving Human Subjects* (WMA Declaration of Helsinki) (1964; latest update 2004)
- *Declaration on Ethical Considerations Regarding Health Databases* (2002)

Box 7.3 (cont.)

- *Statement on Genetics and Medicine* (2005; consolidates and revises earlier statement on genetic counselling and engineering, declaration on human genome project, and resolution on cloning)

Council for International Organisations of Medical Sciences

- *Declaration of Inuyama. Human Genome Mapping, Genetic Screening and Gene Therapy* (1990)
- *International Ethical Guidelines for Biomedical Research Involving Human Subjects* (2002)

of the Convention provides for a right to life, Article 3 for freedom from degrading treatment, Article 8 for the right to private and family life, and Article 14 for freedom from discrimination in the enjoyment of these rights. Antenatal diagnosis, pre-implantation genetic diagnosis, embryo manipulation and therapeutic abortion could all potentially come under renewed scrutiny in the light of these provisions of the Act. So far its impact in these areas appears to have been small, though it has been invoked in a case concerning consent for the storage and implantation of embryos produced by in vitro fertilisation.

The Council of Europe has tended to take a restrictive stance on applications of human genetics but this has found less favour in the UK. Its Convention on Human Rights and Biomedicine (1997) states, for example, that *any* form of discrimination against a person on the grounds of his or her genetic constitution should be prohibited; that *any* genetic test, including a test to detect a predisposition or susceptibility to disease, must be accompanied by genetic counselling; and that the creation of embryos for research purposes should be illegal. Provisions such as these are considered too sweeping (and/or at odds with aspects of national legislation) by many countries including the UK, which has not signed the Convention. Additional protocols to the Convention have also been developed, covering areas such as cloning, transplantation of organs and tissues, and biomedical research.

As the progress of these initiatives has shown, achieving international consensus on policy for genetic science is not easy, and in some areas may be impossible as a result of the very different social, cultural, political and religious influences at work in different countries. A further problem is that the emphasis of most international protocols has been on the rights of the individual alone, with little or no consideration of the public-interest dimension. Public health genetics stresses the need to achieve a balance between society's obligations to the individual, and the individual's responsibilities to society; it is important to ensure that this viewpoint is properly represented on the various committees charged with drawing up international protocols.

Policy for key issues in genetics

We now move our focus back to the UK to consider policy development in some key areas for genetics. In such a broad-ranging discussion we can give only a brief outline of the legislative and regulatory framework relevant to each issue, and our summaries should not be regarded as constituting legal advice or opinion. Readers should refer to the Further reading section at the end of the chapter for more detailed commentaries.

Genetics in reproductive decision-making

One of the most contentious policy questions raised by genetics concerns the extent to which the state should regulate the use of genetic testing in reproductive decision-making. We have discussed the ethical and moral arguments in Chapter 6. Here, we outline the current policy situation in the UK for antenatal genetic testing, pre-implantation genetic diagnosis, population screening and assisted reproduction technologies.

A Human Genetics Commission (HGC 2006a) report published in January 2006 (*Making Babies: Reproductive Decisions and Genetic Technologies*) generally endorsed the current legal and regulatory framework for the use of genetics in reproductive decision-making but recommended improvements in some aspects of counselling and provision of information to couples, and further research on outcomes for children born as a result of use of new reproductive technologies such as pre-implantation genetic diagnosis. One omission from the HGC's report is the issue of consanguinity, which has been the subject of growing discussion, including calls by one Member of Parliament for consanguineous marriages to be banned. This issue must be treated with extreme care. A legal ban on consanguineous marriages is clearly not justified (except, of course, for incestuous marriages, which are already illegal) but a case could be made for a sensitive approach, led by the communities themselves, that included provision of clear and accurate information about the level of risk, which in most cases is low.

Antenatal genetic testing

Antenatal diagnostic genetic testing is not, in itself, currently subject to legal restrictions in the UK. Whether a test is carried out is a matter for decision by the woman or couple concerned, and the professional judgement of the clinician carrying out the test.

If a woman seeks a termination of pregnancy on the basis of a test result, that action is subject to the provisions of the 1967 Abortion Act (UK Government 1967), as amended by the 1990 Human Fertilisation and Embryology Act (UK Government 1990). Under these Acts, abortion is legal up to 24 weeks' gestation provided it is carried out by a doctor, and provided two doctors agree that continuation of the pregnancy would pose a risk to the woman's health (including her mental health) or to the health of any existing children in her family. There is no time limit to the abortion if the fetus is found to be affected by a serious physical or mental handicap.

Questions have been raised about the use of antenatal genetic testing for non-lethal conditions such as deafness, or incompletely penetrant late-onset conditions such as *BRCA1*- or *BRCA2*-related breast cancer. A survey of public opinion by the HGC revealed a mixed response to the issue. The current position is that testing and termination of pregnancy within 24 weeks in such cases is legal provided the provisions of the Abortion Act are met. There is no evidence that antenatal diagnostic testing has so far been requested for such conditions in the UK. Any attempt to institute more restrictive regulation of antenatal genetic testing would be problematic as it could be construed as discriminating against women who had genetic reasons for wishing to terminate a pregnancy.

In the case of late abortions, doctors may need more explicit guidance as to what sorts of conditions (including genetic conditions) constitute a 'serious handicap'. The late abortion of a fetus affected by cleft lip and palate was subject to legal challenge in 2005. The decision was made not to prosecute the doctors concerned, as they were considered to have acted in good faith, but professional organisations including the Royal College of Obstetricians and Gynaecologists have called for clearer guidelines to protect doctors in this situation.

Pre-implantation genetic diagnosis

Statutory regulation does apply to genetic testing by pre-implantation genetic diagnosis (PGD), because it involves in vitro fertilisation (IVF) and therefore comes under the provisions of the 1990 Human Fertilisation and Embryology (HFE) Act (UK Government 1990). The Human Fertilisation and Embryology Authority (HFEA) is responsible for licensing treatments involving PGD. In doing so, it generally applies the criterion, under the HFE Act, that the aim of testing is to enable a couple to avoid the birth of a child with a serious genetic disease. Sex selection by PGD is permitted for couples at risk of transmitting a sex-linked disease but the HFEA does not license the use of PGD for sex selection for 'social purposes' such as family balancing. In some cases, the HFEA permits the use of PGD to test embryos for chromosomal abnormalities before they are used for IVF: aneuploidy screening may be considered for older women (who are at increased risk of having children with chromosomal abnormalities), women with a history of recurrent miscarriage, or women who have experienced repeated IVF failure.

In 2002, the HFEA decided to allow the use of PGD with tissue typing to enable a couple to select an embryo that would be both free of the inherited disease beta-thalassaemia and a tissue match for an affected older sibling. The aim was to use cord blood from the baby to treat the sibling. This decision has survived subsequent legal challenge by a 'pro-life' group. More recently, the HFEA has also permitted PGD to be used solely for tissue matching to an older sibling; in other words, in a case where the embryo itself was not at risk of an inherited disease.

The current regulatory regime for PGD does not meet with universal approval. In March 2005 the House of Commons Select Committee on Science and Technology published a controversial report on human reproductive technologies which recommended removing PGD from regulation by the HFEA and allowing individuals and couples to exercise personal choice on issues such as sex selection and 'saviour siblings'. The Government rejected (UK Government 2005a) this recommendation but agreed that the parameters for PGD should be more clearly defined and stated its intention to seek the public's views on acceptable uses of PGD and the nature and scope of appropriate regulation. Following a public consultation exercise during 2005, the HFEA has decided in principle that it is prepared to license the use of PGD to test embryos for serious but incompletely penetrant late-onset conditions such as hereditary non-polyposis colorectal cancer (HNPCC), or breast cancer related to mutations in the *BRCA1* and *BRCA2* genes. Each request will be considered on its own merits.

There is clearly a discrepancy between the tight regulatory control of PGD and the less stringent restrictions on antenatal genetic testing, despite the fact that many would regard antenatal testing (with the option of abortion) as the more morally problematic of the two. The situation is, however, consistent with a general trend towards tighter regulation of procedures that are technologically complex, make heavy demands on the state's resources and carry a high opportunity cost.

The widespread availability of information over the Internet and the willingness of some individuals and couples to travel abroad if the treatment they seek is not available in their own country have led to a small but growing trend towards 'health tourism' in general, and 'reproductive tourism' in particular. Some couples who were originally denied permission to use PGD with tissue matching sought treatment abroad, and there is evidence that some women are travelling to other countries to seek late abortions. There is little that national governments can do to prevent individuals from evading national regulatory regimes in this way. The existence of a global 'market' in health care also affects the regulation of assisted reproduction technologies, discussed later in this chapter.

Population screening programmes

Current population screening programmes in the UK are outlined in Chapter 5. In Chapter 6 we have discussed some of the ethical and social issues raised by population screening. A review of national policy for population screening in the context of reproductive choice was included in the HGC's 2006 report *Making Babies: Reproductive Decisions and Genetic Technologies* (Human Genetics Commission 2006a). The HGC generally endorsed the availability of antenatal screening for couples who decide that they wish to avoid the birth of a child with a serious genetic condition such as Down syndrome. However, it recognised the concerns of those who feel that screening and abortion of affected fetuses devalues the lives of disabled people. It recommended that the best way to address this issue was to ensure that there is a strong programme of research to find better therapies for genetic conditions, and that high-quality services are available for affected individuals and their families.

The HGC report supported the work of the National Screening Committee in setting rigorous criteria for the introduction of new screening programmes and the evaluation of existing programmes, but identified some problems in the quality of the delivery of screening programmes. It recommended that the Department of Health should commission a review of information, counselling and support services for couples whose fetuses are diagnosed with a serious genetic condition.

Assisted reproduction technologies

The use of IVF technology is regulated by the 1990 Human Fertilisation and Embryology Act, and IVF clinics must be licensed by the HFEA.

As discussed in Chapter 6, the growing use of donated gametes (sperm or eggs) or embryos to assist infertile couples has raised questions about the general right of any resulting children to know about their biological parentage and, in particular, to have access to any relevant genetic information about them. There is also a need for regulation of the donation process to ensure that donors are not coerced and that donated materials meet standards of quality and safety.

Under the Human Fertilisation and Embryology Authority (Disclosure of Donor Information) Regulations 2004, individuals conceived through donations made after 31 March 2005 have the right, from the age of 18, to obtain the donor's identity and certain information about them including their ethnic origin and country of birth. A couple wishing to marry may also find out from the HFEA whether they are related to their intended partner, in order to avoid the possibility of a consanguineous marriage. In practice, it may be difficult to enforce these legal provisions if parents are unwilling to tell their child that they were conceived using donated material. The Human Genetics Commission in January 2006 (Human Genetics Commission 2006a) recommended that greater efforts should be made to ensure that parents are aware of the importance of telling children about their genetic origins, and that counselling should be available to assist them.

The HFEA's code of practice sets out the medical information required from donors in order to reduce the possibility of a serious disease being passed on to the child. This information includes details of family history. Donors are also tested for certain infectious diseases and for carrier status for some recessive conditions. The conditions tested for include cystic fibrosis, Tay Sachs disease or haemoglobinopathies, depending on the racial/ethnic origin of the donor. The requirements for donor screening and testing may be revised in light of the 2004 Sperm Egg and Embryo Donation (SEED) review (Human Fertilisation and Embryo Authority 2004b), which recommended that consolidated guidance should be produced by a joint group involving the main relevant professional bodies.

Fertility clinics using donated gametes or embryos must also comply with the provisions of the UK's Human Fertilisation and Embryology Act (UK Government 1990) and with the EU Tissue Directive (European Parliament and Council 2004a; discussed further later in this chapter), which imposes standards for quality and safety of donated tissues and cells. The SEED review included a review of HFEA procedures as part of preparations for ensuring compliance with the EU Tissue Directive. The Review's recommendations included: gametes donated by an individual should not be used to produce children for more than ten families in the UK; eggs collected from a woman during a single cycle should not be shared with more than two other recipients; donors may receive reasonable reimbursement of expenses incurred by donation; and gametes sourced from abroad should meet the same quality standards as those that apply in the UK.

In late 2005 the Government carried out a public consultation on the Human Fertilisation and Embryology Act (Department of Health 2005d), as part of a wide-ranging review of the Act (UK Government 1990) that may lead to significant changes. Issues explored in the consultation include the extent to which the welfare of the potential child should govern access to fertility treatment, information to be provided to donor-conceived people, surrogacy, sex selection for non-medical reasons, and the criteria for embryo screening and selection by procedures including PGD. The Government may also attempt to regulate internet services supplying gametes.

The use of cloning in assisted reproduction is illegal in the UK under the Human Reproductive Cloning Act (UK Government 2001b). The Government decided that explicit legislation was needed in order to ensure that reproductive cloning was clearly distinguished from 'therapeutic cloning' (the use of cloning technology to produce embryonic stem cells for potential therapeutic use) which, as discussed later in this chapter, is legal under supplementary Regulations (passed in 2001) to the 1990 Human Fertilisation and Embryology Act.

Consent to genetic testing and analysis

As discussed in Chapter 6, in the context of ethical and legal issues in clinical genetics, the main pieces of legislation governing consent to genetic analysis of a human biological sample are the Human Tissue Act 2004 (UK Government 2004c) and the Mental Capacity Act 2005 (UK Government 2005b). In this chapter, we will consider the policy context of this legislation and in particular its effect on genetic and genomic research.

The Human Tissue Act 2004

The Human Tissue Act 2004 (UK Government 2004c) originated as a response to the organ retention scandals at the Liverpool Children's Hospital (Alder Hey) (The Royal Liverpool Children's Inquiry 2001) and the Bristol Royal Infirmary (Bristol Royal Infirmary Inquiry 2001), and to subsequent investigations which revealed that many other hospitals had collections of tissue, ranging from paraffin blocks and histology slides through to whole organs, for which they were not able to demonstrate that adequate consent had been obtained. Existing legislation governing consent for the use of tissue was regarded as inadequate. The Government decided also to use the Human Tissue Act as the vehicle for acting on the Human Genetics Commission's recommendation that non-consensual DNA testing should be a criminal offence.

Under the provisions of the Human Tissue Act it is legal to store and use relevant tissue from the living and to remove, store and use relevant tissue from the dead for a specific set of purposes, provided 'appropriate consent' has been obtained from the donor or, if the donor is dead and has not made his or her wishes clear before death, from a nominated representative, relative or a friend of long standing. There is a specified hierarchy of individuals who are able to give consent in this situation.

Among the purposes requiring consent are research in connection with disorders, or the functioning, of the human body (including genetic research); and obtaining scientific or medical information about a living or deceased person which may be relevant to any other person, including a future person. If the prospective donor is dead, consent is also required for an additional set of purposes: clinical audit, education or training relating to human health, performance assessment, public health monitoring and quality assurance. These activities may be carried out without consent on material from living donors.

As pointed out in Chapter 6, the Human Tissue Act does not regulate the analysis of DNA as such, but makes it an offence to hold a sample of bodily material (that is, material that consists of or includes human cells) with the intention of analysing the DNA contained within it, without consent. Where material from a person is needed for DNA analysis, 'qualifying consent' is required rather than appropriate consent. If the material is from a deceased person the difference, essentially, is that the list of 'qualifying relatives' is unranked (see

Chapter 6, Box 6.2). The provisions relating to DNA analysis apply to the whole of the UK, unlike the rest of the Act which applies only in England and Wales.

The Human Tissue Act specifies some concessions when samples are used to extract DNA for research purposes: consent to use the samples in the context of research is not required provided that the tissue comes from a living person, the research has ethical approval, and the person carrying out the analysis is not able to identify the donor, and is not likely to be able to do so in the future. These provisions cover both irreversibly anonymised samples and coded or 'pseudo-anonymised' samples (see Chapter 6 for definitions), provided that the person holding the encryption key is not a member of the research team.

The Human Tissue Act establishes a new statutory body, the Human Tissue Authority, to provide guidance about the law and oversee compliance. A licence from the Authority is needed to carry out specific activities including the removal, storage and certain uses of tissue from a dead person or storage of human tissue from a living person. In the context of genetic and genomic research, licences may be required to enable tissue to be stored as a precursor to DNA extraction and analysis in England and Wales.

The implementation of the Human Tissue Act is likely to increase both the costs of research and the administrative burden on researchers and the NHS. For example, procedures and documentation for establishing that valid consent has been obtained must be developed by every organisation carrying out activities regulated by the Act. Where activities require a licence, the fact that licences will be site, person and purpose specific is likely to cause difficulties – and considerable expense – for organisations holding multiple collections for different purposes, or samples or collections dispersed between different sites. Training will be required for all staff to ensure that they understand their responsibilities under the Act. Any person operating in breach of the Act is committing a criminal offence and is personally liable to a fine and/or a prison sentence.

Some researchers consider that the provisions of the Human Tissue Act are disproportionate to the problems it was designed to solve, and that the policy balance has shifted too far in the direction of individual rights and autonomy, at the expense of the public interest. The history of the Human Tissue Act illustrates the way in which a powerful political imperative – in this case the Government's need to be seen to be taking rapid action in response to the organ retention scandals – may sometimes overwhelm the gradualist, consultative processes that normally apply in policy development, at least in the UK.

Research on samples from individuals who lack the capacity to consent

The Human Tissue Act also provides for regulations to be made deeming consent to use of material from those lacking capacity to consent, pending the commencement of the Mental Capacity Act in 2007. The Regulations, implemented on 1 September 2006, provide that an individual may be deemed to have consented to the use of material for certain purposes provided that the research has the approval of a research ethics committee and that research of comparable effectiveness cannot be carried out on individuals who are able to give consent, or on anonymised material. These purposes include obtaining information for the benefit of others – provided that this is in the best interests of the patient – and use in clinical trials.

The Mental Capacity Act establishes more comprehensive regulation of genetic and genomic research using material from those lacking competence to consent. It sets out the basis for ethical approval of intrusive research involving those lacking capacity and establishes a requirement to consult a carer or nominee for advice as to whether an incompetent person should participate in a particular research project, taking account of what that person's wishes and feelings would be if they were competent.

This is an area in which the law is rapidly evolving. Regulations and Codes of Practice to the Human Tissue Act and the Mental Capacity Act are not yet finalised and it is unclear how these will interrelate.

Privacy and confidentiality of genetic information

In Chapter 6 we discussed the ethical principles underlying the use of genetic information, and the ethical and legal framework for confidentiality in the clinical genetics setting. In this chapter we consider the regulation of other uses of genetic information, particularly in the context of medical research, and explore the policy debate about whether there should be specific legal protection for genetic information.

The legislative framework for the use of medical information in research

The growing burden of regulation governing the use of personal information has had a profound impact on all medical research but particularly on epidemiological research that requires the use of medical and other data about many hundreds or even thousands of people. The large genetic association studies and population biobank projects that are designed to tease out the contribution of common genetic variants to disease risk, and to help understand gene–environment interactions (see Chapter 3) come into this category. As discussed in Chapter 6, there are also many disease-based databases: collections of information, held by individual researchers or groups of researchers, about people suffering from specific diseases, including genetic diseases and diseases with a genetic component.

In the UK and most other western developed nations, the response to concerns about the mass of information now held about many individual citizens, particularly information held on computers and computer networks, has been a drive towards the development of statutory controls. This has left little room for manoeuvre in the debate about what level of regulation ought to be applied in this area, and has led to confusion among health professionals and others about the legality of some long-standing practices.

Researchers working with medical data relating to living identifiable individuals, or health professionals who are asked to provide such data for research projects must work within a regulatory framework that includes both legal requirements and health service codes of practice (summarised in simplified form in Box 7.4). The key piece of legislation affecting use of personally identifiable information is the Data Protection Act 1998 (DPA) (UK Government 1998), which incorporates into UK law the provisions of the 1995 EU Data Protection Directive. Any research that involves the use of identifiable data on NHS patients must also obtain approval from an NHS research ethics committee and from a 'Caldicott Guardian' – a person nominated by the relevant NHS Trust as having responsibility for ensuring proper use and confidentiality of patients' health data. Health professionals asked to disclose records for use in research also have a duty of confidentiality to patients under the common law.

The DPA applies to all personally identifiable data about living individuals. It sets out eight data protection principles for the fair and lawful 'processing' of data, where 'processing' means essentially anything that might be done with the data, including obtaining, storing, altering, disclosing or destroying them. Data may only be used for lawful purposes that are specified by the data controller. The data controller has certain obligations which include ensuring that the data are accurate and up-to-date, held securely, and not kept for longer than is necessary.

Special provisions apply to 'sensitive' personal data, including health data. In most circumstances, in order to meet the requirement for lawful processing, the *explicit* consent of the data subject (the person to whom the data relate) must be obtained, unless the processing can be shown to be necessary for one of a specific set of purposes. One of these is 'medical purposes', which includes medical research. In practice, researchers and health professionals responsible for medical records have generally been advised to seek explicit consent wherever possible, because of the difficulty of proving the *necessity* of proceeding without consent. (We shall discuss current debate about how the legal requirements for consent should be interpreted later in this section.)

Explicit consent is not required under the DPA if data can be completely anonymised so that they are no longer personally identifiable. If data are key-coded or pseudo-anonymised, the custodians of the key-coding system must comply with the DPA. However, for some research purposes anonymisation may not be possible, as information such as the age, sex and place of birth of the

Box 7.4 The legal and regulatory framework in England and Wales for use of medical information in research

1. Legal requirements

Data Protection Act 1998 – The eight data protection principles state that data must be:

- Processed fairly and lawfully (including more stringent consent requirements for 'sensitive' personal information)
- Processed only for specified lawful purposes and not used for any purpose other than those specified
- Adequate, relevant and not excessive in relation to the purpose for which it is being processed
- Accurate and up-to-date
- Not kept longer than necessary
- Processed in accordance with the rights of the data subject
- Protected by appropriate security
- Not transferred outside the EU without adequate protection.

Human Rights Act 1998 – Article 8 sets out an individual's 'right to respect for private and family life'.

Common law duty of confidentiality – a breach of confidence under the common law may occur if information that is communicated in circumstances entailing an obligation of confidence (for example, in the course of a medical consultation) is disclosed without consent. The courts recognise some situations in which disclosure is justified; for example, if there is a legal obligation to disclose the information, or there is an over-riding duty to the public in disclosing it.

Section 60 of the Health and Social Care Act 2001 – allows the Secretary of State for Health (advised by the Patient Information Advisory Group) to make Regulations allowing the processing of identifiable 'patient information' without explicit consent, for specific 'medical purposes' (defined as in the *Data Protection Act*) that are in the interests of improving patient care or in the public interest. The Secretary of State and Patient Information Advisory Group must be satisfied that it is not possible/practicable to anonymise information or obtain consent. Permission must be reviewed annually.

2. Health service codes of practice

Caldicott Guardians – each NHS Trust has to appoint a senior health professional whose key responsibilities are to oversee the use of personal health information and ensure that patients' confidentiality is respected. Caldicott Guardian approval is needed to access patient-identifiable information held by the Trust.

NHS Code of Confidentiality – summarises the legal requirements for data protection, interpretation of the law and NHS procedures for compliance.

Research Ethics Committee – the role of research ethics committees is to protect the rights, dignity and welfare of people participating in research. All NHS research projects require approval from a research ethics committee.

individual may be needed as part of the project; such information, combined with readily available public records, may be sufficient to identify an individual.

The need for explicit consent to use personally identifiable medical information is waived for certain purposes specified in Section 60 of the Health and Social Care Act (UK Government 2001a, which applies in England and Wales). These purposes must be approved by the Secretary of State for Health, who is advised by a body called the Patient Information Advisory Group (PIAG). They must be purposes for which it is impossible to use anonymised information, and for which it would not be practicable to obtain explicit consent. Purposes that have been granted this waiver include cancer registries, communicable disease surveillance and a variety of epidemiological research projects.

Regardless of whether explicit consent is required, those using or disclosing medical information for research purposes must comply with the DPA's requirement for 'fair' processing of the information. In practice, this means that individuals whose data are to be used must be *informed* of the fact and provided with certain information, including who will be using the data and for what purpose. Individuals must be free to opt out if they are not willing to allow their data to be used. The Information Commissioner has issued guidance on the nature and amount of information required in different circumstances. In some situations, for example, it may be acceptable to provide broad, general information about the nature of the research if it is not possible to specify every potential future use of the data. There are also circumstances in which it could be acceptable to use general forms of communication such as leaflets or posters as a way of providing information about a proposed use of medical data, rather than individual letters to each person concerned.

The NHS National Programme for IT Connecting for Health, which includes a programme for development of an electronic care record for all NHS patients, also contains plans for developing robust procedures for seeking patient consent, and for anonymisation of patient data for use in audit and research. The Section 60 provisions of the Health and Social Care Act, and the PIAG, are intended as temporary measures pending the implementation of this system.

In summary, under the current legal framework medical researchers, or custodians of medical data required for research, should seek explicit consent or use irreversibly anonymised data if possible, and must inform individuals if their data are to be used.

The interpretation of data protection law

The requirements for data protection in medical research are regarded by many researchers as very onerous. The source of much of the difficulty lies not in the DPA itself but in the spotlight it has thrown on the health professional's common law duty of confidentiality: the DPA requires that data must be processed 'lawfully', that is in compliance with the common law and other relevant statutes, and the common law imposes a duty of confidentiality unless explicit consent is obtained.

As we have already outlined, the DPA contains provisions for the use of personal data without consent in some circumstances, and there has always been a public-interest defence against a breach of confidentiality. These principles have rarely been tested in the courts, however, and in recent years lawyers have tended to advise medical professionals and others responsible for holding medical records that they should not put themselves at risk. Several professional bodies, including the General Medical Council (2002), the Medical Research Council (2000) and the British Medical Association (1999, 2005a), have issued guidance on the use of medical information in research; these guidelines have tended to recommend a very cautious approach.

Some commentators, including a working party set up by the Academy of Medical Sciences (AMS), have suggested that this degree of caution is not warranted. The AMS 2006 report argues that identifiable medical data can legally be used for research without consent, provided that the use 'is necessary and is proportionate with respect to privacy and public interest benefits'. For example, in the case of epidemiological research requiring access to many thousands of records, where seeking consent may be very expensive and may bias the results of the study, and where there is no conceivable harm to those whose data are used, the use of data without consent may be justifiable under both the DPA and the common law. The report calls for improvements in and simplification of the process for approving research proposals. It also suggests a need for more research on public attitudes to research using personal data.

The 2006 AMS report also recommends that the Department of Health should ensure that research needs are fully considered during the development of the electronic care record under the Connecting for Health programme. It is likely that a new regulatory body will be set up to oversee use of patient data and to seek a balance between individual rights and society's interest in facilitating medical research.

Federal legislation in the US

In the US, regulations were introduced in 2002, under the Health Insurance Portability and Accountability Act (US Congress 1996), to protect medical records and other personal information held by bodies such as health maintenance organisations, healthcare providers and health insurers. Usually referred to as the Federal Privacy Rule, the Standards for Privacy of Individually Identifiable Health Information (US Congress 2002) are similar in many respects to the provisions of the DPA in respect of medical information: consent of the data subject is the cornerstone principle, but disclosure without consent is permitted in certain situations, which include 'public interest and benefit activities'. This category includes research. Information protected by the Privacy Rule can be disclosed for use in research without consent under certain conditions, for example if an Institutional Review Board agrees that a waiver on consent is required. Some of the provisions of the Federal Privacy Rule have proved controversial: some civil liberty groups regard the provisions for disclosure without consent (especially to government agencies) as too sweeping, while researchers have found achieving compliance with the Rule onerous and sometimes confusing.

Specific protection for genetic information

An important policy question concerns whether additional measures are needed to protect *genetic* information, beyond those that apply to medical information in general. We have discussed definitions of 'genetic information' and the theoretical arguments for and against 'genetic exceptionalism' in Chapter 6. So far there is no specific legislative protection for genetic information in the UK.

The Human Genetics Commission (HGC) considered this and other issues in an extensive review of genetic information published in its 2002 report *Inside Information: Balancing Interests in the Use of Personal Genetic Data*. The HGC concluded that genetic information was particularly sensitive when it was highly predictive, and when it carried serious implications for other family members. It followed, then, that not all genetic information needed the same level of protection and that requirements for consent and confidentiality would differ according to the circumstances. The report stressed, as a general principle, the need to achieve an optimum balance between the right and wish of people to keep their genetic information private, and their obligations to other family members and to society as a whole to share that information under some circumstances.

Various international bodies have given specific consideration to policy for genetic information, including UNESCO's International Bioethics Committee (*International Declaration on Human Genetic Data*, adopted by UNESCO's General Conference in 2003) and the World Health Organization (2003a) (*Genetic Databases: Assessing the Benefits and the Impact on Human and Patient Rights*). In general, the recommendations of these bodies are based on the premise that genetic data have a special status on the basis of their potential predictive power, implications for families and possible cultural significance for individuals and groups, and the possibility that genetic information about an individual may turn out to have significance not recognised at the time when the original biological sample was collected.

While documents such as the UNESCO Declaration articulate some important values, there is a danger that they fuel a genetic exceptionalist attitude that puts all genetic information, whatever its predictive power, in a single category, and hamper the development of a rational approach in which genetic factors take their rightful place as an important determinant of health along with environmental and lifestyle factors. Most individual countries have so far shied away from introducing specific legal protections for genetic information.

Genetic information and current data protection law

The Article 29 Data Protection Working Party (2004), an EU expert group whose role is to advise the European Commission on matters relating to data protection and to promote uniform application of current data protection legislation throughout the EU, commented on the issues raised by genetic data in a 'working document' issued in 2004 (Article 29 Data Protection Working Party 2004). The Working Party confirmed that genetic data should be regarded as 'sensitive' personal data as defined by the Data Protection Directive. In general it appeared content that the Directive provides adequate protection for genetic data but it noted that the Directive does not address issues raised by the familial nature of these data.

The Working Party suggested that in the context of genetic data it might be relevant to consider a biologically related family group as a 'new legal entity'. However, it was unable to resolve the potentially conflicting rights of different individuals within the group, suggesting only that each situation should be considered on a case-by-case basis. By this reasoning, it could be permissible – at least under data protection legislation – for an individual to demand access to genetic information about a close relative if the information had direct and serious implications for the individual's health (as discussed in Chapter 6 in the context of clinical genetics practice), but he or she would not have rights over the processing of less serious information such as low-penetrance genetic polymorphisms associated with increased susceptibility to a common disease.

A related question, for which there is also as yet no clear legal answer, concerns family history data, a type of genetic information that by definition contains medical information about an individual's close relatives. An example might be the information that an individual's mother, who is still living, had a diagnosis of breast cancer at age 50. It is not clear whether data protection law and all it entails (for example, the obligation to seek explicit consent for processing the data) extends to any living relatives specified by family history information. The Joint Committee on Medical Genetics' 2006 report on *Consent and Confidentiality* suggests that most family history information that is used to construct a pedigree 'is likely to be known to a wide circle of people' including the patient concerned, implying that it is in some sense in the public domain. It stresses that family history and pedigree information is held in confidence by the genetics centre but states that guidance from the Information Commissioner indicates that such information can be passed between health professionals without explicit consent from all those concerned, provided that the processing is for medical purposes.

Protection against unfair discrimination

Calls are often made to outlaw discrimination against people on the basis of their genetic make-up. Discrimination, meaning treating people differently on the basis of their different characteristics, is not necessarily wrong in itself; rather, it becomes so if the discrimination is unfair or contravenes human rights. The difficulty, not unique to genetics, is in deciding what is unfair. An added difficulty is deciding exactly what constitutes 'genetic discrimination'.

In the western developed world, many aspects of discrimination against disabled people are regarded as unfair and are not permitted. The UK's Disability Discrimination Act (UK Government 2005c) outlaws discrimination against disabled people in areas such as employment, access to public transport and access to goods and services. The Act applies to people who have a current disability, so it covers those who have a symptomatic genetic disease but not someone whose genetic make-up may increase their risk of future disability. This exclusion has been criticised by some disability rights campaigning groups.

There is currently no specific legislation in the UK that protects individuals or groups against discrimination based on genetic characteristics. In 2005 the Government set up The Equalities Review 'to investigate the causes of persistent discrimination and inequality in British society'. Alongside The Equalities Review (2005), the Government established a Discrimination Law Review to carry out a comprehensive review of current law and policy on discrimination, with a view to working towards a single, overarching Equality Act and establishing an independent Commission for Equality and Human Rights. In *Interim Report for Consultation* (2005), The Equalities Review identified genetic discrimination as a potential problem. In addition, the possibility of legislating against the use of genetic tests in employment and insurance is being considered as part of the Discrimination Law Review, which is due to publish a Green Paper for consultation during 2006.

The HGC has a Genetic Discrimination Working Group that is considering these issues. In a response to The Equalities Review consultation, the HGC expressed its view that the potential for unfair discrimination resulting from the misuse of personal genetic data must be recognised, and any trends in this direction carefully monitored. However, it also pointed out the difficulty of defining 'genetic test' and 'genetic information', and the illogicality of protecting people from discrimination on the basis of DNA test results but having no protection against misuse of results from non-DNA-based tests that might be more highly predictive.

There have been many attempts in the US to introduce federal legislation outlawing 'genetic discrimination'. As in the UK, the current disability discrimination legislation, the Americans with Disabilities Act (US Congress 1990), applies only to those with a current disability. Some individual US States have enacted legislation banning 'genetic discrimination', defined in various ways but usually applying specifically to information from DNA tests. Although several Bills to ban genetic discrimination have been introduced to Congress in recent years, none has so far been passed into law.

It is essential that clarity of thinking should prevail in any future development of anti-discrimination legislation. The salient criteria should be the predictive power of any personal medical information (DNA based or otherwise), the seriousness of the condition to which it relates, and whether its use in particular circumstances is fair or unfair.

Insurance

The concept of fairness is frequently invoked in the context of the use of genetic information in insurance. As we have argued in Chapter 6, it is debatable whether the use of genetic information in risk-rated insurance can really be considered unfair in principle, but governments and policy makers have nevertheless had to take into account widespread public unease about the issue. In the UK, a five-year voluntary moratorium on the use of predictive genetic test results in underwriting decisions was negotiated in 2001 between the Government and the Association of British Insurers (ABI) (Box 7.5). In 2005 it was announced that the moratorium would be extended for a further five years beyond its original expiry date (Department of Health and Association of British Insurers 2005).

Insurers can still use family history information in assessing insurance applications but the HGC and others have questioned whether this information is being used fairly by insurers. While the moratorium is in operation, research is being undertaken to assess the absolute levels of risk associated with a family history of various common conditions such as heart disease and bowel cancer, with the aim of encouraging the industry to apply evidence-based standards of practice. Other researchers are attempting to assess the real risk of adverse selection: that is, whether there is evidence to support the contention that people who know they are at increased risk because of a genetic factor will tend to exploit this situation by taking out insurance or seeking high levels of cover.

Box 7.5 The UK voluntary moratorium on use of predictive genetic test results in insurance

A voluntary moratorium on the use of predictive genetic test results in insurance underwriting was negotiated in 2001 between the Government and the Association of British Insurers. The moratorium is currently scheduled to run until 2011 (UK Government and Association of British Insurers 2005).

Under the terms of the moratorium, the ABI's members undertake not to use predictive genetic test results in assessing applications for life insurance policies up to a value of £500 000, for critical illness policies up to a value of £300 000, or for income protection policies paying annual benefits of up to £30 000. When assessing applications for policies above these values, insurers will only use the results of tests approved by the Government's independent Genetics and Insurance Committee (GAIC). GAIC assesses the reliability and actuarial relevance of specific tests in relation to specific types of insurance product. GAIC has so far approved only tests for Huntington's disease in respect of life insurance. Insurers may agree to use results of predictive genetic tests that are in the customer's favour.

Employment

So far, there has been little pressure for imposition of statutory controls on the use of genetic information in the context of employment. The HGC considered the issue in its report *Inside Information* (2002). It found scant evidence to justify use of genetic testing by employers in the UK, either for health and safety purposes or in recruitment decisions; equally, there was little evidence that employers have any interest in introducing genetic testing for such purposes. The HGC's predecessor group, the Human Genetics Advisory Commission, reached similar conclusions in a report published in 1999. The Government, replying to the HGC report, requested that the HGC work with the Disability Rights Commission, the Health and Safety Executive and other interested parties to keep the situation under review. In a further monitoring exercise in 2006 (*Genetic Testing and Employment* 2006b) the HGC found that little had changed since 2002.

The Information Commissioner (2005a, b) has developed an *Employment Practices Code* that includes guidance on compliance with the Data Protection Act in the use and retention of sensitive personal information (including information related to health) by employers. Part 4 of the Code covers information about workers' health. Genetic testing is specifically discussed: employers are advised to use genetic testing only where the genetic condition in question would pose a serious danger to the worker or to others, and if the danger cannot practicably be avoided by changing the working environment. Only scientifically validated tests should be used, full consent should be obtained, and workers should

Box 7.6 Genetic testing and employment: the Burlington North and Santa Fe Railway case

In 2001 the United States Equal Employment Opportunity Commission (EEOC) successfully invoked the Americans with Disabilities Act (ADA) to stop the Burlington North and Santa Fe Railway (BNSF) carrying out genetic testing on employees who had submitted claims for work-related carpal tunnel syndrome. There was no scientific justification for the use of the test (which detected a very rare chromosomal deletion highly unlikely to be relevant to the employees' condition), valid consent for genetic testing was not obtained, and it was alleged that some employees were threatened with dismissal if they refused to submit a blood sample. The EEOC succeeded in having the testing programme stopped. The BNSF denied that it had violated the ADA or discriminated against employees but agreed in a mediated settlement in 2002 to pay total damages of $2.2 million to the employees concerned.

not be required to disclose the results of previous genetic tests. Genetic testing should not be used in an attempt to obtain information about a predisposition to future ill health. The advice is sensible, if somewhat premature given the current rudimentary evidence base for such use of genetic tests.

In the US, genetic testing in insurance and employment are often linked issues, as many people's health insurance coverage is tied to their employment contract, so the concern is that employers have an interest in ensuring that they do not recruit employees who are at increased risk of developing a disease that will lead to time off work and/or a claim on the health plan. An executive order (US President 2000) signed by President Clinton in 2000 forbids use of genetic information in employment decisions (recruitment or promotion) but the order applies only to federal departments and agencies. Although some have called for this protection to be extended to all workers, there is no clear evidence that existing legislation preventing unfair discrimination in recruitment and promotion is inadequate. A notorious case in 2001 highlighted an indefensible use of genetic testing by a US employer, but also the successful use of existing legislation to curb it (Box 7.6).

Regulating the availability of genetic tests

Many new genetic tests are likely to be developed over the coming decades, including pharmacogenetic tests and tests designed to indicate genetic susceptibility to common disease. Some of these tests will have demonstrable clinical value but others will not. In deciding how to regulate the availability of genetic tests, policy makers face the challenge of attempting to protect the interests of patients and the public, while avoiding unnecessary regulation and preserving at least an element of individual choice.

Many clinicians agree that a medical test (including a genetic test) should only be carried out when it leads to the potential for an improved health outcome – in other words, if clinical utility can be demonstrated (see Chapter 4) – but there is less consensus on what constitutes an improved health outcome and what evidence is needed to document benefit. For example, there is evidence that the *APOE4* polymorphism increases risk of coronary heart disease, so it could be argued that individuals who carry this variant would benefit from knowing their genotype because they would have a particular incentive to reduce their risk through drug treatment or lifestyle modification. However, this knowledge might lead to a fatalistic attitude with a poorer health outcome. Moreover, *APOE4* carriers are also at increased risk of Alzheimer's disease but in the absence of any effective preventive action this information could be harmful. Who should decide whether an individual should be allowed to be tested for *APOE4*: the actual individual, a clinician, or those who fund healthcare services?

The approach to answering questions such as this will affect the availability and use of genetic tests. A test manufacturer will attempt to assess the potential market for a test and will be influenced by the nature of the regulatory regime to which they will have to adhere. Healthcare systems (such as the NHS) and healthcare providers will have expectations regarding the clinical evidence base for a test's use, its cost-effectiveness and other considerations. Patients will be interested in safety and perhaps also in their freedom to exercise individual autonomy.

The regulation of genetic tests can be seen as a set of strategies to enable a consistent decision-making process for the various stakeholders. A wide variety of regulatory strategies is available, ranging from statutory regulation to no regulation at all. Different strategies will be appropriate for different types of test. The context of regulation must also be considered; for example, strategies that are effective in the context of professional medical care may be different from those that will be needed to regulate the availability of genetic tests direct to the public.

Statutory and other explicit regulatory controls may be applied at any stage of the pathway from development and pre-market review of a test through to conditions attached to its use or availability (Box 7.7).

Market authorisation

Statutory regulation of medical tests at the market authorisation stage is in place in most western countries. In the UK and the rest of Europe this tier of regulation has tended so far to be concerned mainly with ensuring the analytical validity of tests; in the US and Canada, an assessment of clinical validity is also included.

In the UK, all medical tests, including genetic tests, are subject to regulation under the *Medical Devices Regulations* (UK Government 2002), which incorporate into UK law the provisions of the EU In Vitro Diagnostic Devices Directive

Box 7.7 Strategies for regulating the availability of genetic tests

- **Market authorisation** – ensures that commercially available tests meet legally required standards for technical performance and that tests marketed direct to consumers perform safely in that setting.
- **Laboratory regulation** – laboratories carrying out tests are required to meet specified standards including quality control, reporting standards, staffing, training and laboratory accommodation.
- **Regulation of advertising and consumer protection** – manufacturers marketing tests direct to the public are required to meet standards for truthfulness in advertising and are subject to product liability laws.
- **Regulatory mechanisms within healthcare services** – organisations commissioning or paying for healthcare services fund tests for which there is evidence of health benefits (clinical utility).
- **Professional and practice guidelines** – health professionals ordering tests use practice guidelines and clinical judgement to ensure that tests are appropriate for the patient.

(European Parliament and Council 1998a). An executive agency of the Department of Health, the Medicines and Healthcare Products Regulatory Agency (MHRA) is responsible for ensuring that tests comply with the Regulations in safety, quality and performance. Tests that directly inform medical action, and for which the consequences of a false result are serious, are subject to more stringent requirements under the Regulations than lower-risk tests. Self-test kits, used by a consumer/patient without direct medical supervision, form a special category: manufacturers have to show that the test performs adequately and safely in this setting.

So-called home brew kits (tests both developed and used within a laboratory, using its own reagents and protocols) are exempt from the legislation as long as they are manufactured and used on the same premises, or premises in the immediate vicinity, for purposes that are intrinsic to the purposes of the health institution to which the laboratory belongs; for example, to diagnose a genetic disease in the context of the clinical genetics service. The exemption applies even if an NHS laboratory uses a home-brew kit to test samples sent by another NHS Trust. As many such tests are in use as part of the UK's national genetic testing network, the exemption is an important one.

In the US, the Food and Drug Administration (FDA) is responsible for premarket review of medical tests but only a small number of genetic tests have come under its scrutiny, mainly because tests offered as a service by the laboratory that developed them (home-brew tests) are not included. Under the Clinton administration, the Secretary's Advisory Committee on Genetic Testing (2000) recommended a detailed review procedure for genetic tests. With the change of administration in 2000, this advisory committee was disbanded and its recommendations were not implemented. Its successor body, the Secretary's Advisory Committee on Genetics Health and Society (2006), has decided to maintain a watching brief on the issue rather than actively to push for further regulation at this level.

Laboratory regulation

Regulation of laboratories carrying out molecular genetic testing is in place in many countries including European countries, the US, Canada and Australia. In the UK, DNA and cytogenetic testing laboratories in the NHS are obliged to be accredited by the United Kingdom Accreditation Service and the Clinical Pathology Accreditation Co Ltd. Standards of staffing, training, laboratory accommodation, reporting and quality assurance are imposed. UK DNA testing laboratories also participate in the European Molecular Genetics Quality Network, a European Commission-funded initiative to provide external quality assessment for laboratories and encourage best practice. The professional group representing laboratory genetics professionals, the Clinical Molecular Genetics Society, also publishes best practice guidance for laboratory procedures and undertakes audit of the activities of all NHS laboratories.

Similar regulatory oversight of laboratories in the US is provided by the federal Consolidated Laboratory Improvement Amendment (CLIA); specific requirements for laboratories carrying out genetic tests are being developed.

In May 2005 the Organisation for Economic Cooperation and Development published a survey of molecular genetic testing in 18 countries. The report discusses the availability and extent of molecular genetic testing services in these countries, their quality assurance procedures and their policies on sampling and data handling, including transfer of samples and data across international borders. Recommendations included harmonisation of standards for laboratory accreditation, better access to international networks for rare-disease tests, standardisation of measures of clinical validity and utility, and the development of international guidelines for sample storage and security.

Advertising and over-the-counter tests

Much of the current concern about genetic testing has been in the context of genetic tests available directly to the public, often via the Internet. In the UK, while advertising of medicines direct to the public is illegal, advertising of tests is not. Some companies have marketed tests claiming, for example, to assess genetic susceptibility to deep vein thrombosis, or analysing polymorphisms proposed to be related to dietary needs. Consumer interest in these testing services has so far been very low. While the evidence base underlying such tests is sometimes poor and they may have little or no clinical value, views differ as to how they should be regulated: some advocate an outright ban, while others feel that consumer education about the shortcomings of the tests would be a more appropriate path to follow.

In posing this question, we need to consider the purpose of regulation: is it to protect the public from harm, or should it aim to go further by outlawing products or services that offer no real health benefit but are otherwise 'safe'? Interestingly, consumer groups in the UK and the US have taken opposing positions on this question: the UK's Consumers' Association has argued for strict controls on genetic tests (Consumers' Association and GeneWatch UK 2002), while in the US, freedom of consumers to make their own judgements is considered the paramount value.

The HGC investigated the issue of over-the-counter genetic tests in its 2003 report *Genes Direct. Ensuring the Effective Oversight of Genetic Tests Supplied Directly to the Public.* The Commission rejected the two extreme options of either allowing a free-for-all or banning direct-to-public/consumer tests altogether, opting instead for a mixture of voluntary and statutory controls. Tests for single-gene disease, which may have serious clinical, psychological and social consequences for individuals and their families, should, it suggests, only be administered by qualified professionals and in most cases accompanied by genetic counselling. Susceptibility tests, however, may merit no tighter regulation than, say, cholesterol testing or blood pressure measurement. Whether current consumer protection legislation is adequate for genetic tests remains to be seen.

General legislation regarding truthfulness of advertising governs the direct-to-public marketing of genetic tests (and other medical tests and products) in the US. Additional oversight of advertising comes from the FDA for the products it regulates and from the Federal Trade Commission for other products such as dietary supplements; both have attracted some criticism for being insufficiently rigorous. At the instigation of the Secretary's Advisory Committee on Genetics, Health and Society (SACGHS), inter-agency working groups have been set up to monitor advertising claims made by companies marketing tests direct to consumers, and to assess the public health impact of direct-to-consumer test marketing.

Regulatory mechanisms within healthcare services

Within the context of professional medical care, it can be argued that a range of mechanisms are available that fall short of statutory control but can have the effect of achieving appropriate use of genetic tests. One powerful mechanism is the allocation of healthcare resources. Health-economic implications of genetics are discussed in more detail later in this chapter. In the specific context of genetic testing, the opportunity costs of tests that are expensive and of low clinical utility are likely to motivate healthcare funders to exclude such tests and to demand demonstration of clinical utility as a prerequisite for funding tests. This will be particularly important in situations where tests must be accompanied by extensive counselling and/or medical follow-up, thus increasing the associated healthcare costs.

In the NHS, evaluation of genetic tests (see Chapter 4) has assumed increasing importance as the number of available tests for single-gene diseases and chromosomal disorders increases rapidly, and stronger emphasis is placed on evidence-based medicine. As discussed in Chapter 5, the 2000 report *Laboratory Services for Genetics* recommended (Department of Health 2000c), among other measures, that the Department of Health should establish a coordinated mechanism for evaluating new tests and testing technology. Two developments followed: the designation of two National Genetics Reference Laboratories, and the establishment of the UK Genetic Testing Network. The responsibilities of the National Genetics Reference Laboratories include health technology assessment in the area of genetic testing, development of quality systems, and advice to government and other bodies. The UK Genetic Testing Network, overseen by a steering group under the auspices of the Genetics Commissioning Advisory Group (see also Chapter 5, Box 5.1), has undertaken to evaluate all DNA tests offered by NHS genetic testing laboratories, using the criteria of analytical validity, clinical validity and clinical utility, with the aim of assembling a directory of tests that merit funding by the NHS.

In the US the SACGHS published a report in February 2006 recommending improvements to the current provision of genetic testing services and policies concerning coverage and reimbursement in both the public and private health sectors. The report suggested that a task force should be set up to assess current evidence on the evaluation of genetic tests and to identify areas where further evidence is required.

Practice guidelines

In the past, expert opinion has guided the application of genetic testing in clinical practice. It has been argued by some that, at least in the case of rare single-gene diseases and chromosomal disorders, the gold standard of evidence-based medicine – controlled clinical trials on large numbers of people – will never be attainable. Instead, basic science and clinical observation together may provide sufficient evidence of positive clinical outcomes that depend on the use of information from genetic test results. As an example of a test that satisfies this criterion, prophylactic thyroidectomy is beneficial in people shown by a genetic test to be presymptomatic for multiple endocrine neoplasia type 2. It is less easy, however, to document clear clinical benefit when the result of a genetic test is information alone, though the provision of information remains one of the cornerstones on which the profession of clinical genetics is built.

It is unlikely that this view of the clinical utility of genetic tests can survive the possible translation of genetic tests into mainstream medical practice. Rather, there is likely to be increasing pressure from healthcare planners and funders for an evidence-based approach, particularly in the evaluation of genetic susceptibility and pharmacogenetic tests. Any claimed benefits, for example in disease prevention, will have to be backed up by evidence of better health outcomes.

The NHS's Health Technology Assessment Programme and National Institute for Health and Clinical Excellence and the US Preventive Services Task Force are likely to be key players in the development of practice guidelines for genetic testing, but all such groups will need better data on outcomes associated with genetic testing. There is also a need for consensus-building processes, to integrate clinical opinion with views of patients and the wider public and so achieve a robust approach to policy development for genetic testing. The US CDC Office of Genomics and Disease Prevention is leading a project (EGAPP) to support a coordinated process for evaluating genetic tests and other genomic applications that are in transition from research to clinical and public health practice.

Pharmacogenetics

Regulation of pharmacogenetic tests

Many of the policy questions raised by the development of pharmacogenetic tests are the same as those for other types of genetic test. Perhaps the most important of these is the question of whether regulatory authorities should be concerned only with the analytical validity of tests, or should also demand evidence of clinical validity and utility. In the case of a pharmacogenetic test to determine the optimum dose of a drug, for example, demonstration of clinical utility would require evidence that the test led to better outcomes for patients than standard clinical approaches such as careful post-prescription monitoring and dose adjustment. Health-economic considerations (discussed later in this chapter) would also be part of the assessment.

In cases where a pharmacogenetic test is available that can inform prescribing of an existing drug, the US Food and Drug Administration (FDA) has used drug labelling requirements to indicate whether testing is required for achieving safety and efficacy. If the drug is safe and effective without testing, but testing may be helpful in determining the therapeutic strategy or dosing schedule, then an 'informative label' to this effect is approved. This, in effect, leaves the decision of whether to use the test as a matter for clinical judgement. If the drug is safe and effective only in the patient subgroup defined by testing, then testing is required before prescription and the drug label must include an explicit statement to that effect. This is the case for the drug Herceptin®, where the label states that testing should be used to evaluate a patient's tumour for over-expression of the HER2 protein.

Pharmacogenetics in drug development

Pharmaceutical companies are increasingly using pharmacogenetic and pharmacogenomic approaches as part of their drug development programmes. In most cases their goal is not to develop a test–drug combination for bringing to the market, but to produce better drugs that are safe and effective in a broad range of people. Drug candidates that are found to be metabolised by pathways that are known to be subject to substantial pharmacogenetic variation may be abandoned for that reason.

Pharmacogenetic testing may also be used during drug development to ensure that clinical trial groups contain a balance of the relevant genotypes, or that late-stage clinical trials can be targeted at good responders. These uses of pharmacogenetics require a policy response from the regulatory authorities responsible for drug licensing. Questions include:

- What pharmacogenetic information should such authorities require pharmaceutical companies to submit as part of a licence application?
- What weight should be given to this information in the regulatory process?
- If the drug is licensed, is an accompanying pharmacogenetic test either advisory or mandatory?

In March 2005 the FDA released guidance on the collection and submission of pharmacogenetic data by pharmaceutical companies. The guidance recognises that in many cases pharmacogenetic data 'may not be well enough established scientifically to be suitable for regulatory decision making' but it encourages voluntary submission of such data on the grounds that it will help industry by improving the FDA's understanding of pharmacogenetic approaches and therefore the quality of any future regulatory decisions.

The guidance sets out different requirements for applications at different stages of the drug development and licensing pathway. For example, an 'investigational new drug' (IND) application is required when drug development reaches the stage of clinical trials in humans. The guidance states that pharmacogenetic data must be submitted as part of an IND application if the test results are to be used for making decisions in relation to a clinical trial (for example, selection of patients); or the test results are being used to support claims relating to drug characteristics such as its mechanism of action, safety or dosing schedule; or the test constitutes a 'known valid biomarker' for clinical outcomes in humans. Voluntary submission is suggested where, for example, pharmacogenetic information has been obtained from exploratory studies or its validity is not clearly established.

When clinical trials are complete, a new drug application (NDA) must be made to acquire market authorisation for the drug. The guidance suggests that pharmacogenetic data used to support the interpretation of clinical trial results on drug dosing, safety or patient selection should be submitted to the FDA, as should any test results that the company proposes using in drug labelling, or any tests that are needed to achieve the dosing, safety or effectiveness described in the labelling.

The FDA is developing its policy for pharmacogenetics in partnership with the pharmaceutical industry. This approach has been criticised by some as being too industry-friendly and insufficiently rigorous. The FDA believes, however, that the partnership approach will achieve robust regulation without stifling a field of science that is still in the early stages of development.

In the European Union, market authorisation for a new drug may be obtained either from the regulatory authorities in the separate member states (for example, the MHRA in the UK) or from the European Medicines Agency (EMEA). A company may submit a single application to the EMEA's Committee for Medicinal Products for Human Use. If the evaluation is positive, market authorisation is granted that is valid in all the countries of the EU. The EMEA has accepted the need to include pharmacogenetic assessment in the procedure for drug evaluation and has set up a Pharmacogenetics Working Party to prepare guidelines for regulatory submissions, catalyse training for those involved in pharmacogenetics assessment, and recommend ways of maintaining consistency in assessment.

Broader policy considerations

Pharmaceutical companies are currently showing little interest in developing pharmacogenetic tests for existing drugs, or new test–drug combinations, because of concerns about market fragmentation and poor financial viability. Some in the industry are also concerned that companies could be vulnerable to litigation if testing failed for some reason and a serious adverse event occurred.

However, if pharmacogenetics does have anything to offer clinical medicine then it is in the public interest that such tests are developed. It may therefore be necessary for governments to provide incentives for test development, particularly for large-scale clinical studies which are often financially beyond the means of the small- to medium-sized biotech companies that might be interested in test development.

Policy measures may also be needed to counteract some of the ethical and social problems that could potentially arise from pharmacogenetics. For example, there is a possibility that market segmentation could leave some minority population subgroups under-served. Existing provisions for 'orphan drug' development, which provide incentives for research and development on drugs with a small target market, might come into play in this situation, but to date most of the major pharmaceutical companies have shown little interest in orphan drug development.

Concern has also been raised about the possibility that pharmacogenetic variants could be predictive of other characteristics such as disease susceptibility. There is some disagreement here between experts who think that panels of 'anonymous' single nucleotide polymorphisms (SNPs) can be developed that would have no implications for characteristics other than response to a specific drug, and those who think that at least some of the most informative SNPs will almost inevitably be in genes involved in physiological processes relevant to disease susceptibility, and may well turn out to have causal significance for these diseases. If the latter is the case, issues of informed consent to testing arise, as well as a need for robust security of databases storing pharmacogenetic information.

The development of pharmacogenetics has health-economic implications. It has been suggested that pharmacogenetics could lower drug development costs by streamlining clinical trials and possibly enabling resurrection of promising drug candidates that have been abandoned because of rare adverse reactions, allowing development costs to be recouped. For the payer (the health service), there would be obvious financial benefits from greater efficiency and less wastage in drug prescribing, and from avoiding the costs of treating the clinical consequences of inappropriate dosage or adverse reactions.

However, heavy research and development costs may have to be recouped over a smaller market for each pharmacogenetically tailored drug, causing drug costs to rise. In some cases, pharmaceutical companies may be forced to respond to pharmacogenetic tests developed by competitors or by the diagnostics industry.

In practice, the economic case for pharmacogenetic testing will have to be made individually for each test/drug combination. Relevant variables include the price of the test, the prices of the drug with and without testing, the effectiveness of the drug as represented by a measure such as quality-adjusted life years (QALYs), the size of the patient population, the ratio of responders to non-responders and the costs of adverse reactions.

The introduction of pharmacogenetics into health services raises also questions of service organisation, capacity, and education and training of health professionals. These issues have been considered in Chapter 5.

Regulation of gene-based and cellular therapies

So far in this chapter we have been concerned mainly with policy issues related to genetic testing: informed consent for the use of tissue, regulation of the tests themselves, and policy for regulating the uses to which genetic information derived from testing may be put. We now turn to the issue of policy for new medical interventions based on genetics and genetic technologies.

An example are therapies, such as gene therapy and stem cell therapy, that involve transfer of genetic or cellular material to a patient to treat disease or repair damaged tissue. The transferred material may be genetically manipulated in order, for example, to ensure that a therapeutic gene is expressed in the target tissue or, if the material is cellular, that the cells it contains are expressing the correct genetic programme.

The development of these new therapeutic approaches, although still largely at the research stage, has created challenges for ensuring safe clinical use and for granting market approval for commercial therapeutic products. In the case of embryonic stem (ES) cells, additional regulatory issues arise because the starting material is human embryos.

Policy for embryonic stem cell research

The 1990 Human Fertilisation and Embryology Act (UK Government 1990) is the cornerstone of UK policy on the use of embryos both in medical treatments [such as in vitro fertilisation (IVF) and pre-implantation genetic diagnosis] and research. The basic principles underlying the legislation were set out in the 1984 Warnock report on human fertilisation and embryology. Under the 1990 Act, it is legal to carry out research on human embryos up to 14 days after fertilisation for specific purposes mostly related to improving the understanding or treatment of infertility or miscarriages, or to the development of new methods of contraception. Controversially, the Act also made it legal to create embryos specifically for research.

A new statutory authority, the Human Fertilisation and Embryology Authority (HFEA), was set up to oversee compliance with the Act and to license laboratories wishing to carry out embryo research. The legislative framework was extended in 2001 with the introduction of the HFE (Research Purposes) Regulations (UK Government 2001c), following recommendations from a working party chaired by the Chief Medical Officer and a separate inquiry by the Nuffield Council on Bioethics (2001). These regulations extended the list of purposes for which embryo research could be licensed to include research aimed at understanding the development of embryos, or understanding or treating serious disease. The main reason for the introduction of these regulations was to enable ES cell research (including the use of cloning technology to derive ES cells) and its regulation by the HFEA.

The House of Lords passed the Regulations on condition that the government consider the results of an inquiry into stem cell research by a special Committee of the House of Lords; that inquiry supported the Regulations (House of Lords Stem Cell Research Committee 2002). The authority of the HFEA to authorise research

Box 7.8 The UK Stem Cell Bank

The UK Stem Cell Bank, hosted by the National Institute for Biological Standards and Control, has two functions: as a repository for all stem cell types (adult, fetal and embryonic) and as a supplier of cell lines for basic research and clinical applications. The Bank accepts stem cell lines developed in the UK and appropriately accredited lines created in other countries. The Medical Research Council maintains a register of cell lines that have been deposited.

An independent Steering Committee evaluates all applications to deposit and to access cell lines. Requests for deposits or access must show that all ethical approvals, licences and authorisations are in place. A Management Committee oversees the operation of the bank itself.

The Bank's *Code of Practice for the Use of Human Stem Cell Lines* (UK Stem Cell Bank Steering Committee 2005) outlines the criteria that should be observed when deriving and using human stem cell lines, including requirements for consent from donors. The Code will be updated in the future to take account of requirements arising from the implementation of the Human Tissue Act (UK Government 2004c) and the EU Tissue Directive (European Parliament and Council 2004a).

For further information, see the UK Stem Cell Bank website at www.ukstemcellbank.org.uk.

on embryos created by cell nuclear replacement was challenged in the courts by a 'pro-life' group on the grounds that such embryos are not created by fertilisation. This challenge was eventually rejected by the House of Lords. The UK's liberal laws on embryo and ES cell research are regarded as placing it in the 'advance guard' among countries attempting to develop regulatory regimes for stem cell research.

The House of Lords' report (House of Lords Stem Cell Research Committee 2002) on stem cells recommended the setting up of a national Stem Cell Bank to manage stem cell resources under an ethical framework (Box 7.8). The HFEA has made compliance with the *Bank's Code of Practice* (UK Stem Cell Bank Steering Committee 2005) a condition of a licence for ES cell research, and requires a sample of all ES cell lines produced in the UK to be deposited in the Bank.

The Government's 2005 consultation (Department of Health 2005d) on the HFE Act indicated possible changes to some parts of the legislation governing stem cell research. For example, opinions were solicited on whether the creation of chimeric embryos by placing a human nucleus in an animal oocyte, currently illegal but now seen as a potential research tool that could spare the use of human eggs, should be allowed. Some amendments will also be needed to implement the EU Tissue Directive (European Parliament and Council 2004a) into national law.

Stem cell and embryo research are taking place within an increasingly globalised 'landscape' for biomedical research. For example, cell lines are crossing national boundaries as laboratories collaborate and materials are deposited in and accessed from stem cell banks. The sourcing of reproductive cells, particularly human eggs, is also occurring at an international level. However, national policies for embryo and stem cell research vary widely. In the US, for example, a Presidential order (US President 2001) forbids the use of federal funds for research on human embryonic stem cell lines other than a specified set that were derived before the date of the order (2001); however, embryonic stem cell research is going ahead with private funding and, in some cases, with state-level funding. Within Europe, national policies vary from the relatively permissive (but regulated) policies of countries such as the UK and Belgium, and policies that impose a complete ban on all embryo research (for example, Austria).

Some countries implacably opposed to research involving embryos and cloning technology have attempted to achieve international condemnation of this research. For example, attempts were made in the United Nations to pass a declaration banning all forms of human cloning, including cloning for derivation of embryonic stem cells; eventually, a non-binding declaration was passed in 2005 (United Nations General Assembly 2005) that has been rejected by many countries.

In the European Union, there has been protracted wrangling over the use of EU research funds for embryonic stem cell research. During research Framework Programme 6 (FP6), a pragmatic solution was eventually reached that enabled research applications to be considered on a case-by-case basis (European Commission 2002b). The procedure included a scientific assessment of the 'necessity' for the research; satisfactory ethical review to ensure, for example, that embryo donors had given adequate consent and not received payment; and approval by an EU regulatory committee including representatives from all member states. Approval could only be given where it did not contravene the national laws of the country in which the research was to be carried out. The issue has re-ignited with the transition from FP6 to FP7; although the European Commission and Parliament favour continuation of the existing procedures, Ministers from some member states may block this decision.

Recognising the difficulties divergent national policies cause for the governance of stem cell research, an international group of scientists, regulators, ethicists and journal editors published a consensus statement (Hinxton Group 2006) in February 2006 calling for the development of a set of international ethical standards for stem cell research and established a consortium, the Hinxton Group, to take this work forward.

Regulation of therapeutic cell- and tissue-based materials

The UK Stem Cell Bank and the Medicines and Healthcare Products Regulatory Agency (MHRA) are developing policies to ensure that clinical-grade therapeutic cells and tissues are safe, high quality, ethically sourced and traceable. Codes of practice for tissue banks are being updated and harmonised with the provisions of new UK and European legislation, particularly the Human Tissue Act 2004 (UK Government 2004c) and the EU Tissue Directive (European Parliament and Council 2004a). The Human Tissue Authority is responsible for licensing therapeutic tissue banks as required by the EU Tissue Directive and has issued information about licensing arrangements and fees.

The 2004 EU Tissue Directive sets 'standards of quality and safety for the donation, procurement, testing, processing, preservation, storage and distribution of human tissues and cells'. The Directive requires that all cellular material intended for clinical transplant must be traceable to a voluntary donor who has given informed consent to this use of their tissue, and for whom medical information has been obtained. Safety and quality are addressed in a set of rules on product recall, preservation, storage, labelling, packaging and adverse incident reporting.

While the Tissue Directive outlines the information that should be provided to tissue donors, it largely leaves standards of consent to national laws. In the UK, consent procedures are specified by the Human Tissue Act (for cells and tissue other than embryos and gametes) and the Human Fertilisation and Embryology Act (for embryos and gametes). The current statutory bodies with responsibility for this area are the Human Fertilisation and Embryology Authority and the Human Tissue Authority (due to merge to form the Regulatory Authority for Tissue and Embryos in 2008).

Market authorisation of 'advanced therapies'

Difficulties have been encountered in fitting gene therapy and cellular therapy products into the existing framework for market approval, which separates 'medicinal products' from 'medical devices'. Gene therapy products and somatic cell therapy products have been classified as 'medicinal products' and the Directives related to medicinal products have been amended to clarify the relevant definitions.

However, 'tissue engineering products' (cells combined with a non-biological matrix or capsule to aid their integration into host tissue) fell outside this framework. In recognition of this problem, the European Commission is developing, in addition, a new regulatory regime for 'Advanced Therapy Medicinal Products' (available online at the European Commission DG Enterprise and Industry Website), which essentially covers market authorisation of all types of therapy that involve transfer of human biological material (genes, cells or tissues) to a recipient. The Regulation, which will be binding on member states of the EU as soon as it has been finalised, will be accompanied by guidelines setting out detailed standards for good manufacturing practice (GMP) and good clinical practice (GCP) for advanced therapies. The European Medicines Agency will be responsible for evaluation and market authorisation of advanced therapy products, working through a new Committee for Advanced Therapies that will work under the supervision of the Committee for Medicinal Products for Human Use. The challenge for the new regulatory regime will be to protect patients while at the same time stimulating the development of advanced therapies and harmonising market access for companies developing these therapies.

EU member states will be responsible for implementing the Regulation through their own national regulatory bodies. In the UK, the Medicines and Healthcare Products Regulatory Agency (MHRA) fulfils this role.

In the US, the Food and Drug Administration (FDA) is responsible for the market authorisation of gene-based and cellular therapy products. The FDA pays particular attention to the safety characteristics of gene therapy constructs and protocols. No commercial product has yet been licensed by the FDA for human use.

Clinical trials and research governance

The clinical development of gene-based and cellular therapies is closely linked to regulation governing the conduct of clinical trials. The clinical stages of pharmacogenetic and pharmacogenomic research are also subject to this aspect of the regulatory regime.

In the US, the FDA oversees clinical trials of products for gene therapy and cellular therapy. Draft guidance for the conduct of clinical trials involving gene transfer technology was issued in August 2005 (Food and Drug Administration [US] 2005): the guidance recommends long-term follow-up of trial participants in order to monitor for any delayed adverse events.

In the UK, the Medicines for Human Use (Clinical Trials) Regulations 2004 (UK Government 2004b) implement the EU Clinical Trials Directive, replacing the clinical trials provisions in the 1968 Medicines Act. The MHRA is the body responsible for implementing the Regulations.

The new Regulations place on a statutory basis some aspects of the conduct of clinical trials that were formerly based on non-statutory guidance in the UK. These include the role of research ethics committees, additional protections for minors and mentally incompetent adults participating in trials, and a requirement for all clinical trials to be conducted according to the principles of good clinical practice. In addition, all Phase 1 trials on healthy volunteers now need authorisation both from an ethics committee and the MHRA. Medicinal products that are being investigated must be manufactured to the standards of good manufacturing practice, and each trial must have an identified sponsor to take responsibility for all aspects the trial's set-up and conduct.

The new Clinical Trials Regulations have proved controversial in the research community. Some regard them as merely cementing good practice while others consider that they place an unacceptable degree of responsibility on trial sponsors, particularly when the trial is being run through a university and sponsored through the not-for-profit sector.

In the case of gene therapy trials in the UK, a specialist body, the Gene Therapy Advisory Committee (GTAC) fulfils the role of the research ethics committee for the purposes of the Clinical Trials Regulations. GTAC assesses all gene therapy research proposals and clinical trials involving humans, taking into account their scientific merit, their ethical implications and their likely risks and benefits. In a move that would echo the bringing together of all gene-based and cellular therapies within a single category of advanced therapies for the purpose of market authorisation in the EU, it has been suggested that GTAC should metamorphose into a new Cell Therapy Advisory Committee with an expanded remit to include responsibility for trials of all cellular therapies.

General governance of clinical research

At a more general level, sound research governance in all aspects of clinical research is needed to ensure high-quality research and maintain public confidence, though excessive regulation is stifling and expensive.

The Department of Health has a Research Governance Framework which was revised in 2005 (Department of Health 2005e) in the light of several recent pieces of legislation including the Human Tissue Act, the Mental Capacity Act and the Clinical Trials Regulations. In addition to complying with these statutory requirements, all proposed research studies involving NHS patients must obtain approval from a research ethics committee, which is charged with ensuring that the proposed research safeguards the dignity, rights, safety and well-being of the participants. The research ethics committee system has been criticised as being too slow and cumbersome, inconsistent between different committees, and lacking sufficient scientific expertise. A Department of Health (2005c) review of the system published in 2005 recommended streamlining application procedures, creating a national network of research ethics committees, providing more training for lay research ethics committee members, and a better understanding of ethical issues by scientists submitting proposals for consideration.

Intellectual property and patents

The system of intellectual property rights and patent protection has evolved as a way of encouraging innovation by protecting the financial interests of inventors and other creators of intellectual property, while ensuring that the fruits of their work enter the public domain and can thus contribute to the public good. In the context of genetics and genomics, the most important forms of intellectual property protection are copyright, database protection and patents.

The most contentious area has been that of patents. A patent is a right that enables the holder to prevent others making commercial use of an invention for a specific time period (usually 20 years) and in a specific jurisdiction (for example, the UK). A patent can only be granted to an invention that fulfils specific criteria, which may vary in different jurisdictions.

In the UK, patent law is set out in the Patents Act 1977 (UK Government 1977) and by the Patents Regulations (UK Government 2000), which is the legal instrument by which the UK complied with the 1997 EU Directive on the Legal Protection of Biotechnological Inventions (European Parliament and Council 1998b). Aspects of UK patent law have also been informed by the European Patent Convention (European Patent Office 1973) and the World Trade Organisation's 1994 Trade-Related Aspects of Intellectual Property Rights (TRIPS) agreement, which constituted an attempt to achieve some international harmonisation in this field.

An applicant seeking to patent an invention in the countries that are parties to the European Patent Convention can apply to the European Patent Office for a patent valid in all EPC countries. Patents valid in specific countries can be obtained by applying separately to the patent authorities in each country.

Box 7.9 summarises (in simplified terms) the requirements for a patentable invention in the UK and other countries that have adopted the EU directive.

At first sight, several of the provisions summarised in Box 7.9 would seem to preclude the patenting of many research advances in genetics. For example, DNA sequences may be thought to come under the heading of 'elements of the human body', while a genetic test is clearly a method of diagnosis. It is important

Box 7.9 Requirements for a patentable invention under the EU Directive on the legal protection of biotechnological inventions

A patentable invention must:

- Be novel
- Involve an inventive step that is not obvious to someone 'skilled in the art'
- Be capable of industrial application
- Be disclosed in sufficient detail.

There are various exclusions from patentability. Those most relevant to genetics are:

- Inventions whose application would run counter to public morality
- The human body and its elements in their natural state
- 'Essentially biological' processes for producing plants or animals
- Methods of treatment/diagnosis or surgery for humans or animals.

to appreciate, however, that in patent law these terms are given very specific and restricted meanings, and the presumption by patent examiners has been in favour of granting rather than rejecting a patent application. For example, although a DNA sequence inside a cell in the body cannot be patented, that same sequence, when extracted from cells (and perhaps reproduced by polymerase chain reaction or molecular cloning), can be. Similarly, a 'method of diagnosis' means one that is directly carried out on the human body and does not apply to a test on extracted blood, for example.

The permissive interpretation of patent law over the past 20–30 years has led to the patenting of thousands of DNA sequences, including those of genes, such as *BRCA1* and *BRCA2*, that are of known clinical importance. Moreover, not only is the sequence itself patented, but often also any future uses of the sequence; those applying for patents tend to aim for as wide a scope as possible for the protection. This situation has led to objections from scientists, clinicians and others, who claim that commercial monopolies over information that should be in the public domain have been granted on sometimes very tenuous grounds. Companies, on the other hand, argue that they will not be able to invest in research that could bring benefits to human health unless patent protection is available to prevent others exploiting their work.

Disagreement on the scope of patent protection for DNA sequences has led to differences in the implementation of the EU Directive in some European countries. France and Germany, for example, have stipulated in their legislation that where inventions concern material isolated from the human body, the scope of patent protection only extends to purposes disclosed in the patent application; this is not the case in the UK, for example. The European Commission has announced that it intends to monitor any economic consequences of divergence between the legislation in different member states.

Divisions have also become apparent within Europe on the issue of whether inventions involving embryonic stem cells can be patented. Inventions may be excluded from patentability if the granting of a patent would be contrary to public policy or morality. The European Patent Office has taken the view (currently subject to appeal) that embryonic stem cell lines and products derived from them are not patentable because the invention was developed through the use of human embryos and cannot be repeated without the use of embryos. However, the UK Patent Office is willing to grant patents claiming pluripotent cell lines from embryos, provided the claims do not expressly claim rights over the use of embryos; *processes* for obtaining stem cells from human embryos are not patentable because such inventions involve 'use of human embryos' and so fall within the prohibited category.

There are signs that some of the difficulties encountered in devising a fair patenting system for inventions involving DNA sequences may be beginning to resolve themselves. There have been moves in several jurisdictions towards more stringent interpretation of the requirements for novelty, inventiveness and utility. The entire reference sequence of the human genome is now in the public domain. In addition, many of the sequences patented in the early days of recombinant DNA protection are now, 20 years later, coming off patent, and the patent holders have in many cases decided that, in the absence of any imminent profitable use of the sequence, the value of keeping the patent protection is not worth the fees incurred.

Various avenues are also available for counteracting the restrictive effects of patents, whether by direct challenge or some other means. Successful challenges have been mounted in Europe against patents on aspects of the sequences of the *BRCA1* and *BRCA2* genes that had been granted to the US company Myriad Genetics: some of these patents have been revoked or restricted in scope (though appeals are ongoing). Governments in some jurisdictions may also make use of provisions for compulsory licensing if they feel that patent holders are adopting an unreasonably restrictive stance by charging exorbitant licence fees.

Exemptions for Crown use (that is, use for governmental purposes upon payment of compensation to the patent holder) or research use (where there is no commercial involvement) may also be invoked in some countries. In practice, the Crown use provision has very rarely been used in the UK, at least by the Department of Health. The research use exemption can prove problematic in that it may not always be easy to be sure that a particular research activity, such as a clinical trial, has a purely academic research purpose and no element of treatment or potential to lead to a commercial development.

The difficulties in deciding how to apply patent law in the area of genetics and biotechnology have led the UK Patent Office to issue guidelines aimed at clarifying how the requirements for novelty, inventiveness, industrial application and disclosure are to be interpreted, and how a fair scope for a patent can be determined (UK Patent Office 2005). The general trend of these guidelines is towards more stringent criteria for patentability and scope but the basic assumption remains in favour of granting rather than rejecting applications.

Government faces difficult issues in deciding on its policy priorities for intellectual property protection. Different government departments have different interests; for example, the Department of Trade and Industry wants to create a favourable climate for commercial investment, while the Department of Health and the NHS wish to make the benefits of medical research available to the population as cost-effectively as possible.

Even within the NHS there are opposing forces. The NHS is both a recipient and, through its research and development activities, a generator of intellectual property. The NHS has its own intellectual property policy (Department of Health 2002a), which urges greater attention to the protection of intellectual property generated by the health service. NHS Regional Innovation Hubs have been established to boost the identification, registration and evaluation of NHS intellectual property.

The issues are discussed in the specific context of genetics in the report of a project commissioned by the Department of Health from academic experts in the field of biotechnology patent law. This document (*Intellectual Property Rights and Genetics. A Study into the Impact and Management of Intellectual Property Rights Within the Healthcare Sector*; Cornish *et al.*, 2003) advises the Government to strike an effective balance that is in the overall public interest, by seeking to ensure that patents in genetics and biotechnology (both its own and others') are reasonable in scope and that fair licensing agreements are negotiated to ensure that advances in genetics are enabled to benefit patients while also providing a just reward for industry.

The Organisation for Economic Cooperation and Development (OECD) has focused on improvements to the licensing system for genetic inventions as a means of facilitating the development of genetics-based treatments and technologies, while protecting the interests of patent holders. Guidelines published by the OECD in early 2006 (*Guidelines for the Licensing of Genetic Inventions*) recommend that patent holders should normally grant broad and non-exclusive licences, avoiding 'reach-through rights' (which give the patent holder rights in the licensee's research using the genetic invention) and excessive up-front fees. The OECD also recommends that licensing practices should permit national or local providers to use genetic inventions in order to improve healthcare services.

General policy issues

In the remainder of this chapter we move beyond the realm of legislation and regulation to consider broader policy issues that have a bearing on both the development of new applications based on genetics and genomics, and on the prospects for their implementation in health care. Box 7.10 summarises some of the major recent policy initiatives and 'think tank' reports that have implications for the development of genetics and genomics.

The scientific and clinical research base

The scientific endeavour involved in the pathway from genome sequence to genetic medicine is a large-scale, complex and costly one, requiring high-throughput genomic technology, bioinformatics, population-scale databases and research projects, sophisticated statistical analysis and computing technology. If the promise of genetic science to deliver improvements in human health is to be fulfilled, a sustained programme of research investment is required. Advance on

Box 7.10 Major recent policy initiatives and 'think tank' reports with implications for genetics and genomics

- *Our Inheritance, Our Future: Realising the Potential of Genetics in the NHS* (Department of Health 2003a)
- *Strengthening Clinical Research* (Academy of Medical Sciences 2003)
- *Lambert Review of Business–University Collaboration* (Lambert 2003)
- *Bioscience 2015.* Improving national wealth, improving national health (Bioscience Innovation and Growth Team 2003)
- *Securing Good Health for the Whole Population* (Wanless 2004)
- *Science and Innovation Investment Framework 2004–2014* (HM Treasury, Department of Trade and Industry and Department for Education and Skills 2004)
- *Research for Patient Benefit Working Party* (Department of Health 2004b)
- *Public Health Sciences: Challenges and Opportunities* (Wellcome Trust 2004b)
- *Choosing Health: Making Healthier Choices Easier* (Department of Health 2004d)
- *NHS Improvement Plan: Putting People at the Heart of Public Services* (Department of Health and HM Government 2004)
- *Better Health Through Partnership* (Healthcare Industry Task Force 2004)
- *Creating a Patient-Led NHS* (Department of Health 2005f)
- *Modernising Pathology: Building a Service Responsive to Patients* (Department of Health 2005b)
- *Best Research for Best Health: A New NHS Research Strategy* (Department of Health 2006a)

the scientific front alone will not be sufficient to realise the health benefits promised by advances in genetics. A strong programme of clinical and translational research will be needed to bridge the gap between laboratory and bedside. Research in public health and the population sciences will be needed to ensure that the benefits of genetics, especially in disease prevention, are delivered to the population as a whole.

In the UK, successive Government spending reviews and science budgets in the early years of the new millennium have specifically boosted funding for genetics and genomics research, leading to the establishment of research programmes in post-genomics by the Medical Research Council, the Biotechnology and Biological Sciences Research Council and the Department of Trade and Industry, and a programme of research into ethical, legal and social implications of genomics funded by the Economic and Social Research Council. A £15 million package to establish a network of Genetics Knowledge Parks was part of this funding boost.

Government support for genetic science comes in the context of a substantial boost for spending on science research in general. July 2004 saw the publication of the Government's *Science and Innovation Investment Framework* for the decade to 2014 (HM Treasury, Department of Trade and Industry and Department for Education and Skills 2004). This framework sets, as a target, an increase in public and private sector investment in research and development from 1.9% to 2.5% of gross domestic product.

A 2003 report by the Academy of Medical Sciences, *Strengthening Clinical Research*, makes the case for a concerted strategy involving government departments, government and charitable research funders and industry, to support clinical and translational research. The creation of the UK Clinical Research Collaboration (UKCRC) may go some way towards fulfilling this aim. The UKCRC brings together the Health Departments of England and the devolved administrations, the NHS, the Medical Research Council, medical charities (such as the Wellcome Trust and Cancer Research UK), and industry to take 'strategic oversight of clinical research, identifying gaps and opportunities for action, and working in partnership to take advantage of these opportunities'. The Government is supporting this initiative by substantially increasing the research and development budget for the NHS, and creating a Joint MRC/DH Health Research Delivery Group to coordinate the contributions of government-funded bodies to the UKCRC. An early action of the UKCRC was the establishment, in 2005, of a funding programme for setting up new clinical research facilities and supporting collaborative research projects between basic and clinical scientists and industry.

The NHS Research and Development Strategy, published in January 2006 in the report *Best Research for Best Health* (Department of Health 2006a), has an emphasis on strengthening the infrastructure for clinical trials, increasing industry investment in clinical research in the NHS, and improving the regulatory framework for research. The strategy forms part of the Government's science and innovation framework and builds on the findings of the *Research for Patient Benefit Working Party*, published in 2004 (Department of Health 2004b).

New initiatives include the establishment of a virtual National Institute for Health Research (NIHR) that will include charitable sector and industry 'partners' along with NHS-funded researchers and research centres. The NIHR will be the third member of a trio of institutes that together form the NHS's framework for innovation (NIHR), evaluation (National Institute for Health and Clinical Excellence) and implementation (National Institute for Innovation and Improvement). Building on the model of the National Cancer Research Network, additional disease-based clinical networks will be set up in England, and a Clinical Research Network covering the whole of England. The Clinical Research Network will include a focused network for clinical genetics 'building on the success of the Genetics Knowledge Parks'. Work in partnership with the National Programme for IT (Connecting for Health) will ensure that electronic care records are designed in such a way as to meet research needs for data collection. There is an undertaking to reduce unnecessary bureaucracy in the procedures for ethical approval and research governance, ensuring that procedures are 'proportionate to risk'.

In commitments with direct importance for public health genetics, the NHS research and development strategy explicitly includes support for evidence synthesis and systematic reviews, and for programmes aimed at dissemination of knowledge to researchers and clinical professionals.

In his 2006 Budget speech, UK Chancellor Gordon Brown announced a proposal to merge the Medical Research Council and the NHS Research and Development programme into a single fund, with the aim of providing a more coherent framework for health research and development similar to that provided by the National Institutes of Health in the US.

Research capacity

Despite evidence of government support for bioscience in general, and genetics/genomics in particular, there has been concern that the status of science in society, and of its individual practitioners, has diminished in recent years. Careers in scientific research are insecure and poorly paid and in many western developed countries there is evidence of a decline in the number of young people choosing to study science both at school and at university.

It is essential that governments invest in good-quality science education at all levels, encourage all citizens to engage with science, and take measures to address the poor career prospects of scientists. The UK Government has recognised this challenge in its *Science and Innovation Investment Framework 2004–2014* (HM Treasury, DTI and DfES 2004), initiating measures that aim to boost the supply and quality of science teachers, improve school students' examination results in science subjects, and increase the number of young people studying science.

EU research policy

At the European level, the European Union's Sixth Framework Programme for Research (FP6, for the years 2002–2006) included, for the first time, a strand specifically focusing on life sciences, genomics and biotechnology for health. Around 2.25 billion euros has been allocated for projects in advanced genomics (for example, gene expression and proteomics, structural genomics and bioinformatics), applying advances in genomics and biotechnology to human health (for example, development of new diagnostic technologies) and applying genomic approaches to the treatment of specific diseases including cardiovascular disease, nervous system disease, diabetes and rare diseases. The European Commission's (2002a) strategy document *Life Sciences and Biotechnology: A Strategy For Europe*, and subsequent reports on the progress of the strategy, note a steadily increasing investment in this area. Tensions have emerged, however, among member states with very different social and political stances with respect to genetics and biotechnology; these differences have, in particular, dogged attempts to reach agreement on the funding of embryo research (discussed earlier in this chapter) and aspects of antenatal genetic testing.

The explicit commitment to genomics in FP6 is replaced by the more general theme of 'health' in European Commission proposals for the Seventh Framework Programme, published in April 2005. FP7 will cover the period 2007–2013. The Commission's explanation for this more broadly defined theme is that the intention is to adapt priorities as research needs change. It does, however, say that particular emphasis will be placed on translational research, defined as the translation of basic discoveries into clinical applications. Many genomic applications are likely to fall into this category.

Public health policy

Soaring expenditure on medical treatment has led most western governments to recognise the need for a shift of emphasis towards the promotion of public health and the prevention of disease. Genetics has the potential to play an important role in disease prevention if the role of genes as determinants of health, and the results of their complex interactions with lifestyle and environmental factors, can be unravelled in the coming years. But if the benefits of this research are to be realised, government rhetoric will have to be accompanied by the development of effective policies for fostering public health research and action. This will require a multidisciplinary approach that integrates the expertise of a wide range of disciplines including epidemiology, social science, psychology and economics.

In recent years, public health experts both in the UK and the US have noted a lack of sustained investment in the public health sciences, and fragmentation of many of the structures and relationships within health services that are essential for effective public health action. In the UK, for example, constant structural change within the health service, including establishment of the locally based Primary Care Trusts as the major fund-holding units, have militated against a coherent whole-population perspective on public health.

Serious deficiencies in public health research were highlighted in a 2004 report by an expert working group set up by the Wellcome Trust. The report, *Public Health Sciences: Challenges and Opportunities* (Wellcome Trust 2004b), criticised the lack of an overarching national strategy for public health. It also pointed out barriers to research, including the disruption of effective partnerships between academia and the NHS, inadequate research investment, and a huge and increasing regulatory burden imposed by such legislation as the Data Protection Act (UK

Government 1998), the Human Tissue Act (UK Government 2004c) and the Clinical Trials Regulations (2004b) (all discussed elsewhere in this chapter). These barriers, although resulting from an understandable desire to protect individuals, are preventing the development of a sound evidence base on which to base public health recommendations and may themselves be based on a faulty perception of the public's wishes and priorities. The need for evidence-based public health action was also stressed in the Government-sponsored review of public health set out in the Wanless reports of 2002 and 2004: *Securing our Future Health: Taking a Long Term View*, and *Securing Good Health for the Whole Population*.

In November 2004 the UK government published a White Paper on public health: *Choosing Health: Making Healthy Choices Easier* (Department of Health 2004d). The White Paper focuses almost exclusively on the environmental determinants of poor health and little mention is made of genetics. However, it does acknowledge that the number of public health specialists needs to be increased, and public health genetics is mentioned specifically as a specialty with growing importance.

With the merging of the National Institute for Clinical Excellence and the Health Development Agency in April 2005, a new organisation responsible for public health guidance was created. The National Institute for Health and Clinical Excellence includes, as one of its three constituent bodies, the Centre for Public Health Excellence, which will produce guidance related to both specific public health interventions and broader public health programmes.

The role of the commercial sector

The UK has a strong industrial sector in biotechnology and the pharmaceutical industry and has traditionally been a major world player in bioscience research and development. Pharmaceutical companies develop and manufacture the medicines in use in health services, while companies in the biotechnology sector focus largely on early-stage pharmaceutical research, and novel diagnostics.

The responsibilities and the risks for translating advances in genomic science into commercial products such as new drugs and diagnostics will inevitably be borne mainly by companies in the commercial sector and by their shareholders. The obligation of companies to maximise the return to their shareholders may not always be compatible with public priorities, however. As discussed earlier in this chapter, the development of pharmacogenetics exemplifies some of the sorts of tensions that may emerge: pharmaceutical companies want to produce drugs that have as large a market as possible but the advent of individually tailored drug therapy may narrow the market for many drug products, making some no longer commercially viable and potentially leaving some patient groups without drug treatments.

The need of commercial companies to recoup the huge costs incurred in genomics research and development could also lead to spiralling healthcare costs and difficult decisions for health service funders. Solutions to problems such as these are not easy to find but a productive way forward may involve the fostering of closer partnerships between the public and private sectors. The government would adopt policies that encourage commercial innovation and investment, while industry, in return, would accept obligations to contribute to the public good by, for example, responsible pricing of drugs and diagnostics, and a commitment to ensuring equity of access to medicines both within the UK and more widely.

Recent policy developments in the UK and elsewhere reflect an increasing emphasis on development of public–private partnerships. Examples in the arena of basic research include the international SNP and HapMap consortia, jointly funded by The Wellcome Trust, several universities and public-sector organisations worldwide, and private sector partners in the pharmaceutical and biotech industries. Plans for UK Biobank include provision for companies to access – with appropriate safeguards – information from the database for pharmaceutical and other research.

Reports by a number of government-sponsored advisory bodies and independent 'think tanks' also pursue the partnership theme. In its 2003 report *Bioscience 2015*, the Bioscience Innovation and Growth Team (BIGT) recommended collaboration between the NHS and industry through the establishment of a National Clinical Trials agency, fostering a regulatory and policy environment supportive of innovation, and creation of a Bioscience Leadership Council to provide a forum for government and industry to work together. Similarly, the *Lambert review of Business–University Collaboration* (Lambert 2003) concluded that companies are moving away from independent and often secret research towards a new model in which they seek more open collaboration with both commercial and public-sector partners. Recent initiatives towards the publication of clinical trial results suggest that companies are beginning to acknowledge the importance of improving public trust in their activities.

The 2004 report of the Healthcare Industry Task Force (HITF), a Government sponsored advisory group set up to identify opportunities for closer cooperation between Government and healthcare companies, encapsulates current Government policy. The HITF focused on several key areas in which it considered it could recommend practical measures to bring about improvement. These included:

- Improving the evaluation of new healthcare technologies, devices and procedures
- Stimulating innovation through an Innovation Centre to coordinate the development, dissemination and commercialisation of innovations coming from both the public and private sectors

- Maximising UK influence in regulatory matters in the EU and other international forums to ensure that regulation is appropriate
- Improving public understanding of the risk:benefit profile and the regulatory system for medical devices
- Training and education of NHS staff in the safe and competent use of new technologies.

Government initiatives in recent years have also signalled a move towards greater involvement of the private sector in service provision. The 2004 *NHS Improvement Plan* (Department of Health and HM Government 2004) describes a healthcare system in which services are delivered by a range of providers funded by the NHS and accredited by the Health Care Commission. The HITF report also develops this theme, recommending mechanisms to improve clarity on levels of access by industry, to involve clinicians in decisions on procurement of new technologies, and to encourage input from industry into policy initiatives such as the National Service Frameworks.

These policies are already being implemented in a number of areas relevant to genetics and genomics. For example, the Pathology Modernisation Programme, set out in the reports *Modernising Pathology Services* (Department of Health 2004e) and *Modernising Pathology: Building a Service Responsive to Patients* (Department of Health 2005b), is a strategy that emphasises partnership with the private sector in the provision of diagnostic services, which include genetic tests. The report also recommends the development of services 'closer to the patient', greater emphasis on the clinical and cost-effectiveness of diagnostic tests, development of mechanisms to ensure the assessment and integration of new technologies, and measures to strengthen the skills and capacity of the pathology workforce.

Attempts to reconcile the aims of the private and public sectors will inevitably lead to some tensions: companies push for a lighter regulatory load, greater rewards for risk and innovation, and streamlined access for their products and services to the patient market. Public and political pressures, on the other hand, may tend to emphasise greater safety and protection for consumers (leading to more stringent regulation), and containment of healthcare costs. There has been criticism of current government strategies to encourage direct involvement of the commercial sector in healthcare research, development and provision. Those who do not support this approach claim that the interests of patients and the public are not sufficiently safeguarded and that issues such as ownership of intellectual property, conflicts of interest, quality control and ethical safeguards have not been resolved.

Financial considerations and health economics

It seems inescapable that many of the new diagnostics, treatments and other interventions that are likely to result from advances in genetic science and biotechnology will be expensive. Gene therapy, protein therapy and applications of cell-based therapy including stem cell therapy are obvious examples. Health service planners and commissioners will have difficult choices to make in assigning priorities: every new intervention adopted has an opportunity cost in a cash-limited system such as the NHS.

There is general commitment within the UK to maintaining the core values of the NHS as a tax-funded service, available to all regardless of income or geographical location. However, it may be difficult for the system to survive the pressures arising from the ageing of the population and the ever-expanding possibilities offered by modern medicine. As discussed in the preceding section, there have already been moves towards greater involvement of the private sector in healthcare provision, though so far services remain free at the point of need. Whether the expansion of private provision will eventually lead to erosion of the NHS's key principle of social equity remains to be seen.

Whatever the model for healthcare funding, there is increasing emphasis on ensuring that new interventions are both clinically effective (hence the growth of 'evidence-based medicine' and the advent of bodies such as the National Institute of Health and Clinical Excellence) and cost-effective. Health economic analysis of genetics-based diagnostics, interventions and services is in its infancy and the literature is small. Studies have focused mainly on a handful of topics including population screening programmes for specific genetic diseases, pharmacogenetics and methodological issues. They have predominantly involved investigation of cost-effectiveness, or straightforward cost estimation; there have been few attempts to determine cost–benefit relationships or cost consequences.

Health-economic implications of pharmacogenetic testing have been discussed earlier in this chapter. The likely economic impact of a broader range of applications for genetic tests is unknown. The cost of testing technology itself is likely to fall but there may be substantial costs associated with analysis and secure storage of the information arising from tests. Many other factors also need to be considered, in particular the clinical utility of tests such as those that may eventually be available for assessing genetic susceptibility to disease. Health economists must find ways of including in their analysis some quantification of factors such as the likelihood that people will take effective action to reduce their disease risk (thus reducing costs to the health service) and the possibility that uncertainties in assessing the level of risk revealed by a genetic test might lead to unnecessary treatment of people who would in any case have remained well (thus increasing clinical costs).

There is also a need for rigorous health-economic assessment of existing clinical genetics services. This can be problematic and new methodologies may be needed. In the case of clinical genetics consultation and genetic counselling, one difficulty has been uncertainty about how to quantify the value of an intervention that consists, essentially, of information. Nor is it clear how to incorporate the fact that the 'patient' in genetic services is often not an individual but an extended family. Laboratory services are also coming under scrutiny from a health-economic standpoint. In the early days of DNA testing, the transition from research to service funding of new tests was almost automatic, but such a relaxed system has proved unsustainable in the face of the explosion in the number of possible tests. As discussed elsewhere in this chapter, the clinical value of genetic tests is now being examined with more rigour, and there have been moves to rationalise test provision, with more centralisation of tests for very rare conditions.

Despite increasing need for their expertise, there is a general shortage of health economists, particularly in the public sector. Government and the NHS must address the problem of capacity in this area by, for example, improving training provision, increasing research funding and devising incentives for talented people to remain in the public sector.

Education and training

Although opinions differ about the rate of progress, there is general consensus that genetic science and genetic technology will eventually have a major impact on health care and that health professionals will need to meet the challenge of incorporating genetics into their professional practice. The provision of genetic information will no longer be confined to the controlled and careful environment of the clinical genetics consultation, but will become the responsibility of GPs or practice nurses in the busy environment of the general practice surgery, or of non-geneticist health professionals in hospital clinics.

All clinical professionals will need to prepare for their changing role by equipping themselves with a working knowledge of genetics and with skills in risk assessment and communication. They will also need an understanding of the social and psychological impact of information about genetic risk and to recognise situations where specialist counselling may be appropriate. Clinical professionals may need support (for example, computer-based tools) to help them in interpreting genetic information for their patients, and new formats for patient information and education may also need to be explored.

Non-clinical personnel including civil servants in health departments, hospital managers, commissioners of services, and public health professionals will all need to understand the impact of genetics in order to discharge their responsibility for making funding available for the necessary professional development of health service staff, and for implementing the changes required to support a new paradigm in the delivery of clinical services.

Many surveys have shown that practitioners in all of these professional fields are ill-equipped and lack confidence to take on the challenge posed by advances in genetics. Competencies in genetics will need to be formulated for all professional groups and programmes of education and training made available at all levels from undergraduate training through post-graduate specialisation and continuing professional development.

Recognising the need to make progress in this area, initiatives have been established in several countries, including the UK and the US, to work towards embedding genetics in health-professional education and training. In the US, the National Coalition for Health Professional Education in Genetics (NCHPEG), set up in 1996 by the American Medical Association, the American Nurses Association and the National Human Genome Research Institute, aims to integrate genetics into the knowledge base of health professionals, to develop educational tools and materials, and to attract other organisations to participate in the coalition and subscribe to its goals.

In the UK, the Department of Health and the Wellcome Trust funded a two-year project in 2001–2003 to survey the status of genetics education of a variety of health-professional groups and to recommend a strategy for the future. An important feature of the project was the active involvement of the professional groups themselves and of representatives from patient groups. Key conclusions from the project report, *Addressing Genetics, Delivering Health* (Burton 2003), included the need to:

- Incorporate genetics into major clinical policy initiatives such as the National Service Frameworks
- Relate genetics education directly to clinical practice and current services
- Develop accessible, authoritative and up-to-date learning resources, for example on the web
- Involve patient groups in scoping what practitioners need to know
- Make genetics a compulsory, examinable part of curricula
- Stress the place of genetics as part of an integrated clinical network.

In its 2003 Genetics White Paper, the UK Government (Department of Health 2003a) accepted the need for a coordinated approach to genetics education in the health service, establishing an NHS National Genetics Education and Development Centre in Birmingham with three-year funding. Key objectives of the Centre are to identify core skills in genetics for different groups of staff (particularly GPs), produce materials and courses to enable staff to access genetics education and training and provide support for new service developments.

Developments such as those outlined here are certainly to be welcomed but there remains doubt as to whether governments are committed to the level of funding that is needed to make a real difference to the competence of health professionals in genetics. The report *Addressing Genetics, Delivering Health* (Burton 2003) estimated a need for around £2 million per year in the UK over the next 5–10 years; by contrast, the funding allocated to the NHS National Genetics Education and Development Centre is £600 000 per year for only 3 years. In the absence of sufficient dedicated funding, it will be important to foster 'champions' of genetics within key professional groups to lobby their colleagues for an increasing emphasis on genetics in professional curricula, and to use available resources prudently, perhaps by working first towards 'training the trainer' and promoting sharing of resources.

The public

In a modern democratic and pluralist society such as the UK, policy is no longer determined in an authoritarian manner by government and the civil service acting in isolation, or by the private deliberations of 'quangos' (quasi-autonomous non-government organisations) composed of the 'great and the good'. Increasingly, attempts are made to involve the wider public in policy-making through mechanisms including electronic consultations, focus groups and opinion polls. New bodies have been established such as the Commission for Patient and Public Involvement in Health, and 'Involve', a group devoted to promoting public involvement in health research. Lay members are included on all advisory committees and research ethics committees.

If the public is to play a full and positive role in policy development for genetics, people must have sufficient knowledge and understanding of the subject to enable them to make an informed contribution. There is evidence that the general level of 'genetic literacy' is low and that people have a poor understanding of risk and probability – concepts that are essential to grasp if, for example, genetic testing for disease susceptibility becomes a reality in the future.

Efforts are needed at all levels, not just in formal programmes of education but more widely, to raise the overall level of scientific understanding. Scientists and the media have a particular responsibility: scientists to communicate scientific advances clearly and to avoid hype, and the media to report accurately and responsibly. Journalists must also be alert to the sources of their information and aware of the different vested interests of groups such as scientific researchers, patient advocacy groups and campaigning organisations that take an anti-science stance. While it is important that the public is exposed to all the arguments surrounding a particular issue, it may be difficult for the media to achieve this while at the same time conveying an accurate sense of the balance of opinion in society overall – very vocal special-interest groups can tend to command a disproportionate amount of 'air time'.

Improved scientific literacy, however, is not a guarantee of enthusiasm and acceptance. The 'public knowledge deficit' model, which holds that people will embrace technological development if only they can understand it, is no longer considered valid and those who are enthusiastic about the potential of genetic science must accept that greater public knowledge of and engagement with genetic science will not necessarily lead to blanket endorsement.

Government, advisory bodies and various other organisations have all been involved in developing policy for public engagement in science and technology. The House of Lords Select Committee on Science and Technology (2000), and the Office of Science and Technology and The Wellcome Trust (2000) have published reports on the issue. Several science-based organisations have specific programmes of public engagement and debate. These include the Royal Society's Science in Society programme (and, jointly with the Office of Science and Technology, the COPUS grants scheme), the British Association for the Advancement of Science, the Office of Science and Technology's Public Engagement with Science and Technology (PUSET) programme, and the Royal Institution.

The Government's strategic *Science and Innovation Investment Framework 2004–2014* (HM Treasury, DTI and DfES 2004) recognises the importance of achieving increased public awareness of, and confidence in, scientific research and its applications. The Office of Science and Innovation's Science and Society budget will double over the next few years, to support a new scheme of grants to build capacity for encouraging citizens, scientists and policy-makers to debate emerging regulatory and ethical issues. A strengthened horizon-scanning system will attempt to identify potentially contentious developments at an early stage, so that public engagement and debate can be more proactive.

So far, applications of genetics in health care appear to command public support. The scientific and medical research communities must continue to earn and nurture this trust and to seek ways of achieving societal consensus on the way forward.

Concluding remarks

In Chapter 1 we set out the background to the enterprise that has come to be known as public health genetics, and a vision (Figure 1.4) for its future growth and development. In Chapters 2–6 we have explored the broad scope of the knowledge base that must be brought together and integrated by participants in this enterprise. This knowledge base encompasses an understanding not just of scientific advances across the whole field of genome-based molecular and cell biology (Chapter 2) but also of their relevance at the population level (Chapter 3), their potential application in clinical medicine (Chapter 4), their effect on health service organisation and development (Chapter 5), their ethical and social dimensions (Chapter 6), and the routes by which policy can be developed – across all these areas – to ensure benefits for the whole population (Chapter 7).

There is now a need to build capacity in public health genetics within the public health profession. Leadership in public health genetics within the UK could be provided by training between 10 and 12 specialists in this field. This could be best done by seconding existing public health physicians for specialist training and creating specialist jobs when they return to their home region. The remit for these jobs should include input into the specialist commissioning process and contributions to the establishment of national and regional networks.

At an international level, progress can be accelerated by communication and collaboration. International networks such as the Genome-based Research and Population Health International Network (GRaPH *Int*) and the European group Public Health Genomics European Network (PHGEN) will help to bring the vision of using genome-based knowledge and technology for the benefit of population health closer to reality.

Further reading and resources

Many of the policy documents concerning key issues in genetics have been cited explicitly in the text of this chapter and their bibliographic details are given in the reference list at the end of the book. The Further reading section of Chapter 6 lists books and papers that discuss some of the conceptual background to policy development in the areas of genetics and reproductive choice, privacy and confidentiality of genetic information, genetic discrimination (including insurance and employment) and informed consent for the use of human tissue for clinical genetic analysis. The HumGen database maintained by the Centre de recherche en droit public at the University of Montreal, and the policy database at the Public Health Genetics Unit in Cambridge are useful repositories of policy documents, reports and legislation.

Policy development for genetics in the UK

For readers interested in the development of genetics policy, the following account outlines some of the most influential reports and documents that have been published over the last decade. (For key reports on the development of genetics services, see the Further reading section of Chapter 5.)

The first evidence of UK policy-makers' interest in genetics and its wider implications beyond specialist clinical genetics services came in the mid 1990s, with the publication of the report *Human Genetics: The Science and its Consequences* by the House of Commons Select Committee on Science and Technology (1995) and, in the same year, two special reports on genetics commissioned by the NHS Central Research and Development Committee (1995a, b; *Genetics of Common Disease*, and *Report of the Genetics Research Advisory Group*).

The mid to late 1990s also saw the establishment of the first Government advisory committees devoted to genetics: the Human Genetics Advisory Commission and the Advisory Committee on Genetic Testing. Early reports from these bodies on issues such as genetic testing in insurance and employment, genetic tests supplied direct to the public, and genetic testing for late-onset disorders, are archived on the Department of Health website.

Other non-government organisations, professional bodies and ad hoc expert groups also became interested at around this time in policy issues raised by genetics. Examples include the Institute of Public Policy Research report *Brave New NHS: The Impact of the New Genetics on the Health Service* (Lenaghan 1998), the British Medical Association report *Human Genetics: Choice and Responsibility* (1998) the Office of Health Economics Report *Genomics Healthcare and Public Policy* (Williams and Clow 1999), and the University College London School of Public Policy report *Human Genomics: Prospects for Health Care and Public Policy* (Richmond 1999). In the European Union, the European Group on Ethics in Science and New Technologies was established and released its first reports on topics including human tissue banking and stem cell research.

The Office of Genomics and Disease Prevention was established in the US in 1997, and the Public Health Genetics Unit in the UK in the same year. Key publications detailing the development of thinking in public health genetics/ genomics are outlined in the Further reading section in Chapter 1.

A 1999 Government review of the advisory and regulatory framework for biotechnology (Office of Science and Technology 1999) led to the establishment of the Human Genetics Commission in 2000, replacing the Advisory Committee on Genetic Testing and the Human Genetics Advisory Commission. The year 2000 also saw the publication of *Genetics and Health* (Zimmern and Cook 2000), the report of the Nuffield Trust Genetics Scenario project. This project, for the first time, brought stakeholders together from across the fields of scientific and clinical research, clinical medicine, public health, policy development, ethics and social science, and patient advocacy, to reach a shared vision for the future development of genetics in health services.

The first five years of the new millennium have been a time of intense debate and policy action, both in genetics specifically (culminating in the Genetics White Paper of 2003: *Our Inheritance, Our Future*; Department of Health 2003a), and more broadly across the whole field of biomedical science and its clinical applications. The HGC has explored a variety of issues including over-the-counter genetic tests (Human Genetics Commission 2003) and personal genetic information (Human Genetics Commission 2002). Parliamentary select committees have also been active in considering the implications of genetics: the House of Commons Select Committee on Science and Technology has reported on *Genetics and Insurance*

(2001) and *Developments in Human Genetics and Embryology* (2002), while House of Lords committees have produced highly influential reports on *Human Genetic Databases* (2001) and *Stem Cell Research* (2002). The Nuffield Council on Bioethics has maintained a strong focus on genetics, with investigations on topics including mental disorders and genetics, pharmacogenetics, DNA patenting, and genetics and human behaviour (Nuffield Council on Bioethics 1998, 2002a, 2002b, 2003).

News about current policy developments in genetics is provided by the Public Health Genetics Unit online newsletter.

The international context

Information about UNESCO's work on bioethics, including the work of the International Bioethics Committee and the Intergovernmental Bioethics Committee, is available on a dedicated section of the UNESCO website. References for the reports and declarations listed in Box 7.3 can be found in the reference list at the end of the book. The ethics committee of the Human Genome Organisation, an international group representing scientists and others involved in genomics research, has issued statements on a number of issues including genomic databases, cloning, gene therapy, benefit sharing and DNA sampling. These are available on the HUGO website.

The Genomics Resource Centre web pages of the World Health Organization (WHO) website contain information on WHO's international activities in the field of ethical, legal, social and policy implications of genetics and genomics.

Genetics in reproductive decision-making

The issues raised by the use of genetics and genetic technology in reproductive decision-making and assisted reproduction are set out very clearly in the Human Genetics Commission's (2006a) report. Recommendations and a background document published by the European Society of Human Genetics and the European Society of Human Reproduction and Embryology in 2005 discuss the issues from the perspective of clinical and scientific professionals (European Society of Human Genetics and European Society of Human Reproduction and Embryology 2006; Soini *et al.* 2006). The legal arguments for and against the use of pre-implantation genetic diagnosis with tissue typing can be followed through the successive High Court, Appeal Court and House of Lords judgments in the case brought by Quintavalle [listed in the reference list as *R* (on the application of Quintavalle) v *Human Fertilisation and Embryology Authority*].

Assisted reproduction

Current UK policy on genetic issues in assisted reproduction, such as donor anonymity and testing/screening of gamete and embryo donors, is set out in the

HFEA's *Code of Practice* (Human Fertilisation and Embryology Authority 2003a) and in guidance documents available on the HFEA website. A report published by the European Commission in 2006 provides interesting information on the regulation of reproductive cell (gamete) donation in the member states of the European Union. Petersen (2006) has published an international comparison of policy on the issue of donor anonymity.

Several reports and statements published in the late 1990s discuss the issues raised by the application of cloning technology in human reproduction. Examples include a comprehensive report by the US National Bioethics Advisory Commission (1997); a statement by the Royal Society (1998); and a joint report from the Human Genetics Advisory Commission and the Human Fertilisation and Embryology Authority (1998).

Consent to genetic testing and analysis

The Department of Health has published a guide to the provisions of the Human Tissue Act which is available on their website. The Department of Health web page on the Human Tissue Act also provides links to current draft and consultation documents related to the development of codes of practice.

A paper by Liddell and Hall (2005) provides a detailed commentary on the Human Tissue Act. Several professional organisations commented on difficulties raised by the original Bill, including the Wellcome Trust (2004a), the Medical Research Council, the Academy of Medical Sciences and the Royal College of Physicians (2004). Their responses are available on the respective websites. The Human Tissue Authority's website provides the latest versions of their *Codes of Practice*, together with detailed guidance on licensing including compliance reports and sector-specific guidance. Lowrance's 2006 report for the Medical Research Council and the Wellcome Trust provides up-to-date guidelines for researchers on obtaining human tissue samples or data for research.

Liddell, Menon and Zimmern (2004) published a brief commentary pointing out problems with the Mental Capacity Bill. Guidance for health professionals on the Mental Capacity Act in its final form are available on the Department of Health website.

Protection of medical and genetic information

For a clear and informative discussion of the protection of medical information, and policy for regulating its use in research, an excellent reference is Lowrance's 2002 report *Learning from Experience. Privacy and the Secondary Use of Data in Health Research.* For those needing a brief overview, the Parliamentary Office of Science and Technology (2005a) has produced a useful summary (postnote) on the current legislative position regarding data protection and medical research.

The Department of Health's web pages on patient confidentiality and access to medical records contain the NHS 2003 code of practice on patient confidentiality, and information on the Caldicott guardians and the work of the health services data protection review group.

Lucassen, Parker and Wheeler (2006) have published a very lucid, brief commentary on the implications of data protection legislation for family history. In an article in the same issue of *BMJ*, Schmitz and Wiesing (2006) argue that family history information should have the same legal status as laboratory genetic test results.

Protection against unfair discrimination

Documents concerned with policy development for the use of genetic test information in insurance and/or employment include, in addition to reports by the Human Genetics Commission (2006b) and the Human Genetics Advisory Commission (1999), a 2001 report by the House of Commons Select Committee on Science and Technology. This report, regarded by some commentators as unduly biased against the insurance industry, exemplifies the political pressure that can be brought to bear on policy-makers. The Association of British Insurers has issued a code of practice (Association of British Insurers 1999) on genetic testing in insurance and an information leaflet for patients (Association of British Insurers 2005). The Human Genetics Commission website has some useful pages on genetics and employment. A report on genetic testing in the workplace was published in 2003 by the European Group on Ethics in Science and New Technologies.

Regulation of genetic tests

The issues surrounding genetic test regulation are discussed in detail in a paper by Burke and Zimmern (2004). References on the evaluation of genetic tests are detailed in the Further reading section of Chapter 4. A postnote by the Parliamentary Office of Science and Technology (2003a) succinctly sets out the current regulatory position on medical 'self-test' kits, while an additional postnote discusses the current regulatory environment for genetic tests, also providing briefing information on the wider context including patient confidentiality and consent, genetics and information technology, test evaluation, the provision of genetic tests within current NHS services, and possible future applications (Parliamentary Office of Science and Technology 2004a).

Pharmacogenetics: policy issues

The Royal Society has assessed the prospects for pharmacogenetics, including the need for development of capacity and expertise in the health service workforce, in its 2005 report *Personalised Medicine: Hopes and Realities*. For a discussion of ethical and policy issues raised by pharmacogenetics, The Nuffield Council on Bioethics' 2003 report, *Pharmacogenetics: Ethical Issues* is a valuable reference. *My Very Own Medicine: What Must I Know?* (Melzer *et al.*, 2003) is the report from a Wellcome-Trust-funded project to examine the evidence required for regulatory authorities, clinicians and patients to decide on the appropriate use of new pharmacogenetic tests. Webster and colleagues (2004) have examined some of the conflicting interests and options that will need to be resolved if pharmacogenetics is to become a mainstream element of health services. Ginsburg *et al.* (2005) discuss (from a US perspective) policy barriers to the translation of pharmacogenetics into clinical practice, including the lack of a formal agenda to promote innovation, to develop the necessary information technology, or to address financing issues. A review by Phillips, Veenstra and Sadee (2000) urges the need for more research on societal and economic implications of pharmacogenetics to inform clinical and policy decisions about its development. Veenstra and colleagues (2000) have reviewed the cost-effectiveness of pharmacogenetic tests, including some useful case studies. References on scientific and clinical aspects of pharmacogenetics are outlined in Chapter 4.

Advanced therapies

The 2002 report of the House of Lords Stem Cells Committee sets out clearly the regulatory issues raised by the use of embryos for stem cell research and therapy. A more recent 2005 report by the UK Stem Cell Initiative (known as the Pattison review) summarises the 'state of the art' for stem cell research and therapy, develops a strategic vision for supporting this scientific field in the UK, and discusses options for the regulatory framework in the UK. The legal battle over the authority of the HFEA to regulate human embryonic stem cell research and therapeutic cloning can be followed in the court judgements listed in the reference list as *R* (on the application of Quintavalle) v *Secretary of State for Health*.

The battles within the United Nations and the EU over attempts to ban or restrict funding for research involving human embryonic stem cells and cloning technology can be followed through items in the online newsletter on the Public Health Genetics Unit website.

Some of the policy and regulatory considerations raised by advanced therapies are explored in a paper by Liddell and Wallace (2005), in the context of stem cell medicine. A postnote summary on the regulation of gene therapy and possible future regulatory developments was published by the Parliamentary Office of Science and Technology (2005b).

However, the regulatory environment in this area is changing rapidly and is perhaps best followed at the EU level by referring to the European Commission's

DG Enterprise and Industry website. The reference list contains web links to the 2001 EU Directive on medicinal products and to amendments to the Directive passed in 2003 and 2004, which clarify definitions for gene therapy medicinal products and somatic cell therapy medicinal products.

Clinical trials and research governance

Details on the implementation of the EU Clinical Trials Directive in the UK are available on pages of the website of the Medicines and Healthcare Products Regulatory Agency. Some of the concerns about adverse effects of this legislation on medical research are discussed in an editorial by Nicholson (2004) in the *British Medical Journal.*

Intellectual property and patents

For examples of divergent views on the legitimacy and policy implications of patents on gene sequences, and their effects on innovation, see the papers by Andrews (2002) in *Nature Reviews Genetics*, and by Warburg and colleagues (2003) in *Pharmacogenomics.* Bostyn (2003) has published an excellent though quite specialised review of the issues from a legal perspective. A 'perspectives' article by Van Overwalle *et al.* (2006) in *Nature Reviews Genetics* suggest ways of facilitating access to genetic inventions that have patent protection. The Human Genetics Commission has produced some web information pages on intellectual property and genetics, written for a general audience.

Many professional and other groups have set out concerns about the current situation. For examples see the reports of the Nuffield Council on Bioethics (*The Ethics of Patenting DNA*, 2002a) and The Royal Society (*Keeping Science Open: The Effects of Intellectual Property Policy on the Conduct of Science*, 2003). The World Health Organization (2005) has considered the impact of patenting on developing countries. The European Group on Ethics in Science and New Technologies (2002) has issued an opinion on the ethics of patenting inventions involving stem cells.

General policy issues

For an overview of general policy issues, Zimmern and Cook's 2000 report *Genetics and Health* is a good starting point. A review by Sharp, Yudell and Wilson (2004) discusses the policy 'drivers' for science and how these apply to genomics.

Scientific and clinical research policy, and relationships between the public and private sectors

The reports and other documents cited in the text provide a wealth of reading on policy for scientific and clinical research. For insight into some current US thinking on this issue, an editorial by Zerhouni (2005) in the *New England Journal of Medicine* outlines the US National Institutes of Health's 'new vision' for translational and clinical science. A flavour of the controversy over the role of industry in healthcare research, development and provision can be found in a commentary by Pollock, McNally and Kerrison (2006) on the 2006 NHS Research and Development Strategy, and the 2005 report of the House of Commons Health Committee on *The Influence of the Pharmaceutical Industry*. A 2002 report from the Academy of Medical Sciences exemplifies professional alarm about problems with recruitment and retention of clinical academic researchers.

Health economics

A general discussion of the economic problems that health services may confront as a result of the development of genetic and genomic medicine has been published by Danzon and Towse (2002). Zimmern and Cook's 2000 report *Genetics and Health* also deals in general with financial issues for the health services. Examples of health-economic analysis of population screening programmes for genetic conditions are available in reports published on the Health Technology Assessment programme's website.

Education and training

A 2002 review by Burke and Emery discusses the knowledge and competencies primary care practitioners will need in genetics. A systematic review by Suther and Goodson (2003) synthesises the results from 68 papers surveying the barriers to the provision of genetic services in primary care. The paper by Fears and colleagues (1999) reviews in more general terms the impact of advances in genetics and molecular biology on the education and research training of healthcare professionals. Burke (2005) has reviewed ways in which public health can contribute resources and valuable perspectives to educational programmes in genetics for health professionals; her article is one of a series published in a special issue of the journal *Health Education and Behavior*. Further references on genetics education for health professionals are available on the websites of the NHS National Genetics Education and Development Centre and the (US) National Coalition for Health Professional Education in Genetics.

Public involvement

Mathews and colleagues (2005) have investigated the role and attitudes of scientists in public outreach about genetics. A paper by Jones and Salter (2003) explores the relationship between the development of governance in human genetics, and public trust. The Royal Society (2006) has published a report which concludes that scientists should keep the public interest in mind when communicating the results of their research to the public and the media. A postnote summary from the Parliamentary Office of Science and Techology (2003b) summarises some methods for encouraging public dialogue, and what has been learned from them. The case studies presented for illustration are not specifically concerned with genetics, but the conclusions are general. Additional references on public attitudes to genetics are listed in the Further reading section of Chapter 6.

Challenges for public health genetics

Several references discussing the future challenges for public health genetics are mentioned in the Further reading section of Chapter 1. Additional papers discussing the implications of genomics and genetics for the public health agenda in the coming years, and the debate over strategies for prevention of common disease, have been published by Ojha and Thertulien (2005), Kirkman (2005) and Thomas *et al.* (2005).

Further reading

Books, reports and journal papers

Academy of Medical Sciences (2002). *Clinical Academic Medicine in Jeopardy: Recommendations for Change.* Summary available online at www.academicmedicine.ac.uk/uploads/Academic%20Medicine%20in%20Jeopardy.pdf.

Academy of Medical Sciences (2003). *Strengthening Clinical Research.* Available online at www.acmedsci.ac.uk/images/project/Report.pdf.

Academy of Medical Sciences (2006). *Personal Data for Public Good: Using Health Information in Medical Research.* Available online at www.acmedsci.ac.uk/images/project/Personal.pdf.

Acheson, L. S. and Wiesner, G. L. (2004a). Current and future applications of genetics in primary care medicine. *Prim. Care* **31**, 449–60.

Acheson, L. S. and Wiesner, G. L. eds. (2004b). Genetics for Primary Care Clinicians. *Prim. Care* **31**.

Aderem, A. (2005). Systems biology: its practice and challenges. *Cell* **121**, 511–13.

Advisory Committee on Genetic Testing (1998). *Genetic Testing for Late Onset Disorders.* Available online at www.publications.doh.gov.uk/pub/docs/doh/lodrep.pdf.

Andrews, L. B. (2002). Genes and patent policy: rethinking intellectual property rights. *Nat. Rev. Genet.* **3**, 803–8.

Andrews, L. B., Fullarton, J. E., Hotzman, N. A. *et al.*: Committee on Assessing Genetic Risks, Institute of Medicine (1994). *Assessing Genetic Risks. Implications for Health and Social Policy.* Washington, D.C.: National Academies Press.

Article 29 Data Protection Working Party (2004). Working document on genetic data. 12178/03/EN WP91. Available online at www.datenschutz-berlin.de/doc/eu/gruppe29/wp91/wp91_en.pdf.

Association of British Insurers (1999). *Genetic testing – ABI code of practice.* Available online at www.abi.org.uk/Display/default.asp?Menu_ID=1140&Menu_All=1,946,1140&Child_ID=517.

Association of British Insurers (2005). *Insurance and Genetic Tests. What you Need to Know.* Available online at www.abi.org.uk/Display/File/Child/436/Genetics_guide_2005.pdf.

Banks, E. and Meade, T. (2002). The study of genes and environmental factors in common disease. *Lancet* **359**, 1156–7.

Banks, R. E., Dunn, M. J., Hochstrasses, D. F. *et al.* (2000). Proteomics: new perspectives, new biomedical opportunities. *Lancet* **356**, 1749–56.

Bayat, A. (2002). Bioinformatics. *BMJ* **324**, 1018–22.

Bell, J. (1998). The new genetics in clinical practice. *BMJ* **316**, 618–20.

Bell, J. (2004). Predicting disease using genomics. *Nature* **429**, 453–6.

Beskow, L. M., Khoury, M. J., Baker, T. G. and Thrasher, J. F. (2001). The integration of genomics into public health research, policy and practice in the United States. *Community Genet.* **4**, 2–11.

Bioscience Innovation and Growth Team (2003). *Bioscience 2015.* Available online at www.bioindustry.org/bigtreport/.

Bostyn, S. J. R. (2003). The prodigal son: the relationship between patent law and health care. *Med. Law Rev.* **11**, 67–120.

Brandt-Rauf, P. W. and Brandt-Rauf, S. I. (2004). Genetic testing in the workplace: ethical, legal, and social implications. *Annu. Rev. Public Health* **25**, 139–53.

Breslow, N. E. and Day, N. E. (1980). *Statistical Methods in Cancer Research* (Volume 1). *The Analysis of Case–Control Studies.* Lyon: International Agency for Research on Cancer (IARC), World Health Organisation.

Brice, P. (2004). Array of hope. *Health Serv. J.* **114**, 24–5.

Brice, P. and Sanderson, S. (2006a). Genetics, health and medicine. *Pharm. J.* **277**, 53–56.

Brice, P. and Sanderson, S. (2006b). Use for genetics in pharmacy. *Pharm. J.* **277**, 109–12.

Brice, P. and Sanderson, S. (2006c). Pharmacogenetics: what are the ethical and economic implications? *Pharm. J.* **277**, 113–14.

Bristol Royal Infirmary Inquiry (2001). *Learning from Bristol. The Report of the Public Inquiry into Children's Heart Surgery at the Bristol Royal Infirmary 1984–1999.* London: The Stationery Office. Available online at www.bristol-inquiry.org.uk/final_report/the_report.pdf.

British Medical Association (1998). *Human Genetics: Choice and Responsibility.* Oxford: Oxford University Press.

British Medical Association (1999). *Confidentiality and Disclosure of Health Information.* Available online at www.bma.org.uk/ap.nsf/Content/Confidentialitydisclosure.

British Medical Association (2005a). *Confidentiality as Part of a Bigger Picture. A Discussion Paper.* Available online at www.bma.org.uk/ap.nsf/Content/ConfidentialityBiggerPicture.

British Medical Association (2005b). *Population Screening and Genetic Testing. A Briefing on Current Programmes and Technologies.* Available online at www.bma.org.uk/ap.nsf/Content/Populationscreeninggenetictesting.

Brivanlou, A. H., Gage, F. H., Jaenisch, R., Jessell, T., Melton, D. and Rossant, J. (2003). Stem cells. Setting standards for human embryonic stem cells. *Science* **300**, 913–16.

Brock, D. (2002). Human cloning and our sense of self. *Science* **296**, 314–16.

Buchanan, A. E., Brock, D. W., Daniels, N. and Wikler, D. (2000). *Chance to Choice: Genetics and Justice.* Cambridge: Cambridge University Press.

Burke, W. (2002). Genetic testing. *N. Engl. J. Med.* **347**, 1867–75.

Burke, W. (2003). Genomic medicine: genomics as a probe for disease biology. *N. Engl. J. Med.* **349**, 969–74.

Burke, W. (2004). Genetic testing in primary care. *Annu. Rev. Genomics Hum. Genet.* **5**, 1–14.

Burke, W. (2005). Contributions of public health to genetics education for health professionals. *Health Educ. Behav.* **32**, 668–75.

Burke, W. and Emery, J. (2002). Genetics education for primary-care providers. *Nat. Rev. Genet.* **3**, 561–6.

Burke, W. and Zimmern, R. L. (2004). Ensuring the appropriate use of genetic tests. *Nat. Rev. Genet.* **5**, 955–8.

Burke, W., Khoury, M. J., Stewart, A., Zimmern, R. L.: Bellagio Group. (2006). The path from genome-based research to population health: development of an international collaborative public health genomics initiative. *Genet. Med.* **8**, 451–8.

Burt, R. and Neklason, D. W. (2005). Genetic testing for inherited colon cancer. *Gastroenterology* **128**, 1696–716.

Burton, H. (2003). *Addressing Genetics, Delivering Health.* Available online at www.phgu.org.uk/addressing_genetics.shtml.

Burton, H. (2005). *Metabolic Pathways. Networks of Care.* Cambridge: Public Health Genetics Unit. Available online at www.phgu.org.uk.

Burton, P., McCarthy, M. and Elliott, P. (2002). The study of genes and environmental factors in common disease. *Lancet* **359**, 1155.

Burton, P. R., Tobin, M. D. and Hopper, J. L. (2005). Key concepts in genetic epidemiology. *Lancet* **366**, 941–51.

Calvo, K. R., Liotta, L. A. and Petricoin, E. F. (2005). Clinical proteomics: from biomarker discovery and cell signaling profiles to individualized personal therapy. *Biosci. Rep.* **25**, 107–25.

Cambon-Thomsen, A. (2004). The social and ethical issues of post-genomic human biobanks. *Nat. Rev. Genet.* **5**, 866–73.

Campbell, H. and Rudan, I. (2002). Interpretation of genetic association studies in complex disease. *Pharmacogenomics J.* **2**, 349–60.

Cardon, L. R. and Abecasis, G. R. (2003). Using haplotype blocks to map human complex trait loci. *Trends Genet.* **19**, 135–40.

Cavazzana-Calvo, M., Thrasher, A. and Mavilio, F. (2004). The future of gene therapy. *Nature* **427**, 779–81.

Centers for Disease Control and Prevention (1997). *Translating Advances in Human Genetics into Public Health Action: A Strategic Plan.* Available online at www.cdc.gov/genomics/about/strategic.htm.

Chadwick, R., Levitt, M. and Shickle, D. (1997). *The Right to Know and the Right Not to Know.* Aldershot: Avebury.

Christianson, A. and Modell, B. (2004). Medical genetics in developing countries. *Annu. Rev. Genomics Hum. Genet.* **5**, 219–65.

Chung, D. C. and Rustgi, A. K. (2003). The hereditary nonpolyposis colorectal cancer syndrome: genetics and clinical implications. *Ann. Intern. Med.* **138**, 560–70.

Clarke, A., ed. (1998). *The Genetic Testing of Children.* Oxford: Bios Scientific Publishers.

Clayton, D. and McKeigue, P. M. (2001). Epidemiological methods for studying genes and environmental factors in complex diseases. *Lancet* **358**, 1356–60.

Clayton, E. W. (2003). Genomic medicine: ethical, legal, and social implications of genomic medicine. *N. Engl. J. Med.* **349**, 562–9.

Clinical Genetics Society (1994). *The Genetic Testing of Children.* Available online at www.bshg.org.uk/documents/official_docs/testchil.htm.

Collins, F. S. (1999). Shattuck lecture – medical and societal consequences of the human genome project. *N. Engl. J. Med.* **341**, 28–37.

Collins, F. S. (2003). A vision for the future of genomics research. *Nature* **422**, 835–47.

Committee for the Study of the Future of Public Health, Division of Health Care Services, Institute of Medicine (1998). *The Future of Public Health.* Washington, D.C.: National Academies Press.

Consumers' Association and GeneWatch UK (2002). *Genetic Testing in the High Street.* Available online at www.genewatch.org/HumanGen/tests/Letters/GeneWatch.doc.

Cooke, G. S. and Hill, A. V. (2001). Genetics of susceptibility to human infectious disease. *Nat. Rev. Genet.* **2**, 967–77.

Cordell, H. J. and Clayton, D. G. (2005). Genetic association studies. *Lancet* **366**, 1121–31.

Cornish, W. R., Llewelyn, M. and Adcock, M. (2003). *Intellectual Property Rights and Genetics. A Study into the Impact and Management of Intellectual Property Rights Within the Healthcare Sector.* Available online at www.phgu.org.uk/about_phgu/intellect_prop_rights.html.

Costa, L. G. (2000). The emerging field of ecogenetics. *Neurotoxicology* **21**, 85–9.

Council of Europe (1953). *Convention for the Protection of Human Rights and Fundamental Freedoms.* Available online at http://conventions.coe.int/treaty/en/Treaties/Html/005.htm.

Council of Europe (1997). *Convention on Human Rights and Biomedicine.* Available online at conventions.coe.int/treaty/en/treaties/html/164.htm.

Council for International Organisations of Medical Sciences (1990). *The Declaration of Inuyama. Human Genome Mapping, Genetic Screening and Gene Therapy.* Available online at www.cioms.ch/frame_1990_texts_of_guidelines.htm.

Council for International Organisations of Medical Sciences (2002). *International Ethical Guidelines for Biomedical Research Involving Human Subjects.* Geneva: CIOMS. Available online at www.cioms.ch/frame_guidelines_nov_2002.htm.

Daar, A. S., Thorsteinsdottir, H., Martin, D. K., Smith, A. C., Nast, S. and Singer, P. A. (2002). Top ten biotechnologies for improving health in developing countries. *Nat. Genet.* **32**, 229–32.

Danzon, P. and Towse, A. (2002). The genomic revolution: is the real risk under-investment rather than bankrupt healthcare systems? *J. Health Serv. Res. Policy* **5**, 253–5.

Darnton-Hill, I., Margetts, B. and Deckelbaum, R. (2004). Public health nutrition and genetics: implications for nutrition policy and promotion. *Proc. Nutr. Soc.* **63**, 173–85.

Davey Smith, G. and Ebrahim, S. (2003). 'Mendelian randomization': can genetic epidemiology contribute to understanding environmental determinants of disease? *Int. J. Epidemiol.* **32**, 1–22.

Davey Smith, G. D., Ebrahim, S., Lewis, S., Hansell, A. L., Palmer, L. J. and Burton, P. R. (2005). Genetic epidemiology and public health: hope, hype, and future prospects. *Lancet* **366**, 1484–98.

Department of Health (1993). *Population Needs and Genetic Services: An Outline Guide.* London: HMSO.

Department of Health (2000a). *The NHS Cancer Plan: A Plan for Investment, a Plan for Reform.* Available online at www.dh.gov.uk/PublicationsAndStatistics/Publications/Publications

PolicyAndGuidance/PublicationsPolicyAndGuidanceArticle/fs/en?CONTENT_ID=4009609&chk=n4LXTU.

Department of Health (2000b). *Coronary Heart Disease: National Service Framework for Coronary Heart Disease – Modern Standards and Service Models*. Available online at www.dh.gov.uk/PublicationsAndStatistics/Publications/PublicationsPolicyAndGuidance/PublicationsPolicyAndGuidanceArticle/fs/en?CONTENT_ID=4094275&chk=eTacxC.

Department of Health (2000c). *Laboratory Services for Genetics. Report of an Expert Working Group to the NHS Executive and the Human Genetics Commission*. Available online at www.dh.gov.uk/PublicationsAndStatistics/Publications/PublicationsPolicyAndGuidance/PublicationsPolicy AndGuidanceArticle/fs/en?CONTENT_ID=4118936&chk=2yGYxK.

Department of Health (2000d). *Stem Cell Research. Medical Progress with Responsibility. A Report from the Chief Medical Officer's Expert Group Reviewing the Potential of Developments in Stem Cell Research and Cell Nuclear Replacement to Benefit Human Health*. Available online at www.lucacoscioni.it/cms/documenti/donaldson_eng.pdf.

Department of Health (2001). *The Expert Patient: A New Approach to Chronic Disease Management in the 21st Century*. Available online at www.dh.gov.uk/PublicationsAndStatistics/Publications/PublicationsPolicyAndGuidance/PublicationsPolicyAndGuidanceArticle/fs/en?CONTENT_ID=4006801&chk=UQCoh9.

Department of Health (2002a). *The NHS as an Innovative Organisation. A Framework and Guidance on the Management of Intellectual Property in the NHS*. Available online at www.innovations.nhs.uk/pdfs/77169_doh_nhsnnovative_orgfinal.pdf.

Department of Health (2002b). *Specialised Services National Definition Set: 20. Medical Genetic Services (All Ages)*. Available online at www.dh.gov.uk/PolicyAndGuidance/HealthAndSocialCareTopics/SpecialisedServicesDefinition/SpecialisedServicesDefinitionArticle/fs/en?CONTENT_ID=4001694&chk=LwpMsS.

Department of Health (2003a). *Our Inheritance, Our Future: Realising the Potential of Genetics in the NHS*. Available online at www.dh.gov.uk/PublicationsAndStatistics/Publications/PublicationsPolicyAndGuidance/PublicationPolicyAndGuidanceArticle/fs/en?CONTENT_ID=4006538&chk=enskfb.

Department of Health (2003b). *Confidentiality. NHS Code of Practice*. Available online at www.dh.gov.uk/assetRoot/04/06/92/54/04069254.pdf.

Department of Health (2003c). *Guidance on Commissioning Arrangements for Specialised Services*. Available online at www.dh.gov.uk/PublicationsAndStatistics/Publications/PublicationsPolicyAndGuidance/PublicationsPolicyAndGuidanceArticle/fs/en?CONTENT_ID=4081718&chk=goY90I.

Department of Health (2004a). *National Service Framework for Children, Young People and Maternity Services*. Available online at www.dh.gov.uk/PolicyAndGuidance/HealthAndSocialCareTopics/ChildrenServices/ChildrenServicesInformation/ChildrenServicesInformationArticle/fs/en?CONTENT_ID=4089111&chk=U8Ecln.

Department of Health (2004b). *Research for Patient Benefit Working Party – Final Report*. Available online at www.dh.gov.uk/assetRoot/04/08/26/75/04082675.PDF.

Department of Health (2004c). *The Human Tissue Act 2004. New Legislation on Human Organs and Tissue*. Available online at www.dh.gov.uk/assetRoot/04/10/36/86/04103686.pdf.

Department of Health (2004d). *Choosing Health: Making Healthy Choices Easier.* Available online at www.dh.gov.uk/PublicationsAndStatistics/Publications/PublicationsPolicyAndGuidance/PublicationsPolicyAndGuidanceArticle/fs/en?CONTENT_ID=4094550&chk=aN5Cor.

Department of Health (2004e). *Modernising Pathology Services.* Available online at www.dh.gov.uk/assetRoot/04/07/31/12/04073112.pdf.

Department of Health (2005a). *National Service Framework for Long Term Conditions.* Available online at www.dh.gov.uk/PublicationsAndStatistics/Publications/PublicationsPolicyAndGuidance/PublicationsPolicyAndGuidanceArticle/fs/en?CONTENT_ID=4105361&chk=jl7dri.

Department of Health (2005b). *Modernising Pathology: Building a Service Responsive to Patients.* Available online at www.dh.gov.uk/assetRoot/04/11/97/78/04119778.pdf.

Department of Health (2005c). *Report of the Ad Hoc Advisory Group on the Operation of NHS Research Ethics Committees.* Available online at www.dh.gov.uk/assetRoot/04/11/24/66/04112466.pdf.

Department of Health (2005d). *Review of the Human Fertilisation and Embryology Act. A Public Consultation.* Available online at www.dh.gov.uk/assetRoot/04/11/78/72/04117872. pdf.

Department of Health (2005e). *Research Governance Framework for Health and Social Care.* Available online at www.dh.gov.uk/PolicyAndGuidance/ResearchAndDevelopment/ResearchAndDevelopmentAZ/ResearchGovernance/ResearchGovernanceArticle/fs/en?CONTENT_ID=4002112&chk=PJlaGg.

Department of Health (2005f). *Creating a Patient-Led NHS: Delivering the NHS Improvement Plan.* Available online at www.dh.gov.uk/PublicationsAndStatistics/Publications/PublicationsPolicyAndGuidance/PublicationsPolicyAndGuidance/PublicationsPolicyAndGuidanceArticle/Fs/en?CONTENT_ID=4106506&chk=ftV6vA.

Department of Health (2006a). *Best Research for Best Health: A New National Health Service Research Strategy.* Available online at www.dh.gov.uk/assetRoot/04/12/71/52/04127152.pdf.

Department of Health (2006b). *Review of Commissioning Arrangements for Specialised Services.* Available online at www.dh.gov.uk/PolicyAndGuidance/OrganisationPolicy/Commissioning/CommissioningSpecialisedServices/CommissioningSpecialisedArticle/fs/en?CONTENT_ID=4135174&chk=H2g0oV.

Department of Health and Association of British Insurers (2005). *Concordat and Moratorium on Genetics and Insurance.* Available online at www.dh.gov.uk/PublicationsAndStatistics/Publications/PublicationsPolicyAndGuidanceArticle/fs/en?CONTENT_ID=4105905&chk=Gor9x8.

Department of Health and HM Government (2004). *The NHS Improvement Plan: Putting People at the Heart of Public Services.* Available on line at www.dh.gov.uk/assetRoot/04/08/45/22/04084522.pdf.

Donnai, D. (2002). Genetics services. *Clin. Genet.* **61**, 1–6.

Donnai, D. and Elles, R. (2001). Integrated regional genetics services: current and future provision. *BMJ* **322**, 1048–52.

Downward, J. (2004). RNA interference. *BMJ* **328**, 1245–8.

Emens, L. (2005). Trastuzumab: targeted therapy for the management of HER-2/neu over-expressing metastatic breast cancer. *Am. J. Ther.* **12**, 243–53.

Engel, L. S., Taioli, E., Pfeiffer, R. *et al.* (2002). Pooled analysis and meta-analysis of glutathione *S*-transferase M1 and bladder cancer: a HuGE review. *Am. J. Epidemiol.* **156**, 95–109 [Erratum in: *Am. J. Epidemiol.* (2002) **156**, 492.]

Equalities Review (2005). *Interim Report for Consultation.* Available online at www.theequalitiesreview.org.uk/Sites/www.theequalitiesreview.org.uk/publications/interim_report.aspx.

European Commission (2002a). *Life Sciences and Biotechnology: A Strategy for Europe.* Available online at europe.eu.int/eur-lex/en/com/cnc/2002/com2002_0027en01.pdf.

European Commission (2002b). *Procedural Modalities for Research Activities Involving Banked or Isolated Human Embryonic Stem Cells in Culture to be Funded under Council Decision 2002/834/EC.* Available online at http://ec.europa.eu/research/science-society/pdf/procedural_modalities_en.pdf.

European Commission (2003). Commission Directive 2003/63/EC of 25 June 2003 amending Directive 2001/83/EC of the European Parliament and of the Council on the Community code relating to medicinal products for human use. Available online at europa.eu.int/eur-lex/lex/LexUriServ/LexUriServ.do?uri=CELEX:32003L0063:EN:HTML.

European Commission (2004a). *Ethical, Legal and Social Aspects of Genetic Testing: Research, Development and Clinical Applications.* Luxembourg: Office for Official Publications of the European Communities. Available online at europa.eu.int/comm/research/conferences/2004/genetic/pdf/report_en.pdf.

European Commission (2004b). *25 Recommendations on the Ethical, Legal and Social Implications of Genetic Testing.* Luxembourg: Office for Official Publications of the European Communities. Available online at europa.eu.int/comm/research/conferences/2004/genetic/pdf/recommendations_en.pdf.

European Commission (2005a). *Proposal for a Regulation of the European Parliament and of the Council on Advanced Therapy Medicinal Products and Amending Directive 2001/83/EC and Regulation (EC) no. 726/2004.* Available online at pharmacos.eudra.org/F2/advtherapies/docs/COM_2005_567_EN.pdf.

European Commission (2005b). *Report from the Commission to the Council and the European Parliament. Development and Implications of Patent Law in the Field of Biotechnology and Genetic Engineering.* Available online at www.europa.eu.int/comm/internal_market/en/indprop/invent/com_2005_312final_en.pdf.

European Commission (2006). *Report on the Regulation of Reproductive Cell Donation in the European Union.* Available online at ec.europa.eu/health/ph_threats/human_substance/documents/tissues_frep_en.pdf.

European Group on Ethics in Science and New Technologies (1997). *Ethical Aspects of Cloning Techniques.* Available online at europa.eu.int/comm/european_group_ethics/gaieb/en/opinion9.pdf.

European Group on Ethics in Science and New Technologies (2000). *Ethical Aspects of Human Stem Cell Research and Use.* Available online at europa.eu.int/comm/european_group_ethics/docs/avis15_en.pdf.

European Group on Ethics in Science and New Technologies (2002). *Ethical Aspects of Patenting Inventions Involving Human Stem Cells.* Available online at europa.eu.int/comm/european_group_ethics/docs/avis16_en.pdf.

European Group on Ethics in Science and New Technologies (2003). *Ethical Aspects of Genetic Testing in the Workplace*. Available online at europa.eu.int/comm/european_group_ethics/docs/avis18EN.pdf.

European Parliament and Council (1995). Directive 95/46/EC of the European Parliament and of the Council of 24 October 1995 on the protection of individuals with regard to the processing of personal data and on the free movement of such data. Available online at europa.eu.int/eur-lex/lex/LexUriServ/site/en/consleg/1995/L/01995L0046–20031120-en.pdf.

European Parliament and Council (1998a). Directive 98/79/EC of the European Parliament and of the Council of 27 October 1998 on in vitro diagnostic medical devices. Available online at europa.eu.int/eur-lex/pri/en/oj/dat/1998/l_331/l_33119981207en00010037.pdf.

European Parliament and Council (1998b). Directive 98/44/EC of the European Parliament and of the Council of 6 July 1998 on the legal protection of biotechnological inventions. Available online at europa.eu.int/eur-lex/pri/en/oj/dat/1998/l_213/l_21319980730en00130021.pdf.

European Parliament and Council (2001a). Directive 2001/20/EC of the European Parliament and of the Council of 4 April 2001 on the approximation of the laws, regulations and administrative provisions of the Member States relating to the implementation of good clinical practice in the conduct of clinical trials on medicinal products for human use (the Clinical Trials Directive). Available online at www.wctn.org.uk/downloads/EU_Directive/Directive.pdf.

European Parliament and Council (2001b). Directive 2001/83/EC of the European Parliament and of the Council of 6 November 2001 on the Community code relating to medicinal products for human use. Available online at europa.eu.int/eur-lex/pri/en/oj/dat/2001/l_311/l_31120011128en00670128.pdf.

European Parliament and Council (2004a). Directive 2004/23/EC of the European Parliament and of the Council of 31 March 2004 on setting standards of quality and safety for the donation, procurement, testing, processing, preservation, storage and distribution of human tissues and cells. Available online at europa.eu.int/eur-lex/pri/en/oj/dat/2004/l_102/l_10220040407en00480058.pdf.

European Parliament and Council (2004b). Directive 2004/27/EC of the European Parliament and of the Council of 31 March 2004 amending Directive 2001/83/EC on the Community code relating to medicinal products for human use. Available online at europa.eu.int/eur-lex/pri/en/oj/dat/2004/l_136/l_13620040430en00340057.pdf.

European Patent Office (1973, with subsequent amendments). *European Patent Convention*. Available online at www.european-patent-office.org/legal/epc/.

European Society of Human Genetics (2003). International coverage of all aspects of human genetics. *Eur. J. Hum. Genet.* **11**, suppl. 2.

European Society of Human Genetics and European Society of Human Reproduction and Embryology (2005). *The Interface Between Medically Assisted Reproduction and Genetics: Technical, Social and Ethical Issues (Draft Report)*. Available online at www.eshg.org/BGDocuAfterSevilla030605etAnnexes.pdf

Farrall, M. and Morris, A. P. (2005). Gearing up for genome-wide gene-association studies. *Hum. Mol. Genet.* **14** (Review Issue 2), R157–62.

Fears, R., Weatherall, D. and Poste, G. (1999). The impact of genetics on medical education and training. *Br. Med. Bull.* **55**, 460–70.

Feinberg, A. P., Ohlsson, R. and Henikoff, S. (2006). The epigenetic progenitor origin of human cancer. *Nat. Rev. Genet.* **7**, 21–3.

Fineman, R. (1999). Qualifications of public health geneticists? *Community Genet.* **2**, 113–14.

Firth, H. and Hurst, J. (2005). *Oxford Desk Reference – Clinical Genetics*. Oxford: Oxford University Press.

Food and Drug Administration (US) (2005). *Guidance for Industry. Pharmacogenomic Data Submissions*. Available online at www.fda.gov/cber/gdlns/pharmdtasub.htm.

Fox Keller, E. (2000). *The Century of the Gene*. Cambridge, Mass.: Harvard University Press.

Gelehrter, T. D., Collins, F. and Ginsburg, D. (1998). *The Principles of Medical Genetics*, 2nd edn. New York: Lippincott Williams and Wilkins.

General Medical Council (2002). *Research: The Role and Responsibilities of Doctors*. Available online at www.gmc-uk.org/guidance/library/research.asp.

General Medical Council (2004). *Confidentiality: Protecting and Providing Information*. Available online at www.gmc-uk.org/guidance/library/confidentiality.asp.

Genomics Working Group of the Science and Technology Task Force of the United Nations Millennium Project (2003). *Genomics and Global Health*. Toronto: Canadian Program in Genomics and Global Health, University of Toronto Joint Centre for Bioethics.

Ginsburg, G. S., Konstance, R. P., Allsbrook, J. S. and Schulman, K. A. (2005). Implications of pharmacogenomics for drug development and clinical practice. *Arch. Intern. Med.* **165**, 2331–6.

Grace, J., El Toukhy, T. and Braude, P. (2004) Pre-implantation genetic testing. *Br. J. Obstet. Gynaecol.* **111**, 1165–73.

Green, J. M., Hewison, J., Bekker, H. L., Bryant, L. D. and Cuckle, H. S. (2004). Psychosocial aspects of genetic screening of pregnant women and newborns: a systematic review. *Health Technol Assess.* **8**, 1–109.

Green, M. J. and Botkin, J. R. (2003). 'Genetic exceptionalism' in medicine: clarifying the differences between genetic and nongenetic tests. *Ann. Intern. Med.* **1**, 571–5.

Grice, G. R., Seaton, T. L., Woodland, A. M. and McLeod, H. L. (2006). Defining the opportunity for pharmacogenetic intervention in primary care. *Pharmacogenomics* **7**, 61–5.

Guttmacher, A. E. and Collins, F. S. (2002). Genomic medicine – a primer. *N. Engl. J. Med.* **347**, 1512–20.

Guttmacher, A. E. and Collins, F. S. (2005). Realizing the promise of genomics in biomedical research. *J. Am. Med. Assoc.* **294**, 1399–402.

Gwinn, M. and Khoury, M. J. (2002). Research priorities for the public health sciences in the post-genomic era. *Genet. Med.* **4**, 410–11.

Hadfield, S. G. and Humphries, S. E. (2005). Implementation of cascade testing for the detection of familial hypercholesterolaemia. *Curr. Opin. Lipidol.* **16**, 428–33.

Haga, S. B., Khoury, M. J. and Burke, W. (2003). Genomic profiling to promote a health lifestyle: not ready for prime time. *Nat. Genet.* **34**, 347–50.

Halliday, J. L., Collins, V. R., Aitken, M. A., Richards, M. P. and Olsson, C. A. (2004). Genetics and public health – evolution, or revolution? *J. Epidemiol. Community Health* **58**, 894–9.

Harris, J. (2000). Is there a coherent social conception of disability? *J. Med. Ethics* **26**, 95–100.

Harris, J. and Holm, S., eds. (1998). *The Future of Human Reproduction: Ethics, Choice and Regulation*. Oxford: Clarendon Press.

Hattersley, A. T. and McCarthy, M. I. (2005). What makes a good genetic association study? *Lancet* **366**, 1315–23.

Healthcare Industry Task Force (2004). *Better Health Through Partnership*. Available online at www.dh.gov.uk/assetRoot/04/09/52/23/04095223.pdf.

Hedgecoe, A. (2001). Ethical boundary work: geneticisation, philosophy and the social sciences. *Med. Health Care Philosoph.* **4**, 305–9.

Hernandez, L. ed.: Committee on Genomics and the Public's Health in the Twenty-First Century, Institute of Medicine (2005). *Implications of Genomics for Public Health. Workshop Summary*. Washington, D. C.: National Academies Press.

Hinxton Group (2006). *An International Consortium on Stem Cells, Ethics and Law. Consensus Statement*. Available online at www.hopkinsmedicine.org/bioethics/finalsc.doc.

Hirschhorn, J. N. and Daly, M. J. (2005). Genome-wide association studies for common diseases and complex traits. *Nat. Rev. Genet.* **6**, 95–108.

HM Treasury, Department of Trade and Industry and Department for Education and Skills (2004). *Science and Innovation Investment Framework 2004–2014*. Available online at www.hm-treasury.gov.uk/spending_review/spend_sr04/associated_documents/spending_sr04_science.cfm.

Hodge, J. G. Jr (2004). Ethical issues concerning genetic testing and screening in public health. *Am. J. Med. Genet. C. Semin. Med. Genet.* **125**, 66–70.

Holtzman, N. A. (1989). *Proceed with Caution: Predicting Genetic Risks in the Recombinant DNA Era*. Baltimore: Johns Hopkins University Press.

Holtzman, N. A. (2006). What role for public health in genetics and vice versa? *Community Genet.* **9**, 8–20.

Holtzman, N. A. and Marteau, T. M. (2000). Will genetics revolutionize medicine? *N. Engl. J. Med.* **343**, 141–4.

Hood, L., Heath, J. R., Phelps, M. E. and Lin, B. (2004). Systems biology and new technologies enable predictive and preventive medicine. *Science* **306**, 640–3.

Hopper, J. L., Bishop, D. T. and Easton, D. F. (2005). Population based family studies in genetic epidemiology. *Lancet* **366**, 1397–406.

House of Commons Health Committee (2005). *The Influence of the Pharmaceutical Industry*. London: The Stationery Office. Available online at www.publications.parliament.uk/pa/cm200405/cmselect/cmhealth/42/42.pdf.

House of Commons Select Committee on Science and Technology (1995). *Human Genetics: The Science and its Consequences*. Third Report of the House of Commons Science and Technology Committee. London: HMSO.

House of Commons Select Committee on Science and Technology (2001). *Genetics and Insurance*. Available online at www.publications.parliament.uk/pa/cm200001/cmselect/cmsctech/174/17402.htm.

House of Commons Select Committee on Science and Technology (2002). *Developments in Human Genetics and Embryology*. London: The Stationery Office. Available online at http://www.publications.parliament.UK/pa/cm200102/cmselect/cmsctech/791/79103. htm.

House of Commons Select Committee on Science and Technology (2005). *Human Reproductive Technologies and the Law*. London: The Stationery Office. Available online at http://www.publications.parliament.UK/pa/cm200405/cmselect/cmsctech/7/702.htm.

House of Lords Select Committee on Science and Technology (2000). *Science and Society*. Available online at www.publications.parliament.uk/pa/ld199900/ldselect/ldsctech/38/3801.htm.

House of Lords Select Committee on Science and Technology (2001). *Human Genetic Databases: Challenges and Opportunities*. Available online at www.publications.parliament.uk/pa/ld200001/ldselect/ldsctech/57/5701.htm.

House of Lords Stem Cell Research Committee (2002). *Stem Cell Research*. Available online www.parliament.the-stationery-office.co.uk/pa/ld200102/ldselect/ldstem/83/8301.htm.

Hubbard, R. and Wald, E. (1997). *Exploding the Gene Myth*. Boston: Beacon Press.

Hudson, K. L., Rothenburg, K. H., Andrews, L. B., Kahn, M. J. and Collins, F. S. (1995). Genetic discrimination and health insurance: an urgent need for reform. *Science* **270**, 391–3.

Human Fertilisation and Embryology Authority (2003a). *Code of practice*, 6th edn. Available online at www.hfea.gov.uk/HFEAPublications/CodeofPractice/Code%20of%20Practice%20 Sixth%20Edition%20-%20final.pdf.

Human Fertilisation and Embryology Authority (2003b). *Sex Selection: Report Summary*. Available online at www.hfea.gov.uk/AboutHFEA/Consultations/Final%20sex%20 selection%20summary.pdf.

Human Fertilisation and Embryology Authority (2004a). *Report of the Preimplantation Tissue Typing Policy Review*. Available online at www.hfea.gov.uk/AboutHFEA/HFEAPolicy/Preimplantationtissuetyping.

Human Fertilisation and Embryology Authority (2004b). *Report of the Sperm Egg and Embryo Donation (SEED) Review*. Available online at www.hfea.gov.uk/PressOffice/TheSEEDReview.

Human Fertilisation and Embryology Authority (2004c). *The Human Fertilisation and Embryology Authority (Disclosure of Donor Information) Regulations 2004*. Statutory instruments 2004 1511. London: The Stationery Office. Available online at www.opsi.gov.uk/si/si2004/20041511.htm.

Human Fertilisation and Embryology Authority (2005). *Choices and Boundaries. Should People be Able to Select Embyros Free From an Inherited Susceptibility to Cancer*? Available online at www.hfea.gov.uk/AboutHFEA/Consultations.

Human Genetics Advisory Commission (1999). *The Implications of Genetic Testing for Employment*. Available online at www.advisorybodies.doh.gov.uk/hgac/papers/papergl.htm.

Human Genetics Advisory Commission and Human Fertilisation and Embryology Authority (1998). *Cloning Issues in Reproduction, Science and Medicine*. Available online at www.hfea.gov.uk/AboutHFEA/Consultations/1998%20December%20Cloning%20Issue%20in%20 Reproduction%20 Science%20and%20Medicine%20Report.pdf.

Human Genetics Commission (2001). *Public Attitudes to Human Genetic Information*. Available online at www.hgc.gov.uk/UploadDocs/DocPub/Document/morigeneticattitudes.pdf.

Human Genetics Commission (2002). *Inside Information: Balancing Interests in the Use of Personal Genetic Data.* Available online at www.hgc.gov.uk/UploadDocs/DocPub/Document/insideinformation_summary.pdf.

Human Genetics Commission (2003). *Genes Direct. Ensuring the Effective Oversight of Genetic Tests Supplied Direct to the Public.* Available online at www.hgc.gov.uk/UploadDocs/DocPub/Document/genesdirect_full.pdf.

Human Genetics Commission (2004). *Choosing the Future: Genetics and Reproductive Decision Making.* Consultation document available online at www.hgc.gov.uk/UploadDocs/DocPub/Document/ChooseFuturefull.pdf.

Human Genetics Commission (2005). *Profiling the Newborn: A Prospective Gene Technology?* Available online at www.hgc.gov.uk/uploadDocs/Contents/Documents/final%20Draft%20of%20Profiling%20Newborn%20/Report%2003%2005.pdf.

Human Genetics Commission (2006a). *Making Babies: Reproductive Decisions and Genetic Technologies.* Available online at www.hgc.gov.uk/UploadDocs/DocPub/Document/Making%20Babies%20Report%20-%20final%20pdf.pdf.

Human Genetics Commission (2006b). *Genetic Testing and Employment.* (Letter to Lord Sainsbury, Parliamentary Under-Secretary of State for Science and Innovation). Available online at www.hgc.gov.uk/UploadDocs/Contents/Documents/For%20web%20-%20%20Lord%20Sainsbury%20prevalence%20of%20genetic%20testing%20 response.doc.

Hunt, S. C., Gwinn, M. and Adams, T. D. (2003). Family history assessment: strategies for the prevention of cardiovascular disease. *Am. J. Prev. Med.* **24**, 136–42.

Hunter, A. and Humphries, S. E. (2005). Family history of breast cancer and cost of life insurance: a test case comparison of current UK industry practice. *BMJ* **331**, 1438–9.

Hunter, D. J. (2005). Gene–environment interactions in human disease. *Nat. Rev. Genet.* **6**, 287–98.

Information Commissioner (2002). *Use and Disclosure of Health Data. Guidance on the Application of the Data Protection Act 1998.* Available online at ico-cms.amaze.co.uk/DocumentUploads/use%20and%20disclosure%20of%20health%20data.pdf.

Information Commissioner (2005a). *Employment practices code.* Available online at www.ico.gov.uk/upload/documents/library/data_protection/practical_application/ICO_EmpPracCode.pdf.

Information Commissioner (2005b). *Employment Practices Code. Supplementary Guidance. Managing Data Protection.* Available online at http://www.ico.gov.uk/upload/documents/library/data_protection/practical_application/ico_suppgdnce.pdf.

Ioannidis, J. P., Gwinn, M., Little, J. *et al.* (2006). A road map for efficient and reliable human genome epidemiology. *Nat. Genet.* **38**, 3–5.

Jackson, E. (2001). *Regulating Reproduction: Law, Technology and Autonomy.* Oxford: Hart Publishing.

Janssens, A. C., Pardo, M. C., Steyerberg, E. W. and van Duijn, C. M. (2005). Revisiting the clinical validity of multiplex genetic testing in complex diseases. *Am. J. Hum. Genet.* **74**, 585–8.

Joint Committee on Medical Genetics (2006). *Consent and Confidentiality.* London: British Society of Human Genetics, Royal College of Pathologists, Royal College of Physicians.

Jones, M. and Salter, B. (2003). The governance of human genetics: policy discourse and constructions of public trust. *New Genet. Soc.* **22**, 21–41.

Juengst, E. T. (1995). 'Prevention' and the goals of genetic medicine. *Hum. Gene Ther.* **6**, 1595–605.

Kanehisa, M. and Bork, P. (2003). Bioinformatics in the post-sequence era. *Nat. Genet.* **33**, 305–10.

Kaput, J., Ordovas, J. M., Ferguson, L. *et al.* (2005). The case for strategic international alliances to harness nutritional genomics for public and personal health. *Br. J. Nutr.* **94**, 623–32.

Kelada, S. N., Eaton, D. L., Wang, S. S., Rothman, N. R. and Khoury, M. J. (2003). The role of genetic polymorphisms in environmental health. *Environ. Health Perspect.* **111**, 1055–64.

Kerr, A. and Shakespeare, T. (1999). *Genetic Politics: From Eugenics to Genome (Issues in Social Policy)*. Cheltenham: New Clarion Press.

Kevles, D. J. (1995). *In the Name of Eugenics: Genetics and the Uses of Human Heredity.* Cambridge, Mass.: Harvard University Press.

Khoury, M. J. (1996). From genes to public health: application of genetics in disease prevention. *Am. J. Public Health.* **86**, 1717–22.

Khoury, M. J. (2003). Genetics and genomics in practice. The continuum from genetic disease to genomic information in health and disease. *Genet. Med.* **5**, 261–8.

Khoury, M. J. (2004). The case for a global human genome epidemiology initiative. *Nat. Genet.* **36**, 1027–8.

Khoury, M. J. and Mensah, G. A. (2005). Genomics and the prevention and control of common chronic diseases: emerging priorities for public health action. *Prev. Chronic Dis.* [serial online] April. Available online at www.cdc.gov/pcd/issues/2005/apr/05_0011.htm.

Khoury, M. J., Burke, W. and Thomson, E. J., eds. (2000). *Genetics and Public Health in the 21st Century.* New York: Oxford University Press.

Khoury, M. J., McCabe, L. L. and McCabe, E. R. B. (2003). Genomic medicine: population screening in the age of genomic medicine. *N. Engl. J. Med.* **348**, 50–8.

Khoury, M. J., Little, J. and Burke, W. eds. (2004a). *Human Genome Epidemiology.* Oxford: Oxford University Press.

Khoury, M. J., Little, J. and Burke, W. eds. (2004b). *Human Genome Epidemiology.* Part III. *Methods and Approaches II: Assessing Genetic Tests for Disease Prevention*, pp. 195–301. Oxford: Oxford University Press.

Khoury, M. J., Yang, Q., Gwinn, M., Little, J. and Dana Flanders, W. (2004c). An epidemiologic assessment of genomic profiling for measuring susceptibility to common diseases and targeting interventions. *Genet. Med.* **6**, 38–47.

Khoury, M. J., Davis, R., Gwinn, M., Lindegren, M. L. and Yoon, P. (2005). Do we need genomic research for the prevention of common diseases with environmental causes? *Am. J. Epidemiol.* **161**, 799–805.

King, R. A., Rotter, J. I. and Motulsky, A. G. (2002). *The Genetic Basis of Common Diseases,* 2nd edn. New York: Oxford University Press.

Kirkman, M. (2005). Public health and the challenge of genomics. *Aust. N. Z. J. Public Health* **29**, 163–5.

Knoppers, B. M. and Fecteau, C. (2003). Human genomic databases: a global public good? *Eur. J. Health Law* **10**, 27–41.

Knoppers, B. M., Bordet, S. and Isasi, R. M. (2006). Preimplantation genetic diagnosis: an overview of socio-ethical and legal considerations. *Annu. Rev. Genomics Hum. Genet.* **7**, 201–21.

Krause, D. E. and Van Etten, R. A. (2005). Tyrosine kinases as targets for cancer therapy. *N. Engl. J. Med.* **353**, 172–87.

Kroese, M., Zimmern, R. and Sanderson, S. (2004). Genetic tests and their evaluation: can we answer the key questions? *Genet. Med.* **6**, 475–80.

Kwiatkowski, D. P. (2005). How malaria has affected the human genome and what human genetics can teach us about malaria. *Am. J. Hum. Genet.* **77**, 171–92.

Lambert, D. (2003). *Lambert Review of Business–University Collaboration*. Available online at www.hm-treasury.gov.uk/media/EA556/lambert_review_final_450.pdf.

Last, J. M. ed. (2001). *A Dictionary of Epidemiology*, 4th edn. New York: Oxford University Press.

Laurie, G. (2002). *Genetic Privacy: A Challenge to Medico-Legal Norms*. Cambridge: Cambridge University Press.

Lee, R. G. and Morgan, D. (2001). *Human Fertilisation and Embryology: Regulating the Reproductive Revolution*. London: Blackstone Press.

Lenaghan, J. (1998). *Brave New NHS: The Impact of the New Genetics on the Health Service*. London: Institute of Public Policy Research.

Lerman, C. and Shields, A. E. (2004). Genetic testing for cancer susceptibility: the promise and the pitfalls. *Nat. Rev. Cancer* **4**, 235–41.

Lewontin, R. C., Rose, S. and Kamin, L. (1984). *Not in our Genes*. New York: Pantheon Books.

Liddell, K. and Hall, A. (2005). Beyond Bristol and Alder Hey: the future regulation of human tissue. *Med. Law Rev.* **13**, 137–69.

Liddell, K. and Wallace, S. (2005). Emerging regulatory issues for human stem cell medicine. *Genomics, Society and Policy* **1**, 54–73. Available online at www.gspjournal.com/.

Liddell, K., Menon, D. K. and Zimmern, R. (2004). The human tissue bill and the mental capacity bill. New regulations are needed to make useful research possible. *BMJ* **328**, 1510–11.

Little, J. and Khoury, M. J. (2003). Mendelian randomisation: a new spin or real progress? *Lancet* **362**, 930–1.

Little, J., Bradley, L., Bray, M. S. *et al.* (2002). Reporting, appraising, and integrating data on genotype prevalence and gene–disease associations. *Am. J. Epidemiol.* **156**, 300–10.

Little, J., Sharp, L., Khoury, M. J., Bradley, L. and Gwinn, M. (2005). The epidemiologic approach to pharmacogenomics. *Am. J. Pharmacogenomics* **5**, 1–20.

Lockwood, M. (2001). The moral status of the human embryo. *Hum. Fertil.* **4**, 267–9.

London IDEAS Genetics Knowledge Park (2004). *Reality Not Hype: The New Genetics in Primary Care*. Available online at www.londonideas.org/internet/events/documents/hunter booklet.pdf.

Lowrance, W. W. (2002). *Learning From Experience. Privacy and the Secondary Use of Data in Health Research*. London: The Nuffield Trust. Available online at www.nuffieldtrust.org.uk/ publications/detail.asp?id=0&PRid=45.

Lowrance, W. W. (2006). *Access to Collections of Data and Materials for Health Research*. London: Medical Research Council and Wellcome Trust. Available online at www.mrc. ac.uk/index/strategy-strategy/strategy-science_strategy/strategy-strategy_implementation/ strategy-other_initiatives/strategy-data_sharing/strategy-data_sharing_implementation/ research_collection_ access.htm.

Lucassen, A., Parker, M. and Wheeler, R. (2006). Implications of data protection legislation for family history. *BMJ* **332**, 299–301.

Ludlam, C. A., Pasi, K. J., Bolton-Maggs, P. *et al.* (2005). A framework for genetic service provision for haemophilia and other inherited bleeding disorders. *Haemophilia* **11**, 145–63.

Maier, L. (2002). Genetic and exposure risks for chronic beryllium disease. *Clin. Chest Med.* **23**, 827–39.

Marteau, T. M. and Lerman, C. (2001). Genetic risk and behavioural change. *BMJ* **322**, 1056–9.

Marteau, T. M. and Richards, M. eds. (1999). *The Troubled Helix: Social and Psychological Implications of the New Human Genetics.* Cambridge: Cambridge University Press.

Martin, N. G., Eaves, L. J. and Fulker, D. W. (1978). The power of the classical twin study. *Heredity* **40**, 97–116.

Martinez Arias, A. and Stewart, A. (2002). *Molecular Principles of Animal Development.* Oxford: Oxford University Press.

Mason, K. and Laurie, G. (2006). *Mason and McCall Smith's Law and Medical Ethics.* Oxford: Oxford University Press.

Mathews, K. A., Kalfoglou, A. and Hudson, K. (2005). Geneticists' views on science policy formation and public outreach. *Am. J. Med. Genet.* **137**, 161–9.

McCabe, L. L. and McCabe, E. R. (2004). Genetic screening: carriers and affected individuals. *Annu. Rev. Genomics Hum. Genet.* **5**, 57–69.

McCandless, S. E., Brunner, J. W. and Cassidy, S. B. (2004). The burden of genetic disease on inpatient care in a children's hospital. *Am. J. Hum. Genet.* **74**, 121–7.

McGee, G., Brakman, S. V. and Gurmankin, A. D. (2001). Gamete donation and anonymity. Disclosure to children conceived with donor gametes should not be optional. *Hum. Reprod.* **16**, 2033–6.

McGlennan, T. (2001). *Insurance and Genetic Information.* Association of British Insurers Research Report.

McHale, J. (2004). Regulating genetic databases: some legal and ethical issues. *Med. Law Rev.* **12**, 70–96.

McKusick, V. A. (1998). *Mendelian Inheritance in Man*, 12th edn. Baltimore: Johns Hopkins University Press.

McVean, G., Spencer, C. C. A. and Chaix, R. (2005). Perspectives on human genetic variation from the HapMap project. *PloS Genetics* **1**: e54.

Medical Research Council (undated). *Stem Cell Therapy.* Available online at www.mrc.ac.uk/pdf_stem_cells.pdf.

Medical Research Council (2000, with update in 2003). *Personal Information in Medical Research.* Available online at www.mrc.ac.uk/pdf-pimr.pdf.

Melzer, D. and Zimmern, R. (2002). Genetics and medicalisation. *BMJ* **321**, 863–4.

Melzer, D., Raven, A., Detmer, D. E., Ling, T. and Zimmern, R. L. (2003). *My Very Own Medicine. What Must I Know? Information Policy for Pharmacogenetics.* Cambridge UK: Public Health Genetics Unit. Available online at www.phgu.org.uk/about_phgu/pharmacogenetics.html.

Merikangas, K. R. and Risch, N. (2003). Genomic priorities and public health. *Science* **302**, 599–601.

Meyer, U. A. (2004). Pharmacogenetics – five decades of therapeutic lessons from genetic diversity. *Nat. Rev. Genet.* **5**, 669–76.

Modell, B. and Kuliev, A. (1998). The history of community genetics: the contribution of the haemoglobin disorders. *Community Genet.* **1**, 3–12.

Mount, D. W. and Pandey, R. (2005). Using bioinformatics and genome analysis for new therapeutic interventions. *Mol. Cancer Ther.* **4**, 1636–43.

Mulkay, M. (1997). *The Embryo Research Debate: Science and the Politics of Reproduction.* Cambridge: Cambridge University Press.

Muller, M. and Kersten, S. (2003). Nutrigenomics: goals and strategies. *Nat. Rev. Genet.* **4**, 315–22.

Murray, T. (1997). Genetic exceptionalism and 'future diaries': is genetic information different from other medical information? In *Genetic Secrets: Protecting Privacy and Confidentiality in the Genetic Era*, ed. M. A. Rothstein, pp. 60–73. New Haven: Yale University Press.

Narod, S. A. and Offit, K. (2005). Prevention and management of hereditary breast cancer. *J. Clin. Oncol.* **23**, 1656–63.

National Collaborating Centre for Women's and Children's Health (2003). *Antenatal Care: Routine Care for the Healthy Pregnant Woman.* Available online at www.rcog.org.uk/resources/Public/pdf/Antenatal_Care.pdf.

National Institute for Clinical Excellence and National Collaborating Centre for Primary Care (2004). *Familial Breast Cancer Guidelines.* Available online at www.nice.org.uk/page.aspx?o=203181.

Neil, H. A., Hammond, T., Mant, D. and Humphries, S. E. (2004). Effect of statin treatment for familial hypercholesterolaemia on life assurance: results of consecutive surveys in 1990 and 2002. *BMJ* **328**, 500–1.

Nelkin, D. and Lindee, M. S. (1995). *The DNA Mystique: The Gene as a Cultural Icon.* New York: W. H. Freeman and Co.

NHS Central Research and Development Committee (1995a). *Genetics of Common Disease.* London: Department of Health.

NHS Central Research and Development Committee (1995b). *Report of the Genetics Research Advisory Group.* London: Department of Health.

Nicholson, R. (2004). Another threat to research in the United Kingdom. *BMJ* **328**, 1212–13.

Nowlan, W. (2002). A rational view of insurance and genetic information. *Science* **297**, 195–6.

Nuffield Council on Bioethics (1998). *Mental Disorders and Genetics.* London: Nuffield Council on Bioethics. Available online at www.nuffieldbioethics.org/go/ourwork/mentaldisorders/introduction.

Nuffield Council on Bioethics (2001). *Stem Cell Therapy: The Ethical Issues.* London: Nuffield Council on Bioethics. Available online at www.nuffieldbioethics.org/go/ourwork/stemcells/publication_304.html.

Nuffield Council on Bioethics (2002a). *The Ethics of Patenting DNA.* London: Nuffield Council on Bioethics. Available online at www.nuffieldbioethics.org/go/ourwork/patentingdna/publication_310.html.

Nuffield Council on Bioethics (2002b). *Genetics and Behaviour: the Ethical Context.* London: Nuffield Council on Bioethics. Available online at www.nuffieldbioethics.org/go/ourwork/behaviouralgenetics/introduction.

Nuffield Council on Bioethics (2003). *Pharmacogenetics: Ethical Issues.* Available online at www.nuffieldbioethics.org/go/ourwork/pharmacogenetics/introduction.

O'Connor, T. P. and Crystal, R. G. (2006). Genetic medicines: treatment strategies for hereditary disorders. *Nat. Rev. Genet.* **7**, 261–76.

Office of Science and Technology (1999). The advisory and regulatory framework for biotechnology: report from the Government's review. Available on line at www.ost.gov.uk/policy/issues/biotech_report/index.htm.

Office of Science and Technology and The Wellcome Trust (2000). *Science and the Public: A Review of Science Communication and Public Attitudes to Science in Britain.* Available online at www.wellcome.ac.uk/doc_WTD003420.html.

Ogilvie, C. M., Lashwood, A., Chitty, L., Waters, J. J., Scriven, P. N. and Flinter, F. (2005). The future of prenatal diagnosis: rapid testing or full karyotype? An audit of chromosone abnormalities and pregnancy outcomes for women referred for Down's Syndrome testing. *Br. J. Obstet. Gynaecol.* **112**, 1369–75.

Ojha, R. P. and Thertulien, R. (2005). Health care policy issues as a result of the genetic revolution: implications for public health. *Am. J. Public Health* **95**, 385–8.

Organisation for Economic Cooperation and Development (1980). *Guidelines for the Protection of Privacy and Transborder Flows of Personal Data.* Available online at www.oecd.org/document/18/0,2340,en_2649_34255_1815186_1_1_1_1,00.html.

Organisation for Economic Cooperation and Development (2001). *Genetic Testing. Policy Issues for the New Millennium.* Available online at www.oecd.org/document/16/0,2340,en_2649_37407_1895632_1_1_1_37407,00.html.

Organisation for Economic Cooperation and Development (2005). *Quality Assurance and Proficiency Testing for Molecular Genetic Testing. A Survey of 18 OECD Member Countries.* Available online at http://www.oecd.org/dataoecd/25/12/34779945.pdf.

Organisation for Economic Cooperation and Development (2006). *Guidelines for the Licensing of Genetic Inventions.* Available online at www.oecd.org/document/26/0,2340, en_2649_34537_34317658_1_1_1_1,00.html.

Ott, M. G., Schmidt, M., Schwarzwaelder, K. *et al.* (2006). Correction of x-linked chronic granulomatous disease by gene therapy, augmented by insertional activation of MDS1-EVI1, PRDM16 or SETBP1. *Nat. Med.* **12**, 401–9.

Palmer, L. J. and Cardon, L. R. (2005). Shaking the tree: mapping complex disease genes with linkage disequilibrium. *Lancet* **366**, 1223–34.

Pandor, A., Eastham, J., Beverley, C., Chilcott, J. and Paisley, S. (2004). Clinical effectiveness and cost-effectiveness of neonatal screening for inborn errors of metabolism using tandem mass spectrometry: a systematic review. *Health Technol. Assess.* **8**, no.12. Available online at www.ncchta.org/execsumm/summ812.htm.

Parliamentary Office of Science and Technology (2003a). *Medical Self-Test Kits.* Postnote number 194. Available online at www.parliament.uk/post/pn194.pdf.

Parliamentary Office of Science and Technology (2003b). *Public Dialogue in Science and Technology.* Postnote number 189. Available online at www.parliament.uk/post/pn189.pdf.

Parliamentary Office of Science and Technology (2004a). *NHS Genetic Testing.* Postnote number 227. Available online at www.parliament.uk/documents/upload/POSTpn227.pdf.

Parliamentary Office of Science and Technology (2004b). *Regulating Stem Cell Therapies.* Postnote number 221. Available online at www.parliament.uk/documents/upload/POST pn221.pdf.

Parliamentary Office of Science and Technology (2005a). *Data Protection and Medical Research.* Postnote number 235. Available online at www.parliament.uk/documents/upload/POST pn235.pdf.

Parliamentary Office of Science and Technology (2005b). *Gene Therapy.* Postnote number 240. Available online at www.parliament.uk/documents/upload/POSTpn240.pdf.

Parry, B. (2004). *Trading the Genome: Investigating the Commodification of Bio-Information.* New York: Columbia University Press.

Patrizio, P., Mastroianni, A. C. and Mastroianni, L. (2001). Disclosure to children conceived with donor gametes should be optional. *Hum Reprod.* **16**, 2036–8.

Patterson, S. D. and Aebersold, R. H. (2003). Proteomics: the first decade and beyond. *Nat. Genet.* **33**, 311–23.

Pencheon, D., Guest, C., Melzer, D. and Gray, M. eds. (2006). *The Oxford Handbook of Public Health Practice.* Oxford: Oxford University Press.

Pennisi, E. (2004). Searching for the genome's second code. *Science* **306**, 632–5.

Petersen, K. (2006). The rights of donor-conceived children to know the identity of their donor. In *Globalization and Health. Challenges for Health Law and Bioethics*, eds. B. Bennett and G. F. Tomossy, pp. 151–67. New York: Springer.

Pharoah, P. D., Antoniou, A., Bobrow, M., Zimmern, R. L., Easton, D. F. and Pondes, B. A. (2002). Polygenic susceptibility to breast cancer and implications for prevention. *Nat. Genet.* **31**, 33–6.

Phillips, K. A., Veenstra, D. L. and Sadee, W. (2000). Implications of the genetics revolution for health services research: pharmacogenomics and improvements in drug therapy. *Health Serv. Res.* **35**, 128–40.

Pollock, A., McNally, N. and Kerrison, S. (2006). Best research. *BMJ* **332**, 247–8.

Powell, L. W., Dixon, J. L. and Hewett, D. G. (2005). Role of early case detection by screening relatives of patients with HFE-associated hereditary haemochromatosis. *Best Pract. Res. Clin. Haematol.* **18**, 221–34.

Qureshi, N., Modell, B. and Modell, M. (2004). Timeline: raising the profile of genetics in primary care. *Nat. Rev. Genet.* **5**, 783–90.

R (on the application of Quintavalle) v *Human Fertilisation and Embryology Authority* (2002) EWHC 2785. High Court judgment available online at www.hmcourts-service.gov.uk/judgmentsfiles/j1474/quintavalle_v_human_fertilisation.htm.

R (on the application of Quintavalle) v *Human Fertilisation and Embryology Authority* (2003) EWCA Civ 667. Appeal Court judgment available online at www.bailii.org/cgi-bin/markup.cgi?doc=/ew/cases/EWCA/Civ/2003/667.html&query=Quintavalle&method=all.

R (on the application of Quintavalle) v *Human Fertilisation and Embryology Authority* (2005) UKHL 28. House of Lords judgment available online at www.publications.parliament.uk/pa/ld200405/ldjudgmt/jd050428/quint-1.htm.

R (on the application of Bruno Quintavalle on behalf of Pro-Life Alliance) v *Secretary of State for Health* (2001) EWHC Admin 918. High Court judgment available on line at www.bailii.org/cgi-bin/markup.cgi?doc=/ew/cases/EWHC/Admin/2001/918.html&query=quintavalle&method=all.

R (on the application of Quintavalle) v *Secretary of State for Health* (2002) EWCA Civ 29. Appeal Court judgment.

R v *Secretary of State for Health (respondent) ex parte Quintavalle (on behalf of Pro-Life Alliance) (appellant)* (2003) UKHL 13. House of Lords judgment available online at www.publications.parliament.uk/pa/ld200203/ldjudgmt/jd030313/quinta-1.htm.

Reindal, S. M. (2000). Disability, gene therapy and eugenics – a challenge to John Harris. *J. Med. Ethics* **26**, 89–94.

Richards, M. P. M. (1996). Lay and professional knowledge of genetics and inheritance. *Public Underst. Sci.* **5**, 217–30.

Richards, M. P. M. (1997). It runs in the family: lay knowledge about inheritance. In *Culture, Kinship and Genes*, ed. A. Clark, pp. 175–94. Basingstoke: Macmillan Publishers.

Richards, M. (2001). How distinctive is genetic information? *Stud. Hist. Phil. Biol. & Biomed. Sci.* **32**, 663–87.

Richmond, M. (1999). *Human Genomics: Prospects for Health Care and Public Policy*. London: University College London School of Public Policy.

Ridley, M. (1999). *Genome: The Autobiography of a Species in 23 Chapters*. New York: HarperCollins.

Ridley, M. (2003). *Nature Via Nurture. Genes, Experience and What Makes us Human*. London: Fourth Estate.

Risch, N., Burchard, E., Ziv, E. and Tang, H. (2002). Categorisation of humans in biomedical research: genes, race and disease. *Genome Biol.* **3**: comment2007. Epub 2002 Jul 1.

Romero, R., Kuivaniemi, H., Tromp, G. and Olson, J. (2002). The design, execution, and interpretation of genetic association studies to decipher complex diseases. *Am. J. Obstet. Gynecol.* **187**, 1299–312.

Rose, G. (1985). Sick individuals and sick populations. *Int. J. Epidemiol.* **14**, 32–8.

Rose, P. and Lucassen, A. (1999). *Practical Genetics for Primary Care*. Oxford: Oxford University Press.

Roses, A. D. (2002). Genome-based pharmacogenetics and the pharmaceutical industry. *Nat. Rev. Drug Discov.* **1**, 541–9.

Rothman, K. J. (2002). *Epidemiology: An Introduction*. Oxford: Oxford University Press.

Rothman, K. J. and Greenland, S., eds. (1998). *Modern Epidemiology*, 2nd edn. Baltimore: Lippincott Williams and Wilkins.

Royal College of Physicians (1996). *Clinical Genetics into the Twenty-First Century*. London: Royal College of Physicians.

Royal College of Physicians (1998a). *Clinical Genetic Services: Activity, Outcome, Effectiveness and Quality*. London: Royal College of Physicians.

Royal College of Physicians (1998b). *Retention of Medical Records with Particular Reference to Medical Genetics*. London: Royal College of Physicians.

Royal College of Physicians (1998c). *Commissioning Clinical Genetic Services*. London: Royal College of Physicians.

Royal College of Physicians (2004). *Human Tissue Bill. Response from the Royal College of Physicians*. Available online at www.rcplondon.ac.uk/college/statements/response_htb.htm.

Royal Liverpool Children's Inquiry, The (2001). *The Royal Liverpool Children's Inquiry report*. London: The Stationery Office. Available online at www.rlcinquiry.org.uk/download/index.htm.

Royal Society, The (1998). *Whither Cloning?* Available online at www.royalsoc.ac.uk/displaypagedoc.asp?id=11525.

Royal Society, The (2003). *Keeping Science Open: The Effects of Intellectual Property Policy on the Conduct of Science.* Available online at www.royalsoc.ac.uk/document.asp?tip=0&id=1374.

Royal Society, The (2003). *Stem Cell Research and Therapeutic Cloning: An Update.* Available online at www.royalsoc.ac.uk/displaypagedoc.asp?id=11474.

Royal Society, The (2005). *Personalised Medicine: Hopes and Realities.* Available online at www.royalsoc.ac.uk/document.asp?tip=0&id=3780.

Royal Society, The (2006). *Science and the Public Interest. Communicating the Results of New Scientific Research to the Public.* Available online at www.royalsoc.ac.uk/downloaddoc.asp?id=2879.

Sadee, W. and Dai, Z. (2005). Pharmacogenetics/genomics and personalized medicine. *Hum. Mol. Genet.* **14** Review issue 2, R207–14.

Sakar, S. (1998). *Genetics and Reductionism: a Primer.* Cambridge: Cambridge University Press.

Salanti, G., Sanderson. S. and Higgins, J. P. (2005). Obstacles and opportunities in meta-analysis of genetic association studies. *Genet. Med.* **7**, 13–20.

Salanti, G., Higgins, J. P. T. and White, I. R. (2006). Bayesian synthesis of epidemiological evidence with different combinations of exposure groups: application to a gene–gene–environment interaction. *Stat. Med.* **25**, 4147–63.

Sanchez-Martin, F., Iakovidis, I., Nørager, S. *et al.* (2004). Synergy between medical informatics and bioinformatics: facilitating genomic medicine for future health care. *J. Biomed. Inform.* **37**, 30–42.

Sanderson, S., Emery, J. and Higgins, J. (2005a). CYP2C9 variants, drug dose, and bleeding risk in warfarin-treated patients: a HuGENet systematic review and meta-analysis. *Genet. Med.* **7**, 97–104.

Sanderson, S., Zimmern, R., Kroese, M., Higgins, J., Patch, C. and Emery, J. (2005b). How can the evaluation of genetic tests be enhanced? Lessons learned from the ACCE framework and evaluating genetic tests in the United Kingdom. *Genet. Med.* **7**, 495–500.

Sankar, P. (2003). Genetic privacy. *Annu. Rev. Med.* **54**, 393–407.

Scheuner, M. T., Yoon, P. W. and Khoury, M. J. (2004). Contribution of Mendelian disorders to common chronic disease: opportunities for recognition, intervention, and prevention. *Am. J. Med. Genet. C. Semin. Med. Genet.* **125**, 50–65.

Schmitz, D. and Wiesing, U. (2006). Just a family medical history? *BMJ* **332**, 297–9.

Sconce, E. A., Khan, T. I., Wynne, H. A., *et al.* (2005). The impact of CYP2C9 and VKORC1 genetic polymorphism and patient characteristics upon warfarin dose requirements: proposal for a new dosing regimen. *Blood* **106**, 2329–33.

Secretary's Advisory Committee on Genetic Testing (US) (2000). *Enhancing the Oversight of Genetic Tests: Recommendations of the SACGT.* Available online at www4.od.nih.gov/oba/sacgt/reports/oversight_report.pdf.

Secretary's Advisory Committee on Genetics, Health and Society (2006). *Coverage and Reimbursement of Genetic Tests and Services.* Available online at www4.od.nih.gov/oba/sacghs/reports/CR_report.pdf.

Segal, S. and Hill, A. V. (2003). Genetic susceptibility to infectious disease. *Trends Microbiol.* **11**, 445–8.

Sharp, R. R., Yudell, M. A. and Wilson, S. H. (2004). Shaping science policy in the age of genomics. *Nat. Rev. Genet.* **5**, 311–16.

Singer, P. A. and Daar, A. S. (2001). Harnessing genomics and biotechnology to improve global health equity. *Science* **294**, 2289–90.

Soini, S. *et al.* (2006). The interface between assisted reproductive technologies and genetics: technical, social, ethical and legal issues. *Eur. J. Hum. Genet.* **14**, 588–645.

Spink, J. and Geddes, D. (2004). Gene therapy progress and prospects: bringing gene therapy into medical practice: the evolution of international ethics and the regulatory environment. *Gene Ther.* **11**, 1611–16.

Stears, R. L., Martinsky, T. and Schena, M. (2003). Trends in microarray analysis. *Nat. Med.* **9**, 140–5.

Steinbrook, R. (2006). Egg donation and human embryonic stem-cell research. *N. Engl. J. Med.* **354**, 324–6.

Stevenson, M. (2004). Therapeutic potential of RNA interference. *N. Engl. J. Med.* **351**, 1772–7.

Strachan, T. and Read, A. (2003). *Human Molecular Genetics*, 3rd edn. New York: Garland Science.

Sudbery, P. (2002). *Human Molecular Genetics*, 2nd edn. Harlow: Prentice Hall.

Sulston, J. and Ferry. G. (2002). *The Common Thread. A Story, of Science, Politics, Ethics and the Human Genome*. London: Bantam Press, Transworld Publishers.

Suther, S. and Goodson, P. (2003). Barriers to the provision of genetic services by primary care physicians: a systematic review of the literature. *Genet. Med.* **5**, 63–5.

Suzuki, D. and Knudson, P. (1990). *Genethics*, revised edn. Cambridge, Mass.: Harvard University Press.

Taylor, C. J., Bolton, E. M., Pocock, S., Sharples, L. D., Pedersen, R. A. and Bradley, J. A. (2005). Banking on human embryonic stem cells: estimating the number of donor cell lines needed for HLA matching. *Lancet* **366**, 1991–2.

Teare, D. M. and Barrett, J. H. (2005). Genetic linkage studies. *Lancet* **366**, 1036–44.

ten Have, H. A. (2001). Genetics and culture: the geneticisation thesis. *Med. Health Care Philosoph.* **4**, 295–304.

ten Kate, L. (1998). Editorial. *Community Genet.* **1**, 1–2.

ten Kate, L. (2000). Editorial. *Community Genet.* **3**, 1.

ten Kate, L. (2005). Community genetics: a bridge between clinical genetics and public health. *Community Genet.* **8**, 7–11.

Thomas, J. C., Irwin, D. E., Zuiker, E. S. and Millikan, R. C. (2005). Genomics and the public health code of ethics. *Am. J. Public Health* **95**, 2139–43.

Trujillo, E., Davis, C. and Milner, J. (2006). Nutrigenomics, proteomics, metabolomics, and the practice of dietetics. *J. Am. Diet. Assoc.* **106**, 403–13.

Tucker, G. (2004). Pharmacogenetics – expectations and reality. *BMJ* **329**, 4–6.

Turnpenny, P. and Ellard, S. (2005). *Emery's Elements of Medical Genetics*, 12th edn. Edinburgh: Churchill Livingstone.

Tutton, R. and Corrigan, O. eds. (2004). *Genetic Databases: Socio-Ethical Issues in the Collection and Use of DNA*. London: Routledge.

Tyagi, A. and Morris, J. (2003). Using decision analytic methods to assess the utility of family history tools. *Am. J. Prev. Med.* **24**, 199–207.

UK Government (1967). Abortion Act 1967: Elizabeth II. Chapter 87. London: HMSO.

UK Government (1977). Patents Act 1977: Elizabeth II. London: HMSO.

UK Government (1990). Human Fertilisation and Embryology Act 1990: Elizabeth II. Chapter 37. London: HMSO.

UK Government (1998). Human Rights Act 1998: Elizabeth II. Chapter 42. Reprinted May 2001 and September 2006. London: The Stationery Office. Available online at www.opsi.gov.uk/acts/acts1998/19980042.htm.

UK Government (1998). Data Protection Act. London: The Stationery Office. Available online at www.opsi.gov.uk/acts/acts1998/19980029.htm.

UK Government (2000). The Patents Regulations 2000. London: The Stationery Office. Available online at www.opsi.gov.uk/si/si2000/20002037.htm.

UK Government (2001a). Health and Social Care Act. London: The Stationery Office. Available online at www.opsi.gov.uk/acts/acts2001/20010015.htm.

UK Government (2001b). Human Reproductive Cloning Act. London: The Stationery Office. Available online at www.legislation.hmso.gov.uk/acts/acts2001/20010023.htm.

UK Government (2001c). *Human Fertilisation and Embryology (Research Purposes) Regulations 2001*. London: The Stationery Office. Available online at www.hmso.gov.uk/si/si2001/20010188.htm.

UK Government (2002). *Medical Devices Regulations 2002*. London: The Stationery Office. Available online at www.opsi.gov.uk/si/si2002/20020618.htm.

UK Government (2003) *Government Response to the HGC's Report 'Inside Information Balancing Interests in the Use of Personal Genetic Data'*. Available online at www.dh.gov.uk/PublicationsAndStatistics/LettersAndCirculars/DearColleagueLetters/DearColleagueLettersArticle/fs/en?CONTENT_ID=4005488&chk=iwH9UG.

UK Government (2004a). *The Human Fertilisation and Embryology Authority (Disclosure of Donor Information) Regulations 2004*. Statutory instrument 2004 no. 1511. Available online at www.opsi.gov.uk/si/si2004/20041511.htm.

UK Government (2004b). *The Medicines for Human Use (Clinical Trials) Regulations 2004*. London: The Stationery Office. Available online at www.uk-legislation.hmso.gov.uk/si/si2004/20041031.htm.

UK Government (2004c). Human Tissue Act. London: The Stationery Office. Available online at www.opsi.gov.uk/acts/acts2004/20040030.htm.

UK Government (2005a). *Human Reproductive Technologies and the Law. Government Response to the Report from the House of Commons Science and Technology Committee*. London: The Stationery Office. Available online at www.dh.gov.uk/assetRoot/04/11/78/74/04117874.pdf.

UK Government (2005b). Mental Capacity Act. London: The Stationery Office. Available online at www.opsi.gov.uk/acts/acts2005/20050009.htm.

UK Government (2005c). Disability Discrimination Act. London: The Stationery Office. Available online at www.opsi.gov.uk/ACTS/acts2005/20050013.htm.

UK Government and Association of British Insurers (2005). *Concordat and Moratorium on Genetics and Insurance*. Available online at www.dh.gov.uk/assetRoot/04/10/60/50/04106050.pdf.

UK Patent Office (2003). *Inventions Involving Human Embryonic Stem Cells*. Available online at www.patent.gov.uk/patent/notices/practice/stemcells.htm.

UK Patent Office (2005). *Examination Guidelines for Patent Applications Relating to Biotechnological Inventions in the UK Patent Office*. Available online at www.patent.gov.uk/patent/reference/biotechguide/index.htm.

UK Stem Cell Bank Steering Committee (2005). *Code of Practice for the Use of Human Stem Cell Lines – Version 2*. Available online at ww.mrc.ac.uk/public-use_of_stem_cell_lines.

UK Stem Cell Initiative (2005). *Report and Recommendations*. Available online at www.advisorybodies.doh.gov.uk/uksci/uksci-reportnov05.pdf.

UNESCO (1997). *Universal Declaration on the Human Genome and Human Rights*. Available online at portal.unesco.org/shs/en/ev.php-URL_ID=1881&URL_DO=DO_TOPIC&URL_SECTION=201.html.

UNESCO (2003). *International Declaration on Human Genetic Data*. Available online at unesdoc.unesco.org/images/0013/001361/136112eb.pdf.

UNESCO (2005). *International Declaration on Bioethics and Human Rights*. Available online at portal.unesco.org/shs/en/file_download.php/46133e1f4691e4c6e57566763d474a4dBioethics Declaration_EN.pdf.

UNESCO International Bioethics Committee (2000). *Report on Confidentiality and Genetic Data*. Available online at http://portal.unesco.org/shs/en/file_download.php/48de04a5e6-de8bc 4966add86540d6c71Confidentiality_en.pdf.

UNESCO International Bioethics Committee (2001). *The Use of Embryonic Stem Cells in Therapeutic Research*. Available online at portal.unesco.org/shs/en/file_download.php/64b74abda57372bdc22570b42c1718f1 StemCells_en.pdf.

UNESCO International Bioethics Committee (2002). *Report on Ethics, Intellectual Property and Genomics*. Available online at portal.unesco.org/shs/en/file_download.php/0f8d8bed 17083342b45db84beef431ac FinalReportIP_en.pdf.

UNESCO International Bioethics Committee (2003). *Report on Preimplantation Genetic Diagnosis and Germ-Line Intervention*. Available online at portal.unesco.org/shs/en/file_ download.php/1f3df0049c329b1f8f8e46b6f381cbd1ReportfinalPGD_en.pdf.

United Nations General Assembly (2005). United Nations Declaration on Human Cloning. Available online at http://daccessdds.un.org/doc/UNDOC/GEN/No4/493/06/PDF/No449306.pdf?OpenElement.

US Congress (1990). Americans with Disabilities Act of 1990. Available online at www.usdoj.gov/crt/ada/pubs/ada.txt.

US Congress (1996). *Health Insurance Portability and Accountability Act of 1996*. Available online at www.cms.hhs.gov/hipaa/hipaa1/content/hipaasta.pdf. Explanatory information is available at www.cms.hhs.gov/hipaa/.

US Congress (2002). *Standards for Privacy of Individually Identifiable Health Information*. Final rule. Available online at www.hhs.gov/ocr/hipaa/privrulepd.pdf.

US Equal Employment Opportunities Commission (2001). *EEOC Petitions Court to Ban Genetic Testing of Railroad Workers in First EEOC Case Challenging Genetic Discrimination Under Americans with Disabilities Act*. Press release available online at www.eeoc.gov/press/2-9-01-c.html.

US Equal Employment Opportunities Commission (2002). *EEOC and BNSF Settle Genetic Testing Case Under Americans with Disabilities Act*. Press release available online at www.eeoc.gov/press/5-8-02.html.

US National Bioethics Advisory Commission (1997). *Cloning Human Beings Report and Recommendations*. Available onling at www.georgetown.edu/research/nrcbl/nbac/pubscloning1/cloning.pdf.

US President (2000). *Executive Order to Prohibit Discrimination in Federal Employment Based on Genetic Information*. Available online at www.genome.gov/10002084.

US President (2001). President Bush statement, 9 August 2001. Available at http://www.Whitehouse.gov/news/releases/2001/08/20010809-2.html. Whitehouse fact sheet available at http://www.Whitehouse.gov/news/releases/2001/08/20010809-1.html.

US Preventive Services Task Force (2005). Genetic risk assessment and BRCA mutation testing for breast and ovarian cancer susceptibility: recommendation statement. *Ann Intern. Med.* **143**, 355–61.

Van Overwalle, G., van Zimmern, E., Ver beure, B. and Matthijs, G. (2006). Models for facilitating access to patents on genetic inventions. *Nat Rev. Genet.* **7**, 143–8.

van Rijn, M. J., van Duijn, C. M. and Slooter, A. J. (2005). Impact of generic testing on complex diseases. *Eur. J. Epidemiol.* **20**, 383–8.

Veenstra, D. L., Higashi, M. K. and Phillips, K. A. (2000). Assessing the cost-effectiveness of pharmacogenetics. *AAPS Pharmsci.* **2**; article 29. Available online at www.pharmsci.org.

Wacholder, S., Rothman, N. and Caporaso, N. (2000). Population stratification in epidemiologic studies of common genetic variants and cancer: quantification of bias. *J. Natl. Cancer Inst.* **92**, 1151–8.

Wacholder, S., Garcia-Closas, M. and Rothman, N. (2002). Study of genes and environmental factors in complex diseases. *Lancet* **359**, 1155–6.

Walgren, R. A., Meucci, M. A. and McLeod, H. L. (2005). Pharmacogenomic discovery approaches: will the real genes please stand up? *J. Clin. Oncol.* **23**, 7342–9.

Wanless, D. (2002). *Securing our Future Health: Taking a Long Term View*. Available online at www.hm-treasury.gov.uk/consultations_and_legislation/wanless/consult_wanless_index.cfm.

Wanless, D. (2004). *Securing Good Health for the Whole Population*. Available online at www.hm-treasury.gov.uk/consultations_and_legislation/wanless/consult_wanless03_index.cfm.

Warburg, R. J., Wellman, A., Buck, T. B. and Ligler Schoenhard, A. (2003). Patentability and maximum protection of intellectual property in proteomics and genomics. *Pharmacogenomics* **4**, 81–90.

Warnock, M. (1984). *Report of the Committee of Inquiry into Human Fertilisation and Embryology*. London: The Stationery Office.

Waters, M. D. and Fostel, J. M. (2004). Toxicogenomics and systems toxicology: aims and prospects. *Nat. Rev. Genet.* **5**, 936–48.

Weber, W. W. (1997). *Pharmacogenetics*. Oxford: Oxford University Press.

Webster, A., Martin, P., Lewis, G. and Smart, A. (2004). Integrating pharmacogenetics into society: in search of a model. *Nat. Rev. Genet.* **5**, 663–9.

Weeraratna, A. T., Nagel, J. E., de Mello-Coelho, V. and Taub, D. D. (2004). Gene expression profiling: from microarrays to medicine. *J. Clin. Immunol.* **24**, 213–24.

Wellcome Trust (2004a). *Human Tissue Bill – second reading, 15 January 2004*. Available online at www.wellcome.ac.uk/doc_wtd002742.html.

Wellcome Trust (2004b). *Public Health Sciences: Challenges and Opportunities*. Available online at www.wellcome.ac.uk/assets/wtd003191.pdf.

Wheeler, J. G., Keavney, B. D., Watkins, H., Collins, R. and Danesh, J. (2005). Four paraoxonase gene polymorphisms in 11212 cases of coronary heart disease and 12786 controls: meta-analysis of 43 studies. *Lancet* **363**, 689–95.

Whelan, A. J., Ball, S., Best, L. *et al.* (2004). Genetic red flags: clues to thinking genetically in primary care practice. *Prim. Care* **31**, 497–508.

White, K. L. (1991). *Healing the Schism: Epidemiology, Medicine, and the Public's Health.* New York: Springer-Verlag.

Willett, W. C. (2002). Balancing life-style and genomics research for disease prevention. *Science* **296**, 695–8.

Williams, P. and Clow, S. eds. (1999). *Genomics Healthcare and Public Policy.* London: Office of Health Economics.

Wilson, J. M. G. and Jungner, G. (1968). *Principles and Practice of Screening for Disease.* Public health paper No. 34. Geneva: World Health Organization.

Wolf, C. R., Smith, G. and Smith, R. L. (2000). Science, medicine and the future: pharmacogenetics. *BMJ* **320**, 987–90.

Wolffe, A. P. and Matzke, M. A. (1999). Epigenetics: regulation through repression. *Science* **286**, 481–5.

World Health Organization (1998). *Proposed International Guidelines on Ethical Issues in Medical Genetics and Genetic Services.* Available online at www.who.int/genomics/publications/en/ethicalguidelines1998.pdf.

World Health Organization (2000). *Statement of the WHO Expert Consultation on New Developments in Human Genetics.* Available online at whqlibdoc.who.int/hq/2000/WHO_HGN_WG_00.3.pdf.

World Health Organization (2002). *Human Genetic Technologies. Implications for Preventive Health Care.* Geneva: World Health Organization.

World Health Organization (2003a). *Genetic Databases: Assessing the Benefits and the Impact on Human and Patient Rights.* Available online at www.law.ed.ac.uk/ahrb/publications/online/whofinalreport.doc.

World Health Organization (2003b). *Review of Ethical Issues in Medical Genetics.* Available online at www.who.int/genomics/publications/en/ethical_issuesin_medgenetics%20report.pdf.

World Health Organization (2005). *Genetics, Genomics and Patenting DNA. Review of Potential Implications for Health in Developing Countries.* Available online at www.who.int/genomics/patentingDNA/en/index.html.

World Health Organization Advisory Committee on Health Research (2002). *Genomics and World Health.* Geneva: World Health Organization.

World Medical Association (1964; latest update 2004). *Ethical Principles for Medical Research Involving Human Subjects (WMA Declaration of Helsinki).* Available online at www.wma.net/e/policy/b3.htm.

World Medical Association (2002). *Declaration on Ethical Considerations Regarding Health Databases.* Available online at www.wma.net/e/policy/d1.htm.

World Medical Association (2005). *Statement on Genetics and Medicine.* Available online at www.wma.net/e/policy/g11.htm.

World Trade Organisation (1994). Agreement on trade-related aspects of intellectual property. Available online at http://www.wto.org/english/docs_e/legal_e/27-trips.pdf.

Yang, Q., Khoury, M. J., Botto, L., Friedman, J. M. and Flanders, W. D. (2003). Improving the prediction of complex diseases by testing for multiple disease susceptibility genes. *Am. J. Hum. Genet.* **72**, 636–49. (Erratum 74, 372).

Yang, Q., Khoury, M. J., Botto, L., Friedman, J. M. and Flanders, W. D. (2005). Revisiting the clinical validity of multiplex genetic testing in complex diseases: reply to Janssens *et al.* *Am. J. Hum. Genet.* **74**, 588–9.

Yoon, P., Scheuner, M. T., Peterson-Oehlke, K. L., Gwinn, M., Faucett, A. and Khoury, M. J. (2002). Can family history be used as a tool for public health and preventive medicine? *Genet. Med.* **4**, 304–10.

Yoon, P., Scheuner, M. T. and Khoury, M. J. (2003). Research priorities for evaluating family history in the prevention of common chronic diseases. *Am. J. Prev. Med.* **24**, 128–35.

Zerhouni, E. A. (2005). Translational and clinical science – time for a new vision. *N. Engl. J. Med.* **353**, 1621–3.

Zimmern, R. L. (2001a). Review. *Community Genet.* **4**, 60.

Zimmern, R. L. (2001b). What is genetic information: whose hands on your genes? *Genet. Law Monitor* **1**, 9–13.

Zimmern, R. L. (2003). Public health genetics. In *Encyclopedia of the Human Genome*, ed. D. N. Cooper. London: Macmillan Publishers Ltd., Nature Publishing Group.

Zimmern, R. L. and Cook, C. (2000). *Genetics and Health.* Policy issues for genetic science and their implications for health services. London: The Stationery Office. Available online at www.archive.official-documents.co.uk/document/nuffield/policyf/genetics.htm.

Zimmern, R. L. and Stewart, A. (2006). Genetics in disease prevention. In *The Oxford Handbook of Public Health Practice*, eds. D. Pencheon *et al.* Oxford: Oxford University Press.

Websites and web pages

Academy of Medical Sciences pages on the Human Tissue Act 2004 www.acmedsci.ac.uk/p48prid34.html

Advisory Committee on Genetic Testing archived web pages www.advisorybodies.doh.gov.uk/genetics/acgt/index.htm

American College of Medical Genetics policy statements and practice guidelines www.acmg.net/resources/policy-list.asp

American Society of Human Genetics policy statements genetics.faseb.org/genetics/ashg/pubs/003.shtml

Association of British Insurers www.abi.org.uk

Bioethics Today www.bioethics-today.org/

BioethicsWeb bioethicsweb.ac.uk/

BioNews www.progress.org.uk/News/

Biotechnology and Biological Sciences Research Council www.bbsrc.ac.uk

Blazing a Genetic Trail. Available from the Howard Hughes Medical Institute at www.hhmi.org/genetictrail

British Association for the Advancement of Science www.the-ba.net/the-ba/

British Society for Human Genetics www.bshg.org.uk

British Society for Human Genetics documents and publications www.bshg.org.uk/documents/official_documents.htm

Central Office for Research Ethics Committees (COREC) www.corec.org.uk/

CLIMB: Children Living with Metabolic Disease www.climb.org.uk/

Clinical Laboratory Improvement Amendments program (US) www.cms.hhs.gov/clia/

Clinical Molecular Genetics Society www.cmgs.org/new_cmgs/

Clinical Pathology (UK) Accreditation Ltd www.cpa-uk.co.uk/

Commission for Patient and Public Involvement in Health www.cppih.org/

Contact a Family www.cafamily.org.uk/

COPUS www.copus.org.uk/

Council of Europe www.coe.int/DefaultEN.asp

Department of Energy (US). Human Genome Project Information website. *Gene Testing.* www.ornl.gov/sci/techresources/Human_Genome/medicine/genetest.shtml

Department of Energy (US). Human Genome Project Information website. *Gene Therapy.* www.ornl.gov/sci/techresources/Human_Genome/medicine/genetherapy.shtml

Department of Health Genetics pages www.dh.gov.uk/PolicyAndGuidance/HealthAndSocialCareTopics/Genetics/GeneticsGeneralInformation/fs/en

Department of Health Genetics, Embryology and Assisted Conception Branch www.dh.gov.uk/PolicyAndGuidance/HealthAndSocialCareTopics/Genetics/GeneticsGeneralInformation/GeneticsGeneralArticle/fs/en?CONTENT_ID=4016202&chk=K6kI4B

Department of Health, Health Services Research Programme in Genetics www.genres.org.uk/hsrp/projects.htm

Department of Health and Human Resources (US), Access Excellence Resource Center. *Understanding Gene Testing.* www.accessexcellence.org/AE/AEPC/NIH/index.html

Department of Health web pages on patient confidentiality and access to health records www.dh.gov.uk/PolicyAndGuidance/InformationPolicy/PatientConfidentialityAndCaldicottGuardians/fs/en

Department of Health web pages on the Human Tissue Act 2004 www.dh.gov.uk/PolicyAndGuidance/HealthAndSocialCareTopics/Tissue/TissueGeneralInformation/TissueGeneralArticle/fs/en?CONTENT_ID=4102169&chk=7yP5JQ

Department of Health web pages on the Mental Capacity Act 2005 www.dh.gov.uk/PublicationsAndStatistics/Bulletins/ChiefExecutiveBulletin/ChiefExecutiveBulletinArticle/fs/en?CONTENT_ID=4108436&chk=z0Ds8/

Department of Trade and Industry web pages on science and technology www.dti.gov.uk/industries_science_technology.html

DNA Learning Centre (Cold Spring Harbor, US) website *DNA From the Beginning* www.dnaftb.org/dnaftb/index.html

Dolan DNA Learning Center, Cold Spring Harbor Laboratory. Eugenics archive www.eugenicsarchive.org/eugenics/

ESRC Genomics Network www.genomicsforum.ac.uk/default.aspx?pageId=43

Ethox Centre www.ethox.org.uk/

European Bioinformatics Insitute www.ebi.ac.uk

European Commission pages on plans for the Seventh Framework Programme for Research europa.eu.int/comm/research/future/themes/index_en.cfm

European Commission DG Enterprise and Industry website pages on advanced therapies at http://ec.europa.eu/enterprise/pharmaceuticals/advtherapies/index.htm

European Group on Ethics in Science and New Technologies http://ec.europa.eu/european_group_ethics/index_en.htm

European Medicines Agency www.emea.eu.int/home.htm

European Molecular Genetics Quality Network www1.emqn.org/index.html

European Nutrigenomics Organisation www.nugo.org

European Patent Office www.european-patent-office.org/index.en.php

European Society of Human Genetics public policy pages www.eshg.org/PPPC.htm

European Society of Human Genetics www.eshg.org/

European Union Sixth Framework Programme for Research http://cordis.europa.eu/fp6/dc/index.cfm? fuseaction=UserSite.FP6HomePage

GeneCards™ bioinformatics.weizmann.ac.il/cards

Generation Scotland project www.generationscotland.org

Genes and Disease www.ncbi.nlm.nih.gov/disease/

GeneTests www.geneclinics.org

Gene Therapy Advisory Committee www.advisorybodies.doh.gov.uk/genetics/gtac/

Genetic Interest Group www.gig.org.uk/index.html

Genetic Science Learning Center website from the University of Utah in the US gslc.genetics.utah.edu/

Genetics and Insurance Committee www.advisorybodies.doh.gov.uk/genetics/gaic/

Genetics Commissioning Advisory Group www.dh.gov.uk/PolicyAndGuidance/HealthAndSocialCareTopics/Genetics/GeneticsGeneralInformation/GeneticsGeneralArticle/fs/en?CONTENT_ID=4117687&chk=ecpwCW

Genetics Home Reference ghr.nlm.nih.gov

Genome News Network www.genomenewsnetwork.org

Genome News Network. *A Quick Guide to Sequenced Genomes*. www.genomenewsnetwork.org/resources/sequenced_genomes/genome_guide_p1.shtml

GRaPH *Int* (Genome based Research and Population Health International Network) www.graphint.org

Guys and St. Thomas' NHS Trust. Tay Sachs programme. http://www.guysandstthomas.nhs.uk/services/managednetworks/childrens/geneticscentre/taysachscarriertesting.aspx

Health Technology Assessment programme www.ncchta.org/

House of Commons Select Committee on Science and Technology www.parliament.uk/parliamentary_committees/science_and_technology_committee.cfm

House of Lords Select Committee on Science and Technology www.parliament.uk/parliamentary_committees/lords_s_t_select.cfm

HuGENet (Human Genome Epidemiology Network) www.cdc.gov/genomics/hugenet

Human Epigenome Consortium Project www.epigenome.org/

Human Fertilisation and Embryology Authority www.hfea.gov.uk

Human Genetics Advisory Commission archived web pages www.advisorybodies.doh.gov.uk/hgac/index.html

Human Genetics Commission www.hgc.gov.uk

Human Genetics Commission web information pages on genetics and employment www.hgc.gov.uk/Client/Content_wide.asp?ContentId=123

Human Genetics Commission web information pages on intellectual property and genetics www.hgc.gov.uk/Client/Content.asp?ContentId=362

Human Genome Organisation (HUGO) ethics committee web pages www.hugo-international.org/committee_ethics_info.htm

Human Genome Program, US Department of Energy www.ornl.gov/sci/techresources/Human_Genome/home.shtml

Human Proteome Organisation www.hupo.org/

Human Tissue Authority www.hta.gov.uk/

HumGen database www.humgen.umontreal.ca/int/index.cfm?lang=1

Institute for the Study of Genetics, Biorisks and Society web pages on BiDil www.nottingham.ac.uk/igbis/reg/bidil.htm#scientific

Journal of Gene Medicine www.wiley.co.uk/genmed/clinical

Kennedy Institute of Ethics National Information Resource on Ethics and Human Genetics at http://www.georgetown.edu/research/nrcbl/nirehg/index.htm.

Khoury, M.J., Beskow, L. and Gwinn, M. *Making The Vision of Genomic Medicine A Reality: The Need for Public Health Research in The 21st Century.* www.cdc.gov/genomics/info/factshts/vision.htm

London IDEAS Department of Health Familial Hypercholesterolaemia Cascade Testing Audit www.fhcascade.org.uk/

Medical Research Council www.mrc.ac.uk

Medical Research Council web pages on the Human Tissue Act 2004 www.mrc.ac.uk/www.mrc.ac.uk/public-human_tissue_consultation.htm

Medicines and Healthcare Products Regulatory Agency www.mhra.gov.uk/home/idcplg?IdcService=SS_GET_PAGE&nodeId=5

Medicines and Healthcare Products Regulatory Agency pages on clinical trials regulation www.mhra.gov.uk/home/idcplg?IdcService=SS_GET_PAGE&nodeId=716

Michigan Center for Genomics and Public Health www.sph.umich.edu/genomics/

National Coalition for Health Professional Education in Genetics www.nchpeg.org/

National Genetics Reference Laboratories www.ngrl.org.uk/Pages/index.htm

National Human Genome Research Institute information about the Human Genome Project www.genome.gov/10001772

National Institute of Environmental Health Sciences (US). *Environmental Genome Project.* www.niehs.nih.gov/envgenom/

National Institute for Health and Clinical Excellence www.nice.org.uk

National Library for Health's specialist library for clinical genetics (GenePool) www.library.nhs.uk/genepool/

National Service Frameworks, Department of Health website www.dh.gov.uk/PolicyAndGuidance/HealthAndSocialCareTopics/fs/en#5295976

Nature Genome Gateway www.nature.com/genomics/

NHGRI health site www.genome.gov/Health

NHS Health Technology Assessment Programme www.hta.nhsweb.nhs.uk/

NHS Institute for Innovation and Improvement www.institute.nhs.uk/default.htm

NHS National Genetics Education and Development Centre www.geneticseducation.nhs.uk/

NHS National Programme for Information Technology (Connecting for Health) www.connectingforhealth.nhs.uk/

NHS Sickle Cell and Thalassaemia Screening Programme www.kcl-phs.org.uk/haemscreening/

North Carolina Center for Genomics and Public Health www.sph.unc.edu/nccgph/

Office of Genomics and Disease Prevention, Centers for Disease Control and Prevention, Atlanta, USA www.cdc.gov/genomics

Office of Genomics and Disease Prevention, US Centers for Disease Control and Prevention. *Family History for Preventive Medicine and Public Health* www.cdc.gov/genomics/activities/famhx.htm

Office of Science and Technology www.ost.gov.uk/index_v4.htm

Office of Science and Technology Public Engagement with Science and Technology (PUSET) website www.dti.gov.uk/ost/ostbusiness/puset/puset.htm

Online Mendelian Inheritance in Man www.ncbi.nlm.nih.gov/entrez/query.fcgi?db=OMIM

Patient Information Advisory Group www.advisorybodies.doh.gov.uk/piag/

PharmGKB The pharmacogenetics and pharmacogenomics knowledge base www.pharmgkb.org/

PHGEN (Public Health Genomics European Network) www.phgen.nrw.de/

Public Health Genetics Unit, Cambridge UK. www.phgu.org.uk

Public Health Genetics Unit online newsletter www.phgu.org.uk/newsletter.php

Public Population Project in Genomics (P3G Consortium) www.p3gconsortium.org/. The P3G Observatory pages may be accessed at www.p3gobservatory.org/welcome.do

Royal Institution of Great Britain www.ri.ac.uk/

Royal Society 'Science in Society' programme www.royalsoc.ac.uk/page.asp?id=1988

Screening Specialist Library. National Electronic Library for Health. www.libraries.nhs.uk/screening/

Scottish Executive web pages on the Adults with Incapacity (Scotland) Act 2000 www.scotland.gov.uk/Topics/Justice/Civil/16360/4927

Secretary's Advisory Committee on Genetic Testing (US) Archived pages available at www4.od.nih.gov/oba/sacgt.htm

Secretary's Advisory Committee on Genetics, Health and Society (US) www4.od.nih.gov/oba/sacghs/sacghsml.htm

UK Accreditation Service www.ukas.com/

UK Biobank www.biobank.ac.uk

UK Clinical Research Collaboration www.ukcrc.org/

UK Genetic Testing Network www.genetictestingnetwork.org.uk/

UK National Screening Committee www.nsc.nhs.uk/

UK Newborn Screening Programme Centre www.newbornscreening-bloodspot.org.uk/

UK Patent Office www.patent.gov.uk

UK Stem Cell Bank www.ukstemcellbank.org.uk

UNESCO bioethics web pages portal.unesco.org/shs/en/ev.php-URL_ ID=1372&URL_DO=DO_TOPIC&URL_SECTION=201.html

unique: Rare Chromosome Disorder Support Group www.rarechromo.org/

University of Washington Center for Genomics and Public Health depts.washington.edu/cgph/

Wellcome Trust Human Genome website www.wellcome.ac.uk/en/genome

Wellcome Trust Sanger Institute www.sanger.ac.uk/

World Health Organization Genomic Resource Centre. www.who.int/genomics/en/

Index

Note: Page numbers in *italics* refer to figures and tables.